Type 1 Diabetes For Dummies®

Cheat Sheet

Essential Tests for People with Type 1 Diabetes

Undergoing tests at the doctor's office is a fact of life for someone who has type 1 diabetes. But with this handy card, keeping track of test results is a snap. You can make copies of this chart and fill in your child's (or your own) results. See Chapter 7 for full details on all the tests listed here.

Test	Frequency	Results
Foot exam	Each office visit	
Blood pressure	Each office visit	
Weight	Each office visit	
Height	Each office visit	
Hemoglobin A1c	Every three months	
Thyroid-stimulating hormone (TSH)	Yearly	
Microalbuminuria	Yearly	
Eye exam	Yearly	
Lipid panel (cholesterol)	Yearly	
Ankle-brachial index	Every five years	

Taking Action if Diabetic Ketoacidosis Strikes

Diabetic ketoacidosis (DKA) occurs when a person's blood glucose is too high. Major symptoms include the following (see Chapter 4 for more information):

- Abdominal pain
- Frequent urination and thirst
- Nausea and vomiting
- Weakness
- Weight loss
- Smell of acetone on the breath
- Confusion or coma
- Cold skin and body temperature
- Rapid, shallow breathing followed by deep, labored breathing

If you suspect that your child has DKA, there are a couple of quick tests you can do at home to verify the diagnosis:

- Check the blood glucose with your home meter (see Chapter 7). With DKA, the meter will generally read greater than 250 mg/dl, but some cases of mild DKA may have a glucose reading under 250 mg/dl.
- Check the urine for ketones (see Chapter 7). With DKA, the reading will be high.

After you verify DKA with a home test, or if you suspect that you or your child has DKA even without a diagnosis of type 1 diabetes, dial 911 and then call your doctor to tell him or her that you're on the way to the hospital.

For Dummies: Bestselling Book Series for Beginners

Type 1 Diabetes For Dummies®

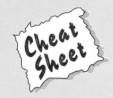
Cheat Sheet

Recognizing and Treating Hypoglycemia

Hypoglycemia occurs when a person's blood glucose level is low (see Chapter 4 for details). Some symptoms of hypoglycemia are

- Whiteness or pallor of the skin
- Sweating
- Rapid heartbeat or palpitations (the sensation that the heart is beating too fast)
- Anxiety
- Irritability
- Numbness in the lips, fingers, and toes
- Sensation of hunger
- Headache
- Loss of concentration
- Vision disorders, like double or blurred vision
- Poor color vision
- Fatigue
- Difficulty hearing
- Confusion and difficulty concentrating
- Feeling of warmth
- Slurred speech
- Dizziness
- Convulsions
- Reduced consciousness or coma

Mild hypoglycemia is marked by a blood glucose of about 75 mg/dl, moderate hypoglycemia by a blood glucose of about 65 mg/dl, and severe hypoglycemia by a blood glucose of less than 55 mg/dl. You can prevent many episodes of hypoglycemia by constantly staying aware of your child's blood glucose and keeping him on a regular schedule; you can adjust his insulin if he's mildly hypoglycemic. Other tips for treating hypoglycemia include the following:

- **Giving your child glucose tablets, which contain 4 mg of glucose.** Two to four tablets is enough for moderate hypoglycemia in most children. If your child has trouble swallowing, give him honey instead of glucose tablets.

- **Giving your child 1½ cups of orange juice.** It effectively raises the blood glucose back to the normal range of 90 to 100 mg/dl.

- **Keeping the child quiet and inactive for 15 to 30 minutes after the reaction.**

- **Checking the blood glucose 20 minutes after treating the hypoglycemia and giving another treatment if the level remains below 100 mg/dl.**

- **Using a prescription glucagon emergency shot for an unconscious child who has severe hypoglycemia.** Just make sure that the glucagon hasn't expired. If the child doesn't wake up in 10 to 15 minutes even though his blood glucose is normal, call 911.

For Dummies: Bestselling Book Series for Beginners

Type 1 Diabetes

FOR

DUMMIES®

by Alan L. Rubin, MD

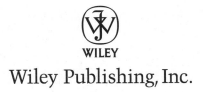

WILEY

Wiley Publishing, Inc.

Type 1 Diabetes For Dummies®

Published by
Wiley Publishing, Inc.
111 River St.
Hoboken, NJ 07030-5774
www.wiley.com

WILEY

About the Author

This is the fifth *For Dummies* book by **Alan L. Rubin, MD.** His previous books, *Diabetes For Dummies, Diabetes Cookbook For Dummies, Thyroid For Dummies,* and *High Blood Pressure For Dummies* (all of which are now in second editions), have been major successes. Letters of praise from numerous readers verify the important role that Dr. Rubin's books have played in their lives. The books have been translated into seven languages and adapted for readers in the United Kingdom, Canada, and Australia. Each of Dr. Rubin's *For Dummies* books provides the latest information on every aspect of its subject while being written in an easy-to-understand format that's full of humor and wisdom.

Dr. Rubin has practiced endocrinology in San Francisco since 1973. He teaches doctors, medical students, and nonprofessionals through classes, lectures, and articles. He has appeared on numerous radio and television shows to answer questions about diabetes, thyroid disease, and high blood pressure. He also serves as a consultant to many pharmaceutical companies and companies that make products for patients with high blood pressure.

Dr. Rubin discusses many health issues in audio "Healthcasts" that may be downloaded at his Web site, www.drrubin.com.

Dedication

This book is dedicated to my new granddaughter Eliana, the beautiful child of my daughter Renee and my son-in-law Marty, who was born on April 9, 2007, just as this book was being born. It is my fervent hope that she will never need the knowledge contained here, but if she should, I hope that it contains everything that she needs to know to live a long, healthy life free of the complications that make life difficult for so many people with diabetes. Eliana: Read this book carefully if you have to. I have tried to include all the available knowledge of this subject that you and your parents need. This book is the answer to the question, "If your granddaughter had diabetes, which book would you recommend?"

Author's Acknowledgments

I wish to thank the numerous people at Wiley Publishing who have made this and all my books such a pleasure to write. The wise people at Wiley understand that type 1 diabetes is, in many ways, a different disease from type 2. Hence the need for this book. It has always been a pleasure to work with my friend Kathy Nebenhaus, Vice President and Executive Publisher of Professional and Trade Publishing at Wiley. Vice President and Publisher Diane Steele has been a valuable resource for the writing of this and all my books. Acquisitions Editor Michael Lewis served as my advocate as we smoothed out the many details that have to be agreed upon before such a project can begin. Project Editor Georgette Beatty offered valuable suggestions and questions that hopefully make this book more understandable and useful to the reader. Copy Editor Elizabeth Rea made sure that my words, my sentences, and my paragraphs followed the rules of the English language. The Technical Editor for this book, Rattan Juneja, MD, checked everything that I wrote so that you, the reader, may be certain that you can trust everything you read to be consistent with modern medical practice. Many other unnamed people are involved from the people who publicize the book to those who take the orders to those who ship out the books. Finally, the booksellers who put the book in your hands deserve my major gratitude. Every one of you is an essential cog in a beautifully running machine.

Publisher's Acknowledgments

We're proud of this book; please send us your comments through our Dummies online registration form located at www.dummies.com/register/.

Some of the people who helped bring this book to market include the following:

Acquisitions, Editorial, and Media Development

Project Editor: Georgette Beatty

Acquisitions Editor: Michael Lewis

Senior Copy Editor: Elizabeth Rea

Editorial Program Coordinator: Erin Calligan Mooney

Technical Editor: Rattan Juneja, MD

Editorial Manager: Michelle Hacker

Editorial Assistants: Joe Niesen, Leeann Harney

Cover Photo: Daniela Richardson

Cartoons: Rich Tennant (www.the5thwave.com)

Composition Services

Project Coordinator: Patrick Redmond

Layout and Graphics: Reuben W. Davis, Alissa D. Ellet, Joyce Haughey, Ronald Terry

Special Art: Illustrations by Kathryn Born, MA

Proofreaders: Todd Lothery, Nancy L. Reinhardt

Indexer: Christine Spina Karpeles

Publishing and Editorial for Consumer Dummies

Diane Graves Steele, Vice President and Publisher, Consumer Dummies

Joyce Pepple, Acquisitions Director, Consumer Dummies

Kristin A. Cocks, Product Development Director, Consumer Dummies

Michael Spring, Vice President and Publisher, Travel

Kelly Regan, Editorial Director, Travel

Publishing for Technology Dummies

Andy Cummings, Vice President and Publisher, Dummies Technology/General User

Composition Services

Gerry Fahey, Vice President of Production Services

Debbie Stailey, Director of Composition Services

Contents at a Glance

Table of Contents

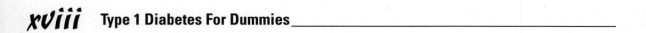

Introduction

* *

*A*lthough they have the same names (but different numbers), type 1 diabetes mellitus (T1DM) and type 2 diabetes mellitus (T2DM) are not the same disease. They share many features, especially the consequences of not controlling the blood glucose (sugar): microvascular complications like eye disease, kidney disease, and nerve disease; and macrovascular complications like heart disease, stroke, and obstruction of blood vessels, especially in the legs and feet.

The big difference is that T2DM is a lifestyle disease; T1DM is not. What exactly does that mean?

- Type 2 diabetes is very often preventable by maintaining a normal weight and doing lots of exercise. And diet and exercise go far in preventing complications of the disease.

- Diet and exercise can't prevent T1DM or its complications. The big difference can be summed up in a single word: *insulin.* This chemical, present in T2DM for long after the disease begins, is partially or completely absent in T1DM from the beginning. T1DM can be cured by restoring insulin so that it's available to the exact extent as in a person who doesn't have diabetes. (Not that food intake and exercise are unimportant in T1DM. But whereas most people with T2DM are middle-aged, heavy, and sedentary, most people with T1DM are young, lean, and active, at least at the time of diagnosis.)

One important fact is true of both types of diabetes: At the present time, although there's not a cure for either type, drugs and equipment are available to control the disease in such a way that your child need never suffer from long-term complications if you're willing to take the time and put forth the effort to make this happen. In fact, your child may grow up to be healthier than friends without diabetes if you follow the recommendations in this book.

About This Book

Each chapter in this book is self-contained, like a short story. That way you can go just where you want and read just what you want. This book isn't meant to be read from cover to cover, although I can't stop you if that's how you want to approach it. You may even want to do that the first time around, and then use it as a reference whenever you want to brush up on a particular subject. If you feel there's an important issue that I haven't addressed or that needs more discussion, please e-mail me at diabetes@drrubin.com.

The subject of diabetes is vast and gets larger daily. Don't believe me? I have an automated update that brings me new articles about diabetes from the National Library of Medicine, and I get three to five new articles every day! This book contains the most important information available on the subject of T1DM, but it can't contain everything. For more on the subject, check the references that I supply at my Web site, www.drrubin.com, by clicking on Diabetes under Related Websites on the home page.

A characteristic of the *For Dummies* series is the use of humor. Readers of my previous books, *Diabetes For Dummies, Diabetes Cookbook For Dummies, Thyroid For Dummies,* and *High Blood Pressure For Dummies,* know that I use humor to get my point across. You may think that there's nothing funny about diabetes, and you'd be wrong. Many patients have sent me humorous stories about their experiences, which I've included in previous books. If you have a funny experience associated with your diabetes, please e-mail it to me at diabetes@drrubin.com.

One important note about the use of this book: Please don't make any changes in your child's treatment (or your own, if you're the patient) based upon what you read in this book without discussing them with your doctor. He or she may have very good reasons, based upon your child's particular situation, for doing something different from what I recommend here. This is exactly the reason I never offer specific advice to people who e-mail me the details of their disease without giving me the opportunity to question them, examine them, and do the tests I feel are appropriate.

Conventions Used in This Book

This book is meant to be read and understood by the non-physician. Therefore, I try to keep scientific terminology to a minimum. Where I must use it, I explain it clearly, and you can also look it up in the glossary at the end of the book. I can't avoid the terminology completely because I want you and your doctor to speak the same language. You should clearly understand the reasons behind everything he recommends, so don't hesitate to ask questions and quote chapter and verse from this book.

In order to save keystrokes, I use some abbreviations throughout the book. The main ones are "T1DM" for "type 1 diabetes mellitus" and "T2DM" for "type 2 diabetes mellitus." You can find these and any others in the book in the glossary. How did these names come about? Good question! People used to refer to diabetes in young people as "juvenile diabetes." In the past, "juvenile diabetes" was understood to mean diabetes due to a lack of insulin, but several years ago, the American Diabetes Association recognized that one result of the epidemic of obesity is the occurrence of T2DM in many juveniles. In addition, a lack of insulin often occurs in adults. Therefore, they changed the name from "juvenile diabetes" to "type 1 diabetes mellitus." T1DM refers to the condition of any patient whose diabetes is due to insulin lack at the very beginning.

Because many T1DM patients are children and young adults, I've geared this book toward parents and caretakers; for the most part, when I say "you," I'm speaking to someone who's caring for a patient. However, adults with T1DM can still apply the information in this book to their own lives; in fact, several topics throughout the book are directed specifically toward adult patients (such as the work and driving information in Chapter 14).

Here are a few more conventions to guide you through this book:

- *Italic* points out defined terms and emphasizes certain words.
- **Boldface** highlights key words in bulleted lists and actions to take in numbered steps.
- Monofont indicates Web addresses.

When this book was printed, it may have been necessary to break some Web addresses across two lines of text. If that happened, rest assured that I haven't put in any extra characters (such as hyphens) to indicate the break. So, when using one of these Web addresses, just type exactly what you see in this book, pretending that the line break doesn't exist.

What You're Not to Read

Shaded areas called sidebars contain material that's interesting but not essential to your understanding. If you don't care to go so deeply into a subject, skip the sidebars. You won't be at any disadvantage.

Foolish Assumptions

In writing this book, I assumed that you know little or nothing about diabetes and T1DM in particular. Forgive me if some of the material is too basic for you, but many of the people who read this, especially the children and young adults, will be learning about diabetes for the first time. I want all my readers to have a sturdy foundation upon which to build a skyscraper of knowledge. If you already know a great deal about T1DM, you'll find new information that adds to your knowledge.

You probably fall into one of the following categories:

- ✔ You're the parent of a child who's newly diagnosed with T1DM, or you just want an introduction to all that's new in this field.
- ✔ You're a child or young adult who's old enough to understand basic ideas about your T1DM.
- ✔ You're an adult who's been recently diagnosed with T1DM. (Don't worry; the information in this book applies to you, too!)
- ✔ You're a friend or family member of a person with T1DM, and you want to understand and help the person.

How This Book Is Organized

The book is divided into six parts to help you find out all that you want to know about T1DM.

Part 1: Defining Type 1 Diabetes

In this part, you discover the central roles of glucose and insulin in T1DM and the way that one, insulin, controls the other. You find out what happens when this control doesn't take place. I also explain who typically gets T1DM, how it's diagnosed, and how to move forward after a diagnosis.

As I say in this introduction, there's more than one kind of diabetes. You find out how to tell them apart in this part. It's not always an easy task, especially when the patient is a child, so the info in this part is essential.

Part II: Considering the Consequences of Type 1 Diabetes

Uncontrolled T1DM has consequences, both short-term, which occur within days or even minutes of loss of control of blood glucose, and long-term, which occur after 10 to 15 years of poor glucose (sugar) control. This part goes in-depth on the topics of short- and long-term complications and also lets you know that your child doesn't have to suffer any of these consequences.

As you find out in this part, in an effort to control glucose, it's possible to overcompensate with insulin, leading to a condition of low blood sugar called hypoglycemia, a significant short-term complication. The long-term consequences or complications can all be detected early in the course of their development. With both short- and long-term complications, it's important to know what they are and what the symptoms are in order to catch them early on and prevent further progression if they do occur.

In this part, I also cover the emotional and psychological difficulties associated with a chronic disease such as diabetes, telling you what they are and how to deal with them.

Part III: Treating Type 1 Diabetes

Treating T1DM requires a lot of effort, as you find out in this part, but I know you and your child can do it. What's involved? For starters, you have to do a great deal of monitoring, which at this time still requires sticking your child's finger four or more times a day. He also has to get certain laboratory tests on a regular basis and go to the doctor for regular checkups.

What your child eats and when he eats is a big part of managing his diabetes. Unlike the person without diabetes, your child needs to arrange his meals and his insulin so that the insulin is in his body when the food is. Then there's exercise, an important part of treatment that lowers the blood glucose because the muscles need sugar to work. As I explain in this part, many patients use exercise in place of insulin and end up taking very few units of insulin.

The subject of insulin requires two chapters in this part. One chapter tells you what insulin is and how to use it properly. The other discusses a new and important device that supplies insulin 24 hours a day, the insulin pump.

Recently, other drugs have become available for treating T1DM. In this part, I make sure that you know about these and the role they can play in controlling your child's blood glucose as well as the effect of drugs that interact with his insulin. I also address other methods of treating diabetes that involve attempts to replace the cells that make insulin and therefore cure the disease.

Part IV: Living with Type 1 Diabetes

The chapters in this part delve into a number of special considerations for the person with T1DM. If he goes to school, his teachers need to know some basic management strategies, such as how to deal with low blood glucose. At work, there are still some jobs for which the person with T1DM isn't welcome. And there are insurance issues that a person with a chronic disease needs to consider.

In addition to these considerations, this part also tells you about how minor illnesses like colds may throw off diabetic control and how to accommodate the special needs of the traveler with T1DM.

Women and the elderly are two special populations when it comes to living with T1DM. In this part, I discuss how women can control their diabetes during menstruation, how a woman with T1DM should be in excellent control of her T1DM prior to conceiving a baby and throughout her pregnancy, and how menopause brings new considerations including whether or not to use hormone replacement therapy. I close this part with a chapter on the elderly population with T1DM and the unique problems that they face in treating their condition.

Part V: The Part of Tens

The Part of Tens is a staple in all *For Dummies* books; in this book, it provides an opportunity to emphasize some of the key points that I make throughout the book and to provide some material that you may not have found there, including the following:

- T1DM is a disease mostly diagnosed in children, but after a while, the child must take over his complete care. The chapter on ten ways to involve kids in their T1DM management offers suggestions on how to start this process.

- A number of management ideas are essential to good diabetes care. In this part, I point out the ones I consider the top ten.

- Myths about diagnosis and treatment tend to develop around any disease, particularly a chronic disease like T1DM. In this part, I dispel ten of those myths. If you know of any that I don't cover, please e-mail them to me.

- I provide information on the latest and greatest discoveries on T1DM in this part so that you can stay on the cutting edge of treatment.

Part VI: Appendixes

If you come upon a term in the text that you don't understand, turn to the glossary in Appendix A for a definition. And if you want new or extended information on any subject, go to Appendix B, where you can find resources for the latest information and numerous suggestions to further your education.

Icons Used in This Book

Books in the *For Dummies* series feature icons, which direct you toward information that may be of particular interest or importance. Here's an explanation of what each icon in this book signifies:

When you find this alongside information, it's time to dial the doctor for help.

When you see this icon, it means the information is essential. Make sure you understand it.

This icon points out important information that can save you time and energy.

This icon warns against potential problems.

Where to Go from Here

Where you go from here depends on your needs. If you want a basic understanding of what T1DM is and isn't, head to Part I. If you or someone you know has a complication due to T1DM, skip to Part II. For help in treating T1DM using every available tool, turn to Part III. If you're thinking of becoming pregnant, are going into menopause, are elderly, or have a parent with T1DM, Part IV is your next stop. Likewise, go there if you want to know what your options are for school, work, and other activities, or if you want to know how to manage travel or illness. For a bird's-eye view of getting kids involved, key treatment strategies, the mythology that surrounds T1DM, and the latest discoveries, check Part V.

In any case, as my mother used to say when she gave me a present, use this book in good health.

Part I
Defining Type 1 Diabetes

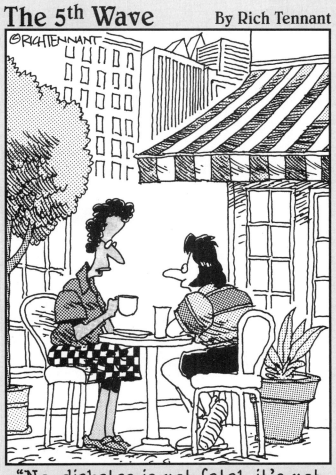

The 5th Wave   By Rich Tennant

"No, diabetes is not fatal, it's not contagious, and it doesn't mean you'll always get half my desserts."

In this part . . .

This part introduces you to type 1 diabetes mellitus. You start with a grand overview of this distinct disease's development. Then you get into the precise symptoms and the diagnosis process followed by an introduction to the diseases commonly confused with type 1 diabetes, especially type 2 diabetes. Luckily, the information in this part helps ensure that you never confuse them again.

Chapter 1

Dealing with Type 1 Diabetes

* *

* *

*1*n 2005, the most recent year for which there are statistics, there were 340,000 people in the United States with type 1 diabetes (T1DM) according to the Centers for Disease Control. About half were children up to age 20. There are 30,000 new cases every year, almost all in children.

Whether you're an older child or young adult able to take care of your own diabetes, or a parent or other caregiver for a young child with this disease, you should be aware that there's a great deal that you can do to minimize both the short- and long-term complications that may develop and live a long and healthy life with T1DM.

What! You don't believe me! Consider the story of two brothers, Robert and Gerald. Robert is 85 years old and developed T1DM at age 5. Gerald is 90 and developed T1DM at age 16. The physician who follows them, Dr. George L. King, research director of the Joslin Diabetes Center in Boston, studies patients with T1DM who have lived more than 50 years with the disease. He has more than 400 such patients.

Dr. King says that these patients have a lot in common. They

- ✔ Keep extensive records of their blood sugars, their diet, their exercise, their insulin dosage, and their daily food consumption
- ✔ Do a lot of exercise
- ✔ Eat very carefully
- ✔ Have a very positive outlook

These actions form the basis of effective T1DM treatment, which I introduce in this chapter. I also give you an overview of the potential consequences of T1DM and tips for living well with it.

At the present time, there's no way to prevent T1DM, but I believe a change isn't far off and T1DM may be preventable in perhaps in the next five years. The breakthrough will come with the use of stem cells, transplantation, or the elimination of the cause of T1DM. You can read much more about this subject in Chapters 13 and 21.

Understanding What Type 1 Diabetes Is (and Isn't)

T1DM, simply stated, is an autoimmune disease. Immunity is what protects you from foreign invaders like bacteria and viruses. In autoimmunity, your body mistakenly acts against your own tissues. In T1DM, the immune cells and proteins react against the cells that make insulin, destroying them. (Insulin is the chemical or hormone that controls the blood glucose; glucose is sugar that provides instant energy.)

Although it often begins dramatically, T1DM doesn't occur overnight. Many patients give a history of several months of increasing thirst and urination, among other symptoms. Also, T1DM usually begins in childhood, but some folks don't develop it until they're adults. In either case, to verify a diagnosis of T1DM, a sample of blood is taken and its glucose level is measured. If the patient is fasting, the level should be no more than 125 mg/dl; if there's no fast, the level should be no more than 199 mg/dl. For further confirmation, tests should be done at two different times to check for inconsistencies. However, a person with a blood glucose of 300 to 500 mg/dl who has an acetone smell on his breath clearly has T1DM until proven otherwise.

So how is type 1 diabetes different from type 2 diabetes (T2DM)? The central problem in T2DM isn't a lack of insulin but insulin resistance; in other words, the body resists the normal, healthy functioning of insulin. Before the development of T2DM, when a person's blood glucose is still normal, the level of insulin is abnormally high because the person is resistant to the insulin and therefore more is needed to keep the glucose normal.

To complicate matters, a type of diabetes called *Latent Autoimmune Diabetes in Adults* (LADA) is a cross between T1DM and T2DM; a person with LADA exhibits traits of both diseases.

Chapter 2 details the basics of T1DM, including how insulin works, what goes wrong when blood glucose levels are too high, the specific symptoms to watch for, and gathering a team of doctors and other specialists after a diagnosis. Chapter 3 fully explains how T2DM and LADA are different from T1DM.

Handling the Physical and Emotional Consequences of Type 1 Diabetes

What makes diabetes a difficult disease are the physical complications associated with poor control of the blood glucose. These complications are generally divided into short-term complications and long-term complications.

✔ **Short-term complications,** which I cover in Chapter 4, are the result of a blood glucose that's either very low or very high. Low blood glucose (called *hypoglycemia*) can occur in minutes as a result of too much insulin, too much exercise, or too little food, but high blood glucose often takes several hours to develop. Whereas low blood glucose often can be managed at home, severe high blood glucose (called *diabetic ketoacidosis*) is an emergency that's managed by a doctor in the hospital. Nevertheless, it's important that you understand how it develops in order to prevent it. Chapter 4 describes the signs and symptoms associated with both of these complications and the best ways of handling them.

✔ **Long-term complications,** which I cover in Chapter 5, can be devastating. It's much better to prevent them with very careful diabetes management than to try to treat them after they develop. Fortunately, they take 15 or more years to fully develop, and there's time to slow them down if not reverse them if you're aware of them. All long-term complications can be detected in the very earliest stages.

The long-term complications consist of eye disease known as *retinopathy,* kidney disease known as *nephropathy,* and nerve disease known as *neuropathy.* Diabetes is the leading cause of new cases of blindness; new cases of kidney failure requiring dialysis, which cleanses the blood of toxins when the kidneys can no longer do their job; and loss of sensation in the feet as well as other consequences of nerve damage.

Not only does T1DM have short- and long-term physical consequences, but as an autoimmune disease, T1DM also is associated with other autoimmune diseases such as *celiac disease,* an inflammation of the gastrointestinal tract; thyroid disease; and skin diseases. Chapter 5 explains the importance of checking for those diseases and correcting them, if present.

As you may expect, people with T1DM also have significant psychological and emotional needs. It's important, first of all, to realize that T1DM has been present in some very high achievers. (I name names in Chapter 6.) In addition, T1DM is not only a disease of the particular patient but also a disease of the entire family. All family members are affected in one way or another. In Chapter 6, you find out ways that family members can help themselves and help the patient to maintain his self-esteem and a high quality of life.

If you're the patient with T1DM, the people around you need to know that you have diabetes and how to help you when you can't help yourself. Often people with T1DM try to keep their disease secret, as though it's a blot on their character. T1DM isn't your fault. There will be times when you may need the help of others, and it will be a whole lot easier for them to help you if they know about your condition and what to do in different circumstances. (All this is also true for your child with T1DM.)

Treating Type 1 Diabetes Effectively

Part III may be the most important part of this book. Your willingness to do all the things I recommend in that part (which I preview in the following sections) means the difference between living a long and healthy life or dying at a much younger age (whether for your child or yourself if you're the patient).

Undergoing regular testing

There are a number of tests that your child's doctor should be doing on a regular basis. Chapter 7 outlines all these tests, explains what they mean, and discusses how often they should be done. These tests include the following:

- Blood pressure check
- Height and weight check
- Foot exam
- Hemoglobin A1c
- Microalbuminuria
- Eye exam
- Lipid panel
- Thyroid function check
- Ankle-brachial index study

Don't leave it up to your child's doctor to order these tests. On the Cheat Sheet at the front of this book, I provide a chart that lists the tests that need to be done and the frequency for each test; it also has spaces for you to enter the test results. Make copies of the blank chart, fill out a copy, and take it to your child's doctor at every visit to remind him or her to do these tests.

Regular testing outside the doctor's office is crucial, too. Daily self-monitoring of blood glucose may be the most important thing that you and your child can do to control his blood glucose. The available meters are simple to use, highly accurate, and require tiny amounts of blood. The more you know about your child's blood glucose under all circumstances, the easier it is to keep it in the normal range — not too low and not too high. Flip to Chapter 7 for full details on monitoring blood glucose.

Eating wisely

If you're a parent of a child with T1DM, you need to make sure that your child gets the right nutrients for proper growth and that he balances the food intake with insulin at all times. If you're meticulous about the food your child eats, you'll find that controlling his blood glucose is much easier. I have numerous patients whose blood glucose levels improved dramatically after I sent them to a dietitian.

Chapter 8 discusses how to count carbohydrates so that your child takes the right amount of insulin for the food that he eats. I explain how to include the right mix of protein, fat, vitamins, minerals, and water along with carbohydrates; the diet challenges you face when you feed a child of any age; and how to take other food factors into account, such as sugar substitutes and fast food. I also offer advice on coping with eating disorders.

Exercising for more control

Exercise helps to reduce the amount of insulin that your child requires and makes it easier to control his blood glucose. Any exercise is better than no exercise, but 30 minutes a day should be your minimum goal for your child. In Chapter 9, I explain how to take care before your child starts an exercise plan by talking to the doctor and adjusting insulin intake, among other tasks. I show you how to encourage your child to exercise at any age and help him pick an activity (even a competitive sport!). I also give you my picks for the best exercises around: walking and training with weights.

Taking insulin

Chapters 10 and 11 tell you all you need to know about insulin (including types and dosages), and all the old and new ways to administer it.

- ✔ The types of insulin are long-acting, rapid-acting, and some in-between insulins. The insulins that most closely mimic the action of human insulin in the body are clearly the best. Insulin can be taken by shots, using jet injections, and by inhaling it into your lungs. I give you the pros and cons of each method in Chapter 10 and let you choose for yourself.

- ✔ Delivering insulin with a pump deserves to have Chapter 11 all to itself because it's quite different from the methods in Chapter 10. Many patients use pumps to administer their insulin. The clever manufacturers have tried to arrange the pump so that it delivers insulin just like your own pancreas. Unfortunately, the pump currently can't detect the level of glucose in your blood and provide insulin accordingly just like your own pancreas, but modern insulin pumps aren't far from that ideal.

Using other medications and treatments

At one time, insulin was the only drug given to the patient with T1DM. Today, there are some new drugs that can assist insulin in controlling the blood glucose. Chapter 12 looks into these drugs and some promising treatments for people with T1DM, such as acupuncture and biofeedback.

At the other end of the spectrum are drugs that make it even more difficult to control your blood glucose (or your child's). Alcohol and nicotine in cigarettes top the list, but there are a number of illegal drugs that also complicate diabetes management. Avoid these drugs at all costs. In Chapter 12, I explain how they make glucose control so difficult.

Deciding to transplant

Chapter 13 could be called "the chapter of hope." It discusses potential cures for T1DM. I tell you about transplanting a kidney, the entire pancreas, or both at the same time (now that's a neat trick!). I also discuss transplanting only the beta cells that make insulin. I describe the preparation and process for each type of surgery and explain the continuing issues that you have to deal with afterward.

Living Well with Type 1 Diabetes

Unfortunately, type 1 diabetes is a lifelong chronic disease. As you find out in the following sections, it requires your child to make adjustments in his life that many people who don't have diabetes take for granted. But making these adjustments is a small price to pay for being able to live life to the fullest!

Handling school, work, and other daily activities

A number of laws mandate the accommodations that schools must provide for your child with diabetes. Chapter 14 tells you how to get the school authorities on your side with the use of Section 504 Plans and individualized education programs. I also discuss how to handle T1DM in college.

Done with college? If you have T1DM, there are certain jobs that aren't open to you. For example, you can't serve in the military, and you can't fly commercial airliners. There was a time when you couldn't fly a private plane either, but fortunately that time is past. Chapter 14 discusses the jobs you can't have when you have T1DM, what to do if you suspect discrimination at work because of your T1DM, and the ways that employers can integrate their employees with T1DM into the workplace. I also talk about some other issues for adults, including driving with diabetes and obtaining insurance.

Adjusting to sick days and travel

If your child has another illness in addition to T1DM, there are special adjustments that you have to make. He may not feel like eating, and you may think that he needs less insulin as a result. The truth is usually the opposite. Your child's body responds to an acute illness by pouring out hormones that promote the production of more glucose, so his blood glucose rises. He may actually need more insulin during an illness when he can't eat than he'd need when he's healthy. Chapter 15 provides the information you need to manage your child's illness when he also has T1DM.

Another special circumstance that affects diabetes care is travel. When traveling, you and your child may go through different time zones. This complicates taking insulin because each type of insulin has a certain duration of action, and you may lose or gain hours as you travel. In Chapter 15, I share suggestions for handling your child's insulin smoothly and traveling with his supplies safely.

Getting through pregnancy and menopause

Women with T1DM have special needs. Starting with oral contraceptives, Chapter 16 takes you through preparing for pregnancy, getting through the pregnancy, and considering hormone replacement therapy during menopause. The surge of estrogens and progesterones that occurs every month in a menstruating female makes it even harder to control the blood glucose, so you find out the best ways to handle this tricky situation.

As a woman with T1DM, you shouldn't even consider pregnancy without reading Chapter 16. The likelihood that you'll produce a baby with malformations will be much lower if you understand the information that I present here and take care of yourself accordingly. Keeping your diabetes under excellent control throughout the pregnancy ensures a much easier delivery and a healthy child. I can't overstate the importance of diet and exercise throughout the pregnancy. Every mother-to-be wants an easy delivery and a healthy baby; if you keep your blood glucose under control throughout the pregnancy, the healthy baby is guaranteed.

Aging with type 1 diabetes

The elderly person with T1DM deserves special consideration. He may not exhibit the same signs and symptoms as younger people. He usually has other illnesses and afflictions that complicate his diabetes care, including loss of hearing, diminished vision, and maybe even loss of mental function. All these circumstances may make insulin administration very difficult. The dosage of drugs given to the elderly is usually significantly lower than the dosage for the non-elderly. What's a caretaker to do? Chapter 17 has the information that can make caring for the elderly person a lot easier.

Chapter 2

Recognizing Type 1 Diabetes

A wasting disease that was probably type 1 diabetes is mentioned in an Egyptian papyrus dated over 3,500 years. Although they didn't call it type 1 diabetes, over 2,000 years ago the Greeks and Romans described many of the features of the condition exactly as doctors see it today. The difference is that the ancients could do nothing about it. In contrast, today's doctors have all the tools needed to make type 1 diabetes nothing more than a major annoyance.

In this chapter, I provide some basic information about type 1 diabetes, or T1DM for short. You find out how it develops, who gets it, and how it's diagnosed.

Understanding How Type 1 Diabetes Works

Type 1 diabetes is all about *glucose* and *insulin*. What's the difference? Here's what you need to know:

- ✔ **Glucose** is one of many sugars, but it happens to be the specific sugar found in your blood that provides instant energy. Sugar is a carbohydrate, one of the three sources of energy in your body, along with protein and fat.

- ✔ **Insulin** is a chemical known as a *hormone,* which means that it's made in an organ, in this case the pancreas, and carried around the body in the bloodstream. The function of insulin is to act as a key to the "door" in each cell of the body that opens to allow glucose in. However, not every cell requires insulin to get its glucose; some cells and organs take up glucose without using insulin. These include

- The brain
- Nerve fibers
- Red blood cells
- The retinas of the eyes
- The kidneys
- Blood vessels

Figure 2-1 shows the pancreas and its parts along with its location behind the stomach. The insulin-producing and insulin-storing pancreas cells (called *B* or *beta cells*) are found in groups called *islets of Langerhans* throughout the pancreas. Other cells present in the islets of Langerhans include A cells, which produce *glucagon,* a hormone that's very important to patients with diabetes because it raises blood glucose when it gets too low; and D cells, which make *somatostatin,* a hormone that blocks the secretion of other hormones but doesn't have a use in diabetes because it causes high blood glucose.

In people who don't have type 1 diabetes, the presence of insulin helps control the conversion of glucose into energy in the body. People with type 1 diabetes, however, go through a triggering event (most likely a viral infection) that leads to a lack of insulin in the body, which in turn leads to having uncontrolled glucose (and that can cause some bad stuff to happen). I explain how the whole process works in the following sections.

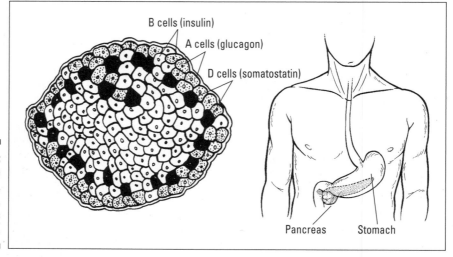

Figure 2-1:
The pancreas, its parts, and its location.

B cells (insulin)
A cells (glucagon)
D cells (somatostatin)

Pancreas   Stomach

Distinguishing between controlled and uncontrolled glucose

The definition of type 1 diabetes is simple: It's the lack of control of glucose in the body due to a lack of insulin. In the following sections, I explain the differences between normally controlled glucose and out-of-control glucose.

Controlling glucose normally

Glucose from the blood gets into most cells (other than those previously listed) when insulin is available to let it in. In the cell, glucose is converted into energy. If there's more than enough glucose to meet the energy needs of the individual, the excess glucose is stored in the liver and in muscle. When the liver and muscle are filled, additional glucose is converted to fat. Your body has an enormous ability to store fat, whether it comes from glucose or from the food you eat.

In a healthy person who diets, the release of insulin declines because glucose is what stimulates insulin to be released. The body then turns to the liver, where glucose is stored as glycogen. The A cells of the pancreas (refer to Figure 2-1) release glucagon, which breaks down the glycogen back into glucose to continue to provide energy.

When the glycogen is used up, the body turns to the other form of stored energy, fat. Fat is converted into compounds called *glycerol* and *fatty acids*.

- **Glycerol** is changed into glucose to provide energy and is used up.

- **Fatty acids** are converted into other compounds called *ketones* in the liver. Except for the brain, the entire body can use fatty acids for energy.

Over time, as the diet continues, the body begins to break down muscle to convert it into glucose.

Losing control of glucose

When the body experiences a complete lack of insulin, as in people with T1DM (see the next section to find out how a lack of insulin is triggered), glucose can't enter cells from the blood with the exception of those it enters passively (as I note earlier in this chapter). These cells continue to take up glucose as long as the glucose inside them is less than the glucose in the bloodstream. When blood glucose is high as a result of inadequate insulin, the cells and organs that can take up glucose continue doing so even though other cells and organs that depend on insulin can't do so. The latter cells and organs suffer the complications of type 1 diabetes that I explain in Chapters 4 and 5.

Sharing some patient stories

For some time, Vincent's parents had noticed that their 8-year-old son didn't have his usual energy. He was drinking more soda than usual and seemed to have an increased appetite. But despite eating more food, he was losing weight. Vincent looked tired, which his parents thought was because he woke up a few times each night to go to the bathroom. He even wet his bed for the first time in years. His concerned parents took him to his pediatrician, who measured Vincent's blood glucose, did a few other tests, and informed Vincent's parents that their son had type 1 diabetes. Vincent's parents were quite upset by the diagnosis, but they began giving him insulin shots and carefully monitoring his food intake. In just a few days, Vincent put on weight, stopped urinating so frequently, and was able to sleep through the night.

Lynn was a 12-year-old girl who loved to play sports. In fact, she was the best soccer player on her team. Because she was so active, she drank a lot of sports drinks and water. One day, she complained to her mother that she was very tired after a particularly strenuous soccer game on a very hot day. Her mother felt this was normal, considering the circumstances. She noticed, however, that her daughter was looking a little thinner. Between soccer games the following

week, Lynn was very thirsty and going to the bathroom frequently, but her parents thought it was normal for an active young girl. However, at her next soccer game, Lynn was too tired to play for very long, and afterward, she went right home and got in bed. Lynn's mother couldn't wake her for dinner, so she called an ambulance and took her daughter to an emergency room. The doctor did an immediate blood glucose test, found it to be 618 mg/dl, and had Lynn admitted to the intensive care unit with a diagnosis of diabetic ketoacidosis caused by type 1 diabetes. Lynn received intravenous insulin and fluids and was awake and alert within 48 hours. She was converted to subcutaneous insulin injections. Lynn and her parents followed up by participating in a diabetes education program, which taught them the skills Lynn would need for the rest of her life.

These two cases are typical of the way type 1 diabetes begins, and the apparent suddenness of the disease in both children obscures the fact that it was probably developing over several months. At one time, Lynn's story was more common in that the condition was unexpected and the child ended up in the intensive care unit. Now, as a result of more awareness of diabetes in the general population, Vincent's story is the more typical one.

Despite there being plenty of glucose in the blood, insulin-requiring cells behave as though there's no glucose. The body therefore begins breaking down fat and turning muscle into glucose for those cells, leading to a large amount of glucose in the body. If this process isn't reversed by giving insulin, the person becomes very sick with diabetic ketoacidosis (see Chapter 4).

Other hormones besides insulin play an important role as control of glucose is lost. Each tries to raise the blood glucose to satisfy the needs of the tissues. I mention one such hormone, glucagon, from the A cells in the pancreas's islets of Langerhans, in the previous section. In addition, the adrenal glands located above the kidneys begin to secrete two important hormones, adrenaline and cortisol. After a while, the pituitary gland in the brain secretes growth hormone. Following is more information on these hormones:

✔ **Adrenaline** works with glucagon on the glycogen in the liver to break it down to produce more glucose. Adrenaline stimulates production of glucose from protein. It also decreases the glucose taken up by muscle and liver cells, thus making it more available to the brain. Adrenaline turns fat into fatty acids as well. Other effects of adrenaline are shakiness, sweating, rapid heartbeat, and hunger.

✔ **Cortisol** increases the production of glucose by stimulating the breakdown of both proteins and fats while decreasing the uptake of glucose by tissues that require insulin, like muscles and the liver, to make it available for the brain.

✔ **Growth hormone** breaks down body fat and decreases the uptake of glucose by blocking the action of insulin where it's necessary to open the cells to glucose, such as in the liver and muscles.

Interestingly, these same hormones play important roles in raising blood glucose when it's too low for any reason (not just a lack of insulin); such a condition is called *hypoglycemia,* and I discuss it in Chapter 4.

Figure 2-2 shows the origins of the different hormones that affect blood glucose.

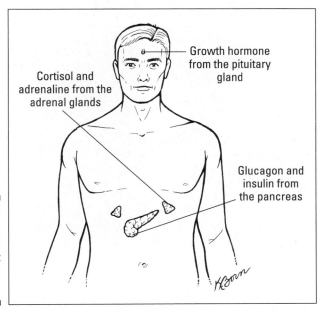

Cortisol and adrenaline from the adrenal glands

Growth hormone from the pituitary gland

Glucagon and insulin from the pancreas

Figure 2-2: The origins of hormones that affect blood glucose.

Triggering type 1 diabetes

Not everyone can get T1DM. It begins with an inherited susceptibility for the disease, which means that chromosomes, the parts of each cell that contain the genetic material, are involved. Specifically, type 1 diabetes is connected to chromosome 6, which has an area called the *HLA complex* (human leukocyte antigen complex). There are many different HLA complexes on the chromosome, but only a few are associated with the development of T1DM. People who develop T1DM all have one or more of several HLA complexes associated with the disease.

If your child has the necessary HLA complex, he needs something in the environment — most probably a viral infection — to trigger T1DM. The viral infection causes his body to produce *antibodies,* protective proteins that try to destroy the virus. Cells that circulate in the blood, called *T cells,* make these antibodies. T cells can kill foreign invaders both by producing antibodies and by acting on them directly. It appears that the *beta cells* that make insulin in the pancreas share some antigens with the virus. Therefore, the T cells in the blood begin to attack and destroy the beta cells that make the insulin because the T cells mistake the beta cells for the virus.

So how does a person reach the point where type 1 diabetes has officially developed? Here's a typical scenario: Your child is born with the HLA complex, and he gets a viral infection when he's 2 years old or at any other age. Over the next six to eight years, the T cells slowly destroy his beta cells. However, he has no symptoms because he has sufficient insulin reserve in his pancreas to maintain normal glucose levels. Finally, enough beta cells have been destroyed that your child can't make enough insulin to keep the glucose level normal. His blood glucose rises and begins to leak into his urine, drawing water with it. After a while, the lack of insulin becomes so severe that he has a condition similar to the ones described in the sidebar "Sharing some patient stories."

How do doctors know all that's happening in the body over such a span of time? They look for T1DM in family members of people with T1DM because the family members may have some of the same genetic material, in this case the gene that led to susceptibility to T1DM. A few years after the viral infection, your child's doctor can measure the antibodies that indicate that the beta cells are being attacked — long before the development of *clinical T1DM,* the point at which symptoms are present. More than 90 percent of patients with new T1DM will have one or more of the antibodies. The most common antibody is called glutamic acid decarboxylase autoantibody, or GAD, and is found in 70 to 80 percent of type 1 patients.

Environmental factors that have antigens similar to the antigens on the beta cells include

- Cow's milk
- Coxsackie B virus

- Enterovirus
- German measles (rubella)
- Mumps virus
- Rotavirus

It's not known which of these, if any, is the precipitating environmental factor for T1DM. Evidence of infection with all these viruses, as well as exposure to cow's milk early in life, has been found in many patients with T1DM. Further evidence for an environmental factor in T1DM comes from the finding that fewer cases are diagnosed in the summer months, when people aren't gathered in small spaces and therefore are less susceptible to catching viruses.

T1DM also tends to develop much more often in people who live in northern climates, where people tend to spend more time indoors. The incidence rate in Finland, for instance, is 40 cases per 100,000 population, whereas the incidence rate in Mexico is less than one case per 100,000 population. (See the following section for more information on who gets type 1 diabetes.)

Checking Out the Statistics on Who Gets Type 1 Diabetes

The folks who develop type 1 diabetes tend to fall into a few distinct groups: They're Caucasians in northern climates, they're typically children, and they have a genetic disposition toward the disease. I discuss these categories in more detail in the following sections.

Rates among different places and races

As I note in the previous section, type 1 diabetes occurs much more often in people who live in northern climates and tend to be Caucasian. The differences between this population and others can be dramatic; following are some facts that illustrate the differences:

- Among youths with diabetes aged 1 to 9, 80 percent have T1DM and 20 percent have T2DM.
- Among youths aged 10 to 19, the percentage who have type 2 diabetes (T2DM) is rising but still isn't as high as the percentage with T1DM. (Statistics are poor in this age group.)
- Canada has 25 new cases of T1DM per 100,000 population per year.
- The United States has 15 new cases of T1DM per 100,000 population per year.

✔ Argentina (in a southern climate and with fewer Caucasians in its population) has seven new cases of T1DM per 100,000 population per year.

✔ Chile, with a similar climate and population makeup to Argentina, has two new cases of T1DM per 100,000 population per year.

Rates in children versus adults

It was with good reason that T1DM used to be called "juvenile diabetes"; the vast majority of new cases are in teenagers and young adults, although the disease may occur at any age. One of the major reasons that T1DM is no longer called "juvenile diabetes," however, is that there's another diabetes on the block: Doctors are seeing more and more type 2 diabetes (T2DM; see Chapter 3) among the juvenile population. T2DM is a different disease requiring a different therapy. Also, doctors are recognizing many more cases of T1DM among the adult population. As many as 5 to 10 percent of cases of diabetes in adults previously thought to be type 2 may actually be type 1.

Of course, kids with T1DM grow up and become adults. But they still appear different from folks with T2DM, a disease that tends to affect overweight, sedentary people. Adults with T1DM usually are normal in weight and are physically active.

Rates in families with members who have type 1 diabetes

A patient with T1DM can have his relatives tested for the HLA complex (see the earlier section "Triggering type 1 diabetes" for more about this complex). The opportunity to do that has led to some valuable insights about T1DM.

✔ Only a small fraction (less than 10 percent) of people with the necessary HLA complex develop T1DM.

✔ Many relatives of people with T1DM who have the HLA complex develop autoantibodies, like GAD, but never develop diabetes.

✔ A small percentage (5 to 10 percent) of patients with type 2 diabetes (see Chapter 3) are found to have autoantibodies and are believed to have a slowly progressing form of T1DM called *latent autoimmune diabetes in adults* (LADA).

These findings indicate that T1DM may be a rapidly progressing disease, it may be a very slowly progressing disease, or it may never occur at all in susceptible individuals. How's that for concrete information?

On the hunt for better names

What's really needed are new names for both T1DM and T2DM that are much more descriptive and clearly separate the two diseases. I believe that referring to them both as types of diabetes suggests that they're extremely similar. It also results in too many instances of confusing studies, where you don't know if the patients were type 1 or type 2 unless it's specified. If you have a suggestion for a name, write me at diabetes name@drrubin.com.

When it comes to the importance of a parent's T1DM in predicting whether the child will get T1DM, if the mother has T1DM, there's only a 3 percent chance that the child will develop it. If the father has T1DM, the child has a 6 percent chance of developing it. If both parents have T1DM, the child's likelihood of developing the disease jumps to 30 percent.

How do siblings factor in? Identical twins have a 60 percent chance of both developing T1DM, but the twin who develops it later often doesn't show it for many years. Fraternal twins, who don't share all the same chromosomes, have only an 8 percent chance of both having T1DM, no greater than that of two children born in different years in the same family.

Making a Diagnosis of Type 1 Diabetes

A number of symptoms signal the possibility of type 1 diabetes, so if your child shows a few of them, it's best to arrange testing right away. After the diagnosis, it's also important to find help from the right doctors and develop some important skills to make sure that your child adjusts to life with type 1 diabetes as smoothly as possible.

Surveying the symptoms and undergoing testing

If T1DM develops rapidly, a number of symptoms suggest this diagnosis. They include the following:

- ✔ Abdominal pain
- ✔ Blurred vision
- ✔ Extreme weakness and tiredness
- ✔ Increased thirst

- ✔ Increased urination
- ✔ Irritability and mood changes
- ✔ Loss of menstruation
- ✔ Nausea
- ✔ Weight loss despite increased food intake
- ✔ Vomiting

If you're a parent or spouse of the person who may have T1DM, you may notice these signs:

- ✔ Acetone-like smell on the breath
- ✔ Dehydration
- ✔ Lethargy or even coma
- ✔ Low body temperature (less than 97 degrees Fahrenheit)
- ✔ Rapid breathing
- ✔ Rapid heart rate
- ✔ Reduced blood pressure (less than 90/60)

As soon as T1DM pops up on a doctor's radar, there's usually little trouble making the diagnosis. To verify it, a sample of blood is taken and its glucose level is measured. If the patient is fasting, the level should be no more than 126 mg/dl; if there's no fast, the level should be no more than 200 mg/dl. For further confirmation, tests should be done at two different times to check for inconsistencies. However, a person who presents with a blood glucose of 300 to 500 mg/dl and has an acetone smell on his breath clearly has T1DM until proven otherwise. The pediatrician or primary doctor usually does these tests and refers the patient to the diabetes specialist after the diagnosis is made.

Gathering a group of the right doctors

Most children who develop T1DM are first seen by their pediatricians (adults who develop T1DM, of course, see their primary care physicians). The pediatrician may have some familiarity with diabetes, but he'll probably refer you to a specialist called an *endocrinologist* or a *diabetologist*. Of course, if a child is very sick with diabetic ketoacidosis (see Chapter 4), he enters the hospital immediately to receive acute care, either from an acute care doctor or diabetes specialist. Once the child is stable, the specialist takes over.

The ongoing care of a child with T1DM is in the hands of many different people in addition to the specialist. They include:

- ✔ **The primary physician,** who is the pediatrician who takes care of day-to-day problems like colds, fevers, rashes, and stomach upsets

- ✔ **The dietitian,** who informs the parents of the food choices that will keep the child growing while avoiding diabetic complications (see Chapter 8 for more about eating a healthy diet)

- ✔ **The diabetes educator,** who teaches the parents and the child what they must know about insulin, complications of diabetes and how to avoid them, handling sick days, and managing travel

  A diabetes educator should be a Certified Diabetes Educator, having been tested by the National Certification Board for Diabetes Educators, and should have a verification of certification to show you. Certified Diabetes Educators must be recertified every five years, so you can be sure that the educator is up-to-date.

- ✔ **The pharmacist,** who ensures that the child gets the right medication and the right materials for testing blood glucose

- ✔ **The mental health worker,** who helps the family get through the mental stresses associated with what will seem like an overwhelming problem at first (see Chapter 6 for more about handling T1DM's emotional and psychological effects)

Later, certain other specialists may be needed such as

- ✔ **An eye doctor** to make sure that diabetes isn't affecting the child's eyes

- ✔ **A foot doctor** to handle minor foot problems before they become worse

- ✔ **A kidney specialist** should the diabetes affect the child's kidneys

You get the names of these other specialists from your diabetes specialist. If you're happy with the diabetes specialist, it's a good idea to work with doctors he or she recommends.

Developing key skills after the diagnosis

In order to help your child to live a long, healthy life free of complications of T1DM, you need a number of skills under your belt. You pick up these skills primarily from the diabetes specialist, the diabetes educator, and the dietitian, but the other professionals listed in the previous section also contribute to your education.

The major skills that you must acquire to help your child and that your child must acquire as he grows are covered throughout this book. They include the following:

- Understanding the diabetes disease process (which I cover earlier in this chapter) and the options for treatment (including ways of administering insulin, diet, exercise, and so forth; see Part III)
- Adjusting to the psychosocial demands of T1DM (Chapter 6)
- Monitoring blood glucose and urine ketones (breakdown products of fat) and using the results to improve glucose control (Chapter 7)
- Managing nutrition (Chapter 8)
- Incorporating physical activity in the child's lifestyle (Chapter 9)
- Using insulin properly (Chapters 10 and 11)
- Preventing, detecting, and treating acute complications (Chapter 4)
- Preventing, detecting, and treating chronic complications (Chapter 5)
- Setting goals to promote health, and problem solving for daily living (Chapters 14 and 15)
- Promoting preconception care and management during pregnancy (Chapter 16)
- Promoting care and management in the elderly (Chapter 17)

If you sign up for a diabetes education program, make sure the curriculum includes all these lessons with the possible exception of the pregnancy information for a young child or a male.

Chapter 3

Excluding Other Types of Diabetes

In This Chapter

▶ Spotting the differences between type 1, latent autoimmune, and type 2 diabetes

▶ Surveying diseases and agents that can cause diabetes

*T*o paraphrase Senator Lloyd Bentsen in a famous vice presidential debate when he told Senator Dan Quayle that he was no Jack Kennedy, I know type 1 diabetes, and type 2 diabetes is no type 1 diabetes. It's unfortunate that type 1 diabetes and type 2 diabetes have the same name except for one digit. One always seems to be confused for the other despite the fact that their differences are numerous. If uncontrolled, both diseases are associated with high levels of blood glucose, leading to the same long-term complications, but even their long-term complications differ in some respects. To mix up matters even more, a form of diabetes called latent autoimmune diabetes in adults (LADA) has features of both type 1 diabetes and type 2 diabetes. This chapter describes type 2 diabetes, latent autoimmune diabetes in adults, and how they differ from type 1 diabetes so you can make sure that you (or your child) are diagnosed with and treated for the correct disease.

In addition, in order to really understand type 1 diabetes (or T1DM), you need to have a handle on other causes of diabetes, specifically conditions like Cushing's syndrome and acromegaly. Fortunately, certain other signs and symptoms identify these conditions, as you find out in this chapter.

Distinguishing Type 2 and Latent Autoimmune Diabetes from Type 1 Diabetes

Type 2 diabetes is the form of diabetes that develops most often in adults and is associated with obesity and lack of exercise. Latent autoimmune diabetes also develops in adults but shares more characteristics with T1DM. The following sections cover these types of diabetes, but for more information about type 2 diabetes, check out my book *Diabetes For Dummies* (Wiley).

Type 2 diabetes

When people talk about diabetes these days, they're generally talking about type 2 diabetes (or T2DM), which used to be called *adult onset diabetes, non-insulin dependent diabetes,* or *insulin independent diabetes.* The vast majority of people with diabetes in the United States have type 2 diabetes, and the numbers are growing. About 21 million people have diabetes in the U.S., and about 20 million of them probably have type 2. In the following sections, I explain how type 2 diabetes works and who's at risk for developing it, and I discuss its diagnosis and treatment.

Understanding how type 2 diabetes works

The central problem in T2DM is not lack of insulin (as it is in T1DM; see Chapter 2 for details) but *insulin resistance.* That is, the body resists the normal, healthy functioning of insulin. Prior to the development of diabetes, when a person's blood glucose is still normal, the level of insulin is abnormally high because the person is resistant to the insulin and therefore more is needed to keep the glucose normal; a shot of insulin doesn't reduce the blood glucose in someone with type 2 diabetes nearly as much as it does in healthy people without insulin resistance. The insulin resistance is caused by a genetic abnormality and is made worse by weight gain and lack of exercise.

When diabetes is present, even though the person actually makes even more than the normal amount of insulin to try to compensate (at least early in the disease), they can't keep the blood glucose in the normal range. It rises to levels greater than 100 mg/dl in the fasting state and 140 mg/dl after eating. This rise results from the body's resistance to its own insulin.

The principal complication that occurs in T1DM but rarely if ever occurs in T2DM is diabetic ketoacidosis (see Chapter 4)

Determining who's at risk for type 2 diabetes

Unlike T1DM, T2DM is strongly inherited. For example, while identical twins with T1DM have a 60 percent chance of both getting T1DM, identical twins with T2DM have a nearly 100 percent chance of both developing T2DM. Nonidentical twins will both develop T2DM 40 percent of the time, but if one has T1DM, there's only an 8 percent chance that the other will develop T1DM.

T2DM also is much more of a lifestyle and environmental disease than T1DM. As lifestyles change and food supplies everywhere have become readily available, the incidence of T2DM has steadily gone up with some exceptions. The countries with the greatest increase in new cases are China and India, places where people previously worked all day in the fields, got around on bicycles, and survived on little food. Today, people in these countries sit in offices, drive cars, and enjoy large meals filled with fat. In other words, they emulate people in the U.S. Another telling example involves Japanese people. In Japan, there's little incidence of T2DM. Japanese who have moved to Hawaii have more cases of T2DM, and those who have moved to the American mainland have the most.

What are the important lifestyle and environmental factors in developing T2DM?

- ✔ **Central distribution of fat:** People with T2DM have apple-shaped rather than pear-shaped bodies. They carry their weight under their belts rather than in their arms and legs. This fat is called *visceral fat* because it settles around the internal organs in the abdomen, or *viscera*. Visceral fat is associated with insulin resistance and the development of diabetes as well as coronary artery disease and heart attacks. Fortunately, visceral fat is often the first to go with diet and regular exercise; you only need to lose 5 to 10 percent of your weight to reduce this fat significantly and your chance of getting T2DM or a heart attack as well.

- ✔ **High body mass index:** Doctors determine *body mass index* (BMI) by looking at weight in relation to height. For example, 150 pounds on a 5 foot 2 inch male is too much weight, whereas 150 pounds on a 5 foot 10 inch male makes him thin.

    You can determine your BMI by multiplying your weight in pounds by 703, dividing the result by your height in inches, and dividing that result by your height in inches again. A BMI greater than 25 is considered overweight, and a BMI over 30 is obese in Caucasians.

- ✔ **Low intake of dietary fiber:** A diet low in dietary fiber (as found in whole grains, fruits, and vegetables) is associated with a greater incidence of T2DM. Fiber protects against T2DM in that, among other things, it slows the uptake of glucose from the intestine into the blood.

- ✔ **Physical inactivity:** Every study that compares physically active individuals with physically inactive individuals finds a higher prevalence of T2DM in the sedentary group.

Because the environment plays such a large role in the development of T2DM, it isn't surprising that spouses of people with T2DM have an increased risk of developing it and should be screened by having their blood glucose measured (see the next section for more about screening).

Table 3-1 is intended to help you clearly see the differences between type 1 diabetes and type 2 diabetes.

Table 3-1	Comparison of T1DM and T2DM	
Feature	*Type 1*	*Type 2*
Internal insulin	Little or none	Normal or increased
Age at diagnosis	Usually children	Mostly adults but increasing in children
Body mass index	Usually normal	Usually overweight or obese
Treatment	Insulin	Diet, exercise, oral agents, insulin
Family history	Uncommon	Common
Relation to HLA	High	None
Presence of antibodies	Usually	Rarely
Condition at diagnosis	Very sick	Mildly ill

Diagnosing type 2 diabetes

Mostly adults are diagnosed with T2DM, although the number of children being diagnosed is increasing. Because T2DM usually presents as a mild illness (whereas folks are usually pretty sick when they're diagnosed with T1DM), the diagnosis depends on finding an abnormal blood glucose either in the fasting state or after food has been eaten. The symptoms of T2DM include fatigue, frequent urination, and thirst, plus vaginal infections in women.

A blood glucose of 126 mg/dl or greater in the fasting state or 200 mg/dl or greater after food consumption is diagnostic of type 2 diabetes. For an accurate diagnosis, these numbers should be found on two occasions separated by a week. The tests are done in the laboratory and are ordered by the primary physician.

The American Diabetes Association recommends that all adults be screened for T2DM beginning at age 45 and every three years thereafter if the initial results are normal. If there's a family history of diabetes or a risk factor such as obesity, the initial screening should take place earlier, as early as age 25. With so much obesity in the U.S. population, I believe that screening should begin in obese children.

Treating type 2 diabetes

Treatment of T2DM begins with lifestyle change. The person with diabetes needs to eat a healthy diet and lose weight, although he or she doesn't have to lose a great deal of weight for the glucose to return to normal. The patient also needs to begin a program of regular exercise, preferably for 30 minutes every day.

If lifestyle change doesn't bring about normalization of blood glucose in the person with T2DM, there are a number of oral agents that can lower the blood glucose. Doctors may consider using the intramuscular drug Byetta either before or after the use of oral agents if the agents aren't successful. Byetta causes weight loss and reverses many of the features of T2DM. If Byetta fails, insulin can be given.

Latent Autoimmune Diabetes in Adults (LADA)

Some folks seem to have features of both T1DM and T2DM when they're screened for diabetes. Some of the characteristics of their condition include:

- Adult onset (over the age of 30), as in T2DM

- Mild at presentation, as in T2DM

- Controlled initially with diet and possibly oral agents, as in T2DM

- Gradual need for insulin, as in T2DM

- Normal weight, as in T1DM

- Doesn't respond to agents that decrease insulin resistance, as in T1DM

- Positive autoantibodies like those found in T1DM (see Chapter 2 for more about antibodies)

- Low levels of substances that indicate the presence of insulin, as in T1DM

- No family history of T2DM, as in T1DM

In adults, this condition presents like T2DM and responds initially to drugs for T2DM, but it also has many features of T1DM. The condition doesn't respond to drugs that treat insulin resistance because this central feature of T2DM isn't present. For this reason, the condition has been called *type 1½ diabetes* in the past, but the current name is *latent autoimmune diabetes in adults* (LADA). It has also been called *late-onset autoimmune diabetes of adulthood* and *slow onset type 1 diabetes.*

Some specialists believe that as many as 20 percent of patients with T2DM actually have LADA. The distinction between T2DM and LADA is important because the treatments differ. Both types improve with better diet and exercise. However, after doctors establish the LADA diagnosis, these patients often receive insulin treatment, although they may need very small doses.

Another feature of LADA patients is that they usually don't have the high cholesterol and high blood pressure often found in people with T2DM. As a result, their tendency to get coronary artery disease and heart attacks is less than that of T2DM patients once the blood glucose is controlled.

A paper in *Diabetes Care* in April 2007 showed that there are at least two different subgroups of LADA:

- ✔ One group has much higher glutamic acid decarboxylase (GAD) autoantibodies and more severe autoimmune diabetes with higher blood glucose levels, lower weight, and less insulin resistance.

- ✔ The other group has lower GAD levels and much milder diabetes. See Chapter 2 for details on GAD autoantibodies.

Delving into Diabetes Caused by Other Diseases and Agents

A number of important hormones help to raise the body's blood glucose when it's too low, whether due to too much insulin, too little food, or too much exercise. Because these hormones can raise the blood glucose when they're present in normal amounts, they also can raise the blood glucose excessively when they're present in abnormally high amounts, like when there's a tumor in the gland that makes the hormones. If the body's blood glucose rises over the levels of 100 mg/dl fasting or 200 mg/dl after eating, diabetes occurs.

Some diseases cause diabetes by destroying pancreatic tissue (the pancreas plays an important role in the development of diabetes because it produces insulin). Drugs also can raise the blood glucose to diabetic levels. In some such cases, the diabetes goes away when the drug is stopped (if stopping the drug is an option).

The following sections focus on the most important and common of these diseases and agents that cause diabetes. It's important point to recognize these diseases and agents and either treat or eliminate them. The diabetes will go away if treatment or elimination can be done successfully, which isn't always possible.

Considering hormone-induced causes of diabetes

Hormones that help to raise the blood glucose when it's too low may cause diabetes when present in very large amounts, such as when a tumor develops on the gland that makes a hormone. The important hormones that bring on diabetes under these circumstances are discussed in this section.

Acromegaly

Acromegaly is the disease that occurs when a benign tumor of the pituitary gland in the brain makes excessive quantities of growth hormone. (In Chapter 2, I discuss the hormones that help to raise the blood glucose when it's abnormally lowered and mention the role of growth hormone.) Growth hormone is essential to normal growth of the bones, but it causes diabetes among other abnormalities when it's present in excessive amounts.

Unfortunately, because acromegaly is relatively rare, it sometimes takes years before the diagnosis is finally considered. Fortunately, excessive growth hormone triggers a number of signs and symptoms that can help point doctors to the diagnosis of acromegaly. Following are some of these signs and symptoms of acromegaly:

- ✔ Carpal tunnel syndrome (tingling and weakness in the hand due to squeezing of nerves in the wrist)
- ✔ Coarsening of facial features (enlargement of facial bones and the nose)
- ✔ Excessive sweating
- ✔ Headaches
- ✔ Infertility in women and erectile dysfunction in men
- ✔ Swelling of hands and feet
- ✔ Tiredness

Diabetes occurs in 40 percent of people with acromegaly, which is usually diagnosed in adults. It appears more like T2DM than T1DM, and it's usually mild and can be managed with oral diabetes agents if necessary.

Doctors diagnose acromegaly by obtaining multiple growth hormone blood tests and finding the average. In unafflicted people, growth hormone measurements throughout the day are usually undetectable, but people with acromegaly have measurable levels of growth hormone in all samples. The diagnosis is confirmed by an X-ray study of the pituitary gland, in which the tumor can be clearly seen.

Acromegaly is treated by surgically removing the tumor. If this can't be done or the patient refuses the procedure, several medications bring the growth hormone down to normal levels. Reducing the growth hormone level to normal will cure the patient's diabetes and either stop the rest of the symptoms from worsening or reverse them.

Cushing's syndrome

Cushing's syndrome, which is usually diagnosed in adults, involves an over-production of the hormone cortisol from the adrenal glands on the kidneys. Cortisol is one of the hormones normally secreted to help raise blood glucose when it's low (see Chapter 2). When present in excessive amounts, cortisol can cause diabetes.

The excessive production of cortisol may be the result of one of these causes:

- In 80 percent of cases, a benign tumor of the pituitary gland produces too much of the hormone adrenocortical stimulating hormone (ACTH), which stimulates the adrenals to make more cortisol.

- In 20 percent of cases, a benign tumor in one of the adrenals stimulates the overproduction of cortisol.

The difference between these two causes is that there's a lot of measurable ACTH in the pituitary gland tumor and none in the adrenal gland tumor. Sometimes a cancer will produce a form of *ectopic* ACTH that stimulates overproduction of cortisol, but ectopic ACTH differs from normal ACTH in that it comes from outside the pituitary.

The most obvious symptoms of Cushing's syndrome, such as a round face and obesity of the trunk with wasting of the arms and legs, are rarely seen today because patients are diagnosed at a much earlier stage. The common signs and symptoms that suggest Cushing's syndrome today are

- Acne

- Depression

- Easy bruising of the skin

- Loss of sexual interest

- Menstrual irregularity

- Weakness and tiredness (weakness and tiredness that come on rapidly and severely suggest that a tumor is secreting ectopic ACTH)

Doctors diagnose Cushing's syndrome by finding high levels of cortisol in the blood both in the morning and at night. In a person without Cushing's, the blood contains much more cortisol in the morning than in the evening. Following the finding of abnormally high cortisol, several tests for ACTH are taken to determine if it's high or low:

- **If the ACTH is high,** X-ray studies of the pituitary gland usually identify a tumor, which can be surgically removed. Radiation therapy to the pituitary also is used in some cases, especially when surgery fails to normalize the cortisol level.

> A number of drugs that block the action of cortisol may be used to pre-
> pare the patient for surgery so that he's in the best condition possible
> and to control the disease until radiation therapy can take effect.
>
> ✔ **If the ACTH is low,** X-rays of the adrenals may point to a tumor in one
> of them, which can be removed surgically to cure the condition.

In people with Cushing's syndrome, X-rays of the chest and abdomen often
reveal the source of ectopic production of ACTH, especially when it's a small
cell carcinoma in the lungs. The carcinoma may or may not be operable.

The diabetes that occurs with Cushing's syndrome tends to be mild, which is
in part due to earlier diagnosis. It presents more like T2DM in that it responds
to oral agents, if necessary, but goes away if the underlying disease is cured.

The most common reason for high levels of cortisol and resultant diabetes
is taking cortisol for its anti-inflammatory action. Cortisol is commonly prescribed to treat a variety of autoimmune diseases and to prevent rejection of
transplanted organs. When the cortisol is essential, the diabetes is treated as
necessary. I discuss other chemicals that may cause diabetes in the later section "Discovering drugs and chemicals that may cause or worsen diabetes."

Other causes

There are a number of other diabetes-causing conditions associated with over-
production of hormones, usually due to tumors. They're rarer than acromegaly
and Cushing's syndrome, which I describe in the previous sections. Here's a
rundown of what these other conditions are and who's most likely to get them:

✔ **Glucagonoma:** This condition results from a tumor of the A cells of the
pancreas, which make glucagon. Glucagon is a hormone that counteracts
insulin and raises the blood glucose (see Chapter 2), and excess glucagon
can cause T2DM. The signs and symptoms of glucagonoma are weight
loss, diarrhea, and anemia. It tends to be malignant 75 percent of the time
but fortunately is very rare. It's found in adults and is treated with surgery.

✔ **Hyperthyroidism:** This disease is caused by excessive production of thyroid hormone, usually due to an autoimmune stimulation of the thyroid
gland. Hyperthyroidism causes increased production of glucose from
amino acids in the liver, more rapid uptake of glucose from the intestine,
and increased insulin resistance. All these effects lead to hyperglycemia
(high blood glucose) and possible diabetes, usually of the type 2 variety.
Control of the hyperthyroidism eliminates the diabetes, and it's rare in
the modern era to see hyperthyroidism go on long enough for T2DM to
develop. Hyperthyroidism may be treated by antithyroid drugs, a dose of
radioactive iodine that destroys the thyroid, or surgical removal of most
of the thyroid. It's seen most often in adults.

✔ **Pheochromocytoma:** This disease is caused by a tumor of the adrenal
gland that causes it to make excessive amounts of norepinephrine.
Excessive norepinephrine causes high blood pressure, headaches, and a

rapid heartbeat, often in recurring episodes. Because this hormone also causes increased blood glucose, type 2 diabetes may be found in patients with pheochromocytoma. It's found in adults, usually, and is treated by surgical removal of the tumor.

Examining diabetes caused by destructive diseases of the pancreas

Several pancreatic diseases, in addition to trauma of the pancreas, can destroy much of the gland, resulting in an absence of insulin much like T1DM. One important difference of diabetes caused by diseases of the pancreas, however, is that the cells that make glucagon (which raises blood glucose when it's too low) are destroyed along with the cells that make insulin, so the drive to make more glucose is diminished. The following sections discuss some of the more prominent examples of destructive diseases of the pancreas.

Pancreatitis

The pancreas has cells that make digestive enzymes as well as insulin and other hormones. The digestive enzymes are carried to the intestine in a tube called the *pancreatic duct,* but if they leak into the tissue of the pancreas, they can digest and destroy the pancreas itself. This is what sometimes happens when the pancreatic duct becomes blocked by a gallstone or when a person drinks large quantities of alcohol.

The resulting inflammation of the pancreas is very painful and makes the patient extremely sick with the following symptoms:

- ✔ Fever
- ✔ Nausea
- ✔ Rapid pulse
- ✔ Severe abdominal pain
- ✔ Swollen and tender abdomen
- ✔ Vomiting

If the patient can't consume any more alcohol or the gallstone passes or is removed, the symptoms subside; however, if the patient has repeated bouts of this same condition or the pancreatitis becomes chronic, a form of diabetes results from the absence of insulin. Treatment is with insulin and avoidance of alcohol. The patient is usually very responsive to insulin, and the diabetes isn't hard to treat, although hypoglycemia may occur.

Other autoimmune diseases associated with T1DM

The occurrence of hyperthyroidism or hypothyroidism (insufficient thyroid hormone) along with T1DM is greater than expected by chance. Many autoimmune diseases occur together in the same person. In particular, celiac disease (intolerance to gluten in wheat and other grains) is found in up to 5 percent of children with T1DM and causes anemia, abdominal discomfort, and diarrhea. Uptake of all foods is decreased in celiac disease, and that includes glucose, leading to more hypoglycemia in these patients.

Cystic fibrosis

As if children with cystic fibrosis (CF) didn't have enough to worry about, as they grow older, about 50 percent of them develop diabetes by age 30. Cystic fibrosis is associated with the following afflictions:

- Frequent lung infections
- Liver disease
- Obstruction of the intestine
- Reduced function of the part of the pancreas making digestive enzymes (see the previous section for more about these enzymes)

CF is an inherited disease that causes the secretion of thick, sticky mucous that clogs the lungs, leading to infection. The mucous also blocks the ducts carrying digestive enzymes, leading to decreased digestion of food in the intestine, increased digestion of the pancreas, and loss of insulin.

The life expectancy of patients with CF used to be very short, and there was little concern about the development of diabetes. With modern methods of CF management, however, many more patients are living to develop diabetes. They're subject to complications similar to those associated with autoimmune T1DM and must be screened for eye disease (see Chapter 5), high blood pressure, and kidney disease in the same way. For example, a study of 38 CF patients in *Diabetes Care* in December 2006 pointed out that the prevalence of eye disease in CF-associated diabetes is similar to autoimmune T1DM of the same duration, about 27 percent of patients. One great difference between autoimmune T1DM and diabetes caused by CF, however, is the absence of coronary artery disease in the latter form because the intestine has trouble absorbing fats.

Treatment for CF may involve lung transplantation. After the transplant, patients receive a drug called cyclosporine to block rejection of the lung. Cyclosporin is known to cause kidney damage, especially in combination with T1DM.

The diabetes associated with CF is treated with insulin and a more liberal diet than is typical for someone with T1DM because of the high calorie requirements in CF.

Discovering drugs and chemicals that may cause or worsen diabetes

There's a long list of drugs and chemicals that may cause diabetes or bring out latent diabetes in a number of different ways. Two of these chemicals are cortisol, which I cover in the earlier section on Cushing's syndrome, and thyroid hormone, which I mention in the earlier section on other hormone-induced causes of diabetes.

Additional common agents that are associated with diabetes are

- **Dilantin:** A drug used for seizures. It has been shown to block the release of insulin, leading to higher blood glucose levels. However, if needed, dilantin can be used as long as the higher blood glucose is managed with other agents.

- **Nicotinic acid:** Commonly used to treat high cholesterol levels. In the 1990s, this agent was found to raise the blood glucose in patients with diabetes treated for high cholesterol, whether type 1 or type 2. More recently, it has been found to cause no deterioration of blood glucose control and can safely be used in people with diabetes.

- **Pentamidine:** An agent used to treat an infection associated with the AIDS virus. It causes destruction of beta cells in the pancreas and insulin deficiency that must be treated by replacing the insulin (like in T1DM).

- **Thiazide diuretics and beta blockers:** Two classes of drugs used to treat high blood pressure. They're associated with the onset of T2DM when used for initial treatment of high blood pressure more often than other drugs for high blood pressure. However, an article in the May 2007 issue of *Current Opinion in Nephrology and Hypertension* points out that there's no evidence in any studies that this initial treatment results in increased coronary artery disease or heart attacks. Because coronary artery disease and heart attacks are the major cause of death in people with diabetes, the authors conclude that "thiazide diuretics are safe to use, even in hypertensive individuals at risk for glucose disorders."

Unless the agent actually destroys the pancreas, the type of diabetes that occurs with the use of these agents generally mimics T2DM. If the agent can't be stopped because it's essential in the treatment of another disease, the diabetes is treated with lifestyle changes (diet and exercise) and the drugs used to treat diabetes.

Part II

Considering the Consequences of Type 1 Diabetes

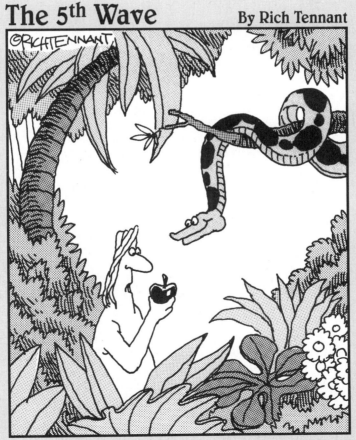

The 5th Wave   By Rich Tennant

"Well, yes, my blood sugar _is_ a little low..."

In this part . . .

People used to die soon after they were diagnosed with type 1 diabetes. This rarely happens today because of the isolation and production of insulin since 1921. Instead of dying from the disease, people with type 1 diabetes are subject to short- and long-term complications, all of which are preventable or manageable. This part tells you all about those complications and how to make them minor annoyances rather than major difficulties.

Many of the consequences of type 1 diabetes are physical, but there's also an emotional price paid for a chronic illness. That important topic is also addressed in this part as I explain how to handle the emotional and psychological effects of type 1 diabetes.

Chapter 4

Overcoming Short-Term Complications

***

In This Chapter

▶ Handling low blood glucose

▶ Taking care of very high blood glucose

***

*L*iving with type 1 diabetes can be very challenging. You or your child will probably have to deal with the short-term complications of the disease that I present in this chapter. The idea is to minimize the frequency of these complications, and arming yourself with knowledge about the causes, symptoms, prevention, and treatment of these complications is a smart move.

One potential short-term complication of type 1 diabetes is low blood glucose, otherwise known as *hypoglycemia*. You may think that you wouldn't have to worry about this given that the problem that sent your child to the doctor in the first place was high blood glucose. Unfortunately, doctors don't yet have the tools to manage blood glucose perfectly, so in an effort to get as close to normal blood glucose levels as possible, which is known to prevent long-term complications of diabetes (see Chapter 5), doctors overshoot the mark on occasion and get levels too low. You find out how to prevent, recognize, and treat hypoglycemia in this chapter.

I also take up diabetic ketoacidosis (very high blood glucose) in this chapter. There are all kinds of events like trauma, infections, and severe stress that precipitate this condition, so you need to be able to recognize it and practice proper management of the diabetes before it occurs. But ketoacidosis is often unstoppable, which makes the hospital your next stop. Diabetic ketoacidosis isn't something you can treat yourself, so you need to know whether you or your child is getting the right treatment from doctors and specialists. I explain it all here.

Managing Low Blood Glucose: Hypoglycemia

If your child has low blood glucose, you'll know it thanks to a number of different symptoms that can result from several possible causes. After you measure the blood glucose and determine the severity of the episode, you can treat it effectively. Better yet, you can (and should) try to prevent hypoglycemia entirely! I explain what you need to know in the following sections.

Make sure that everyone who interacts with your child (or you, if you're the patient) knows that he has T1DM and may develop hypoglycemia. They should know the symptoms to look for and what to do to manage it.

Determining the cause

There are many possible causes for hypoglycemia in T1DM, but it all really comes down to too much insulin (from an external source) and too little glucose in the blood. Even if there's plenty of glucose inside the cells that require insulin, a problem still exists because the brain gets its glucose passively when the glucose in the blood is higher than the glucose in brain cells. If insulin has driven most of the blood glucose into cells that *don't* receive glucose passively, hypoglycemia is present as far as the brain is concerned. And that means that the child becomes confused, sleepy, and even comatose. (Turn to Chapter 2 for a rundown on how insulin and glucose work together in type 1 diabetes.)

Some of the scenarios that may cause hypoglycemia include:

✔ **Too large an injection of insulin:** When you give insulin to your child (or take it yourself), you have to choose a dose that takes care of the carbohydrates in the meal he's about to eat as well as the level of carbohydrates already in his blood. Choosing the correct dose isn't easy. (I explain the basics of taking insulin in Chapter 10.)

✔ **Too little food or a missed meal:** A person with T1DM takes rapid-acting insulin before meals and long-acting insulin once or twice daily. All that circulating insulin has to be balanced with food. If not, the person becomes hypoglycemic.

✔ **Too much exercise using up the glucose:** Exercise acts like insulin to open the cells to glucose. As your child continues to exercise, he uses up his glucose and may become hypoglycemic.

Heavy exercise increases the risk of hypoglycemia for almost 24 hours. As long as your child's glucose doesn't get too low, it's a great way to lower the blood glucose without insulin. I discuss all the benefits of exercise for patients with diabetes in Chapter 9.

✓ **Alcohol intake without food:** Alcohol blocks the liver's release of glucose into the blood.

✓ **Taking the wrong kind of insulin at bedtime:** Intensive treatment of diabetes usually involves a rapid-acting insulin before meals and a long-acting insulin at bedtime. If the patient mistakenly takes the rapid-acting insulin at bedtime, the intense effect of that insulin will produce hypoglycemia.

✓ **More rapid absorption of insulin from a new injection site:** Repeatedly used injection sites may become thickened and release the insulin slowly. A new site releases the insulin into the bloodstream much more quickly, which produces more lowering of glucose by opening more cells to the glucose.

✓ **Poor timing of food and insulin:** Different types of insulin are active at different times. You must know what type your child takes and when it acts in order to keep insulin and glucose in harmony.

✓ **Stomach problem that slows glucose absorption:** Celiac disease, for example, is an autoimmune condition that slows glucose absorption, so the insulin may be in the bloodstream before the food. The insulin lowers the glucose already in the blood, and the glucose in the food isn't there to take its place.

✓ **Loss of hormones that raise blood glucose:** A person with diabetes experiences loss of glucagons, which raises blood glucose. Without glucagon, the response to low blood glucose is severely diminished.

✓ **Drugs that lower blood glucose too much:** Drugs like aspirin that lower the blood glucose in doses greater than the 81 mg commonly taken to reduce heart attacks can produce hypoglycemia.

✓ **Effect of recent low blood glucose:** Recent very low glucose levels lower the sensation of hypoglycemia to very low levels of blood glucose: You may not realize that your blood glucose or your child's is going down because of unawareness (which I discuss later in this chapter in the section "Understanding hypoglycemic unawareness").

✓ **Use of beta blocker drugs for high blood pressure:** These drugs reduce the level at which hypoglycemia symptoms occur, so you or your child may have the condition without knowing it.

Morning highs: The Somogyi effect versus the dawn phenomenon

During sleep, your child's blood glucose may fall from the insulin he took that day, and the hormones that raise blood glucose may be secreted, resulting in a high blood glucose in the morning. This is called the *Somogyi effect* after the doctor who first described it. Some mornings, the blood glucose may be low if it didn't get low enough to trigger hormone secretion, whereas other mornings it may be high. If you fail to realize that the cause is too much insulin and not too little, you may increase your child's insulin and make the situation worse. Before you increase insulin at bedtime, do a blood glucose test in the middle of the night. If the level's low, your child probably has the Somogyi effect, and you should decrease, not increase, the amount of long-acting insulin you give him at bedtime.

Dawn phenomenon, on the other hand, is caused by secretion of too much growth hormone during the night so that, by morning, it has raised the blood glucose to high levels. If your child's morning blood glucose levels are consistently high, nighttime long-acting insulin usually takes care of this problem and provides a more normal morning blood glucose.

Another possible reason for a morning high, unrelated to either of the previously mentioned situations, is that the insulin used at bedtime didn't work long enough to keep the blood glucose from rising overnight. Older forms of insulin such as NPH (see Chapter 10) tend to fall short in this manner, whereas newer long-acting insulins like glargine and detemir do not.

Recognizing the symptoms

The symptoms of hypoglycemia are divided broadly into two categories:

- ✔ **Adrenergic symptoms** result from the secretion of hormones such as adrenaline to increase production of glucose. (I discuss adrenaline in more detail in Chapter 2.)
- ✔ **Neuroglycopenic symptoms** result from the brain not getting enough glucose.

The adrenergic symptoms occur at a slightly higher blood glucose than the neuroglycopenic symptoms. The actual blood glucose levels at which these symptoms occur depends on whether control of the blood glucose has been tight recently (with a lot of glucoses below 100) or loose (with most blood glucoses over 200). For instance, if the adrenergic symptoms come on at a glucose level of 70 mg/dl, the neuroglycopenic symptoms may come on at 65 mg/dl. Secreting the hormones that raise blood glucose first is a way of building up blood glucose before the brain feels the lack.

The major adrenergic signs and symptoms include the following:

- ✔ Anxiety
- ✔ Irritability
- ✔ Numbness in the lips, fingers, and toes
- ✔ Palpitations (the sensation that the heart is beating too fast)
- ✔ Rapid heartbeat
- ✔ Sensation of hunger
- ✔ Sweating
- ✔ Whiteness or pallor of the skin

 The major neuroglycopenic signs and symptoms include:

- ✔ Confusion and trouble concentrating
- ✔ Convulsions
- ✔ Dizziness
- ✔ Fatigue
- ✔ Feeling of warmth
- ✔ Headache
- ✔ Loss of concentration
- ✔ Poor color vision
- ✔ Reduced consciousness or coma
- ✔ Slurred speech
- ✔ Trouble hearing
- ✔ Visual disorders, like double or blurred vision

 Many of these symptoms are similar to those exhibited by a drunk person, and many people with T1DM are arrested for drunk driving when they're actually suffering low blood glucose. To prevent such confusion, wear a necklace or bracelet that indicates that you (or your child) are diabetic. You can find simple jewelry at www.medicalert.com/home/Homegradient.aspx. If you want something more stylish, visit mylifewear.com.

Distinguishing the severity levels of hypoglycemia

 Hypoglycemia is divided into three levels of severity, depending on the symptoms and how difficult it is to get the patient to take some treatment (I discuss treatment in more detail later in this chapter):

✔ **Mild hypoglycemia,** which is marked by a blood glucose of about 75 mg/dl, is easily treated by the patient (or caretaker if the patient is a child). Glucose levels come back to normal with small amounts of carbohydrate. Mild hypoglycemia is usually well-tolerated, and the person can go on with his day after he's raised the blood glucose to normal. The diagnosis is usually made during routine testing of the blood glucose rather than by symptoms.

✔ **Moderate hypoglycemia,** which is marked by a blood glucose of about 65 mg/dl, is treated by the caretaker by giving two to three glucose tablets, waiting 20 minutes, and testing to make sure the glucose is back to normal. If it isn't normal, more glucose is given. It's recognized as the patient begins to feel the adrenergic symptoms, including rapid heartbeat and anxiety. Moderate hypoglycemia leaves the person unable to function; he doesn't recognize the need for glucose and must be helped.

✔ **Severe hypoglycemia,** which is marked by a blood glucose of less than 55 mg/dl, requires the help of someone else to restore the patient's blood glucose. Someone with severe hypoglycemia may be unconscious. It can leave the person with a severe headache and unable to function for lack of glucose in the brain. A shot of glucagon is in order in this situation.

Most people with T1DM have severe hypoglycemia no more than once a year and moderate hypoglycemia no more than twice a week. Mild hypoglycemia occurs about 10 percent of the time as people with T1DM try to keep their blood glucose down.

To interpret a reading accurately, you need to know whether the meter you use to measure blood glucose measures *capillary whole blood* (the entire blood specimen including the liquid and solid parts like the red blood cells) or *plasma* (the fluid left when the solid parts are removed). A plasma reading is 11 percent higher than a capillary whole blood reading. My patients use meters that read capillary whole blood, and that's what I use for glucose levels. If your meter reads plasma glucose, add 11 percent to my numbers. For example, a capillary whole blood reading of 80 mg/dl is equal to a plasma reading of 88.8 mg/dl. You can find the information necessary to understand your reading on the meter box or in the instruction manual; if it's not there, call the manufacturer. (Chapter 7 has full details on measuring your blood glucose.)

If moderate or severe hypoglycemia occurs while the person is driving a car or using complex machinery, the result can be devastating. Check your blood glucose before driving, especially if you're driving more than an hour, and stop and check your levels again every few hours. Keep glucose tablets handy in the car (see the later section "Trying other helpful tips" for more about these tablets). If your child has T1DM and is of driving age, make sure that he follows these recommendations.

Studying the effects of severe hypoglycemia on the brain

A major concern with severe hypoglycemia is the possibility of long-term damage to the brain, especially the brain of a developing child who suffers seizures related to hypoglycemia. Numerous studies have looked at this question of long-term damage, and their results differ. One difficulty is determining whether the decline in brain function, if there is any, is due to low blood glucose or episodes of high blood glucose. Here's a roundup of some prominent studies:

✔ A study from the *Journal of Diabetes and Its Complications* from January 1999 looked at children diagnosed with diabetes before age 10. Eighteen of 55 patients had a history of severe hypoglycemia with seizures. The children were given tests for memory, academic achievement, and fine motor speed/coordination. Their siblings without diabetes were tested for comparison. In most cases, there was no difference in the test performances of the diabetic children and their nondiabetic siblings; their test results were the same and were normal. The exceptions were children with a history of severe hypoglycemia with seizures, who did more poorly on tests of memory skills, short-term memory, and memory of words. The children with severe hypoglycemia without seizures didn't show this abnormality.

✔ A study from *Diabetologia* from January 2002 looked at 64 diabetic children between the ages of 7 and 16 years. They were tested four different times in areas similar to the preceding study. The findings showed a decline in intellectual performance in boys who were diagnosed before age 6 but not in those diagnosed later and not in diabetic girls. However, the decreased intellectual performance wasn't correlated with severe hypoglycemia but rather with poor control of the blood glucose and high glucose readings. The study's authors recommended tighter control of the blood glucose, especially for the younger boys.

✔ A recent, long-term study in *The New England Journal of Medicine* in May 2007 compared tight diabetic control with the much looser control that was the standard of care when another study, called the Diabetes Control and Complications Trial (DCCT), took place between 1983 and 1993. The recent study continued to follow these patients for the next decade. In the original DCCT trial, the patients were between the ages of 18 and 34 and had diabetes from 1 to 14 years. Forty percent of the patients reported having at least one coma or seizure due to hypoglycemia. There was no decline in memory or learning function in either the tightly controlled or loosely controlled groups. After following the DCCT patients for an average of 18 years, "no evidence of substantial long-term declines in cognitive function was found . . . despite relatively high rates of recurrent severe hypoglycemia." This is very good news.

Understanding hypoglycemic unawareness

If your child suffers from hypoglycemic unawareness, he doesn't feel the warning adrenergic symptoms that alert him that his blood glucose is too low. He may have a reduced or no adrenaline response as well as a reduced cortisol and growth hormone response — this means that nothing is raising his blood glucose as it falls. Without the warnings of palpitations, anxiety, and hunger, there's not much between your child and the symptoms associated with lack of glucose in the brain.

Hypoglycemic unawareness occurs in about 25 percent of patients with T1DM. The occurrence of severe hypoglycemia is much more frequent in these patients than in those without the unawareness. It occurs more often when one of these risk factors is present:

- ✔ Many years of diabetes
- ✔ Very tight control of the blood glucose
- ✔ Frequent and repeated hypoglycemia

In order to deal with these frequent and severe hypoglycemic reactions, it may be necessary to allow the blood glucose to be higher than levels that prevent long-term complications, greater than 150 mg/dl, for example. The risk is that long-term complications are more likely to develop, but a person with diabetes who suffers frequent severe hypoglycemia can't function normally and is a danger to himself and others.

Preventing and treating hypoglycemia

Preventing hypoglycemia may be time-consuming, but it's possible and entirely worth the effort! Even if prevention doesn't work and your child still has episodes of hypoglycemia, you can treat it in several different ways, as you find out in the following sections.

Preventing hypoglycemia

The best way to prevent hypoglycemia is to be constantly aware of your child's blood glucose. Meters are being developed that can measure glucose every five minutes and beep if it falls below a set level. (See Chapter 7 for more on these meters and for general information on measuring blood glucose.) Unfortunately, these meters haven't been perfected quite yet, so it's still necessary to stick your child multiple times a day in order to know his blood glucose. But even periodic testing doesn't get around the problem of not knowing your child's glucose for seven to eight hours while he sleeps (unless you set your alarm to wake you for an occasional middle-of-the-night test).

When your child is asleep, he may be unaware of developing hypoglycemia, and you certainly aren't watching him to pick up the cues. One way to avoid hypoglycemia during sleep is to give the child a bedtime snack containing a slowly absorbed source of carbohydrate. Unfortunately, the best food for this purpose, raw cornstarch, isn't very tasty. Even better (or worse!), it needs to be eaten cold to preserve the slow uptake of glucose. Here's a rough guide for how much cornstarch will help your child (or you) fend off hypoglycemia overnight:

- ✔ A 50-pound child needs about 4 tablespoons of raw cornstarch.
- ✔ A 100-pound child or adult needs 7 tablespoons of raw cornstarch.
- ✔ A 150-pound adult needs 10 tablespoons of raw cornstarch.

And here are a couple of ways to make cornstarch somewhat appetizing for your child:

- ✔ Dissolve raw cornstarch in a glass of milk.
- ✔ Ditch the raw cornstarch for a snack called Extend Bar. It contains only 5 g of uncooked cornstarch, considerably less than the recommended 30 g, but children find it more palatable than the raw stuff. A study in *Diabetes Research and Clinical Practice* in September 2001 showed that Extend Bar kept the nighttime blood glucose in a non-hypoglycemic range when eaten by adults at bedtime. (The study results with adults indicate that Extend Bars are an effective option for children.) You can buy Extend Bars at some drugstores or order them online at www.extendbar.com; visit the Web site for more information.

Another way to minimize the occurrence of hypoglycemia is to keep as regular a schedule for your child as you possibly can. If he wakes up at around the same time, eats at around the same time, eats around the same amount of carbohydrates, and exercises around the same amount each day, you'll know how much insulin to give him. Very few people can do this because life intervenes with parties, travel to different time zones, meals eaten away from home, and sleeping late on the weekends. But fear not; I explain how to live well with type 1 diabetes in Part IV.

Adjusting insulin amounts for hypoglycemia

If you're unable to prevent hypoglycemia outright, one thing that you can do to treat it is know which insulin is most responsible for the blood glucose at a given time. If hypoglycemia occurs during that time, you can adjust the insulin down slowly (1 to 2 units a day, and then don't change it again for three to five days) until the hypoglycemia subsides.

Table 4-1 shows you which insulin — rapid-acting or long-acting — is active at certain times of day, assuming that you use the standard therapy of three shots of rapid-acting insulin or three doses of inhaled insulin before meals and one or two shots of long-acting insulin in the morning or both morning and evening.

Table 4-1	Making Adjustments to Insulin Activity	
When Hypoglycemia Occurs	**Relation to Meal Insulin**	**Type of Insulin to Change**
Before breakfast	None	Long-acting
After breakfast	Pre-breakfast shot	Rapid-acting
Before lunch	None	Long-acting
After lunch	Pre-lunch shot	Rapid-acting
Before dinner	None	Long-acting
After dinner	Pre-dinner	Rapid-acting
Bedtime	None	Long-acting
Middle of the night	None	Long-acting

You can see from Table 4-1 that, in general, rapid-acting insulin is responsible for blood glucose for the first couple of hours after meals, whereas long-acting insulin is responsible for all blood glucose the rest of the time. For example, if your child becomes hypoglycemic at about 9 a.m. most mornings, around two hours after breakfast, you need to reduce his pre-breakfast rapid-acting insulin. If the hypoglycemia comes on around 11 p.m., around four hours after dinner, then he's getting too much basal insulin (see Chapter 10 for an explanation of basal insulin).

Unfortunately, things aren't always so clear-cut. Your child may have hypoglycemia one day and hyperglycemia at the same time the next day even if you do everything the same way. In the final analysis, you may have to go back to that old standby, trial and error.

Using a glucose meter with a memory that you can download to a computer data management system is essential in recognizing patterns in your blood glucose. Among other things, the computer can show you all the tests during a given time period, indicating whether your child's glucose levels are typically high or low at that time. Your child's doctor should have this capability. (If you want to be able to download this information yourself, call the meter manufacturer using the 800 number on the meter.)

Trying other helpful tips to treat all severity levels

Some of the practices I recommend here for treating hypoglycemia may seem obvious, but they'll come in handy when your mind goes blank in the middle of a hypoglycemic episode happening to your son or daughter (or to you, if you're the patient). Most of these tips work for treating mild or moderate hypoglycemia (the last one is for severe hypoglycemia):

✔ Glucose tablets, which contain 4 g of glucose and are available over-the-counter, are usually the best way to treat mild to moderate hypoglycemia; two to four tablets is enough for most children and adults. More than that will cause hyperglycemia and you'll be tempted to give rapid-acting insulin to treat it, creating a vicious circle.

If your child has trouble swallowing, give him honey instead of glucose tablets. One teaspoon of honey is about 5 g of glucose, so you need about 3 teaspoons to give the equivalent of three to four glucose tablets.

✔ Don't push large quantities of food into the child. The result will be a high rather than a normal blood glucose. A piece of fruit may be all that's needed.

✔ Giving your child 1½ cups of orange juice effectively raises the blood glucose back to the normal range of 90 to 100 mg/dl. Cartons of juice may be a convenient way to have a quick and satisfying source of glucose to treat hypoglycemia. A cup of apple juice or lemon-lime soda both work as well and may be used when glucose tablets aren't available.

✔ Always check the blood glucose 20 minutes after treating the hypoglycemia and give another treatment if the level remains below 100 mg/dl.

✔ Keep the child quiet and inactive for 15 to 30 minutes after the reaction. Activity tends to lower the blood glucose again.

✔ Use a prescription glucagon emergency shot for an unconscious child who has severe hypoglycemia. Just make sure that the glucagon hasn't expired.

If the child doesn't wake up in 10 to 15 minutes even though his blood glucose is normal, call 911.

Dealing with Very High Blood Glucose: Diabetic Ketoacidosis

Diabetic ketoacidosis (DKA) is a severe diabetic complication that has to be managed in a hospital. It's characterized by high blood glucose (though it need not be very high) associated with an acid condition of the blood due to the production of ketones, which are the products of fat breakdown. The root of the illness is a lack of insulin. Without enough insulin, glucose can't get into insulin-dependent cells like muscle and the liver, so glucose accumulates in the blood, and the body turns to fat for energy.

In the following sections, I outline the causes, symptoms, prevention, and treatment of DKA.

Although it's thought of as an illness of children, DKA occurs more often in adults than in children. Sixty percent of cases occur in people who are 40 years of age or older. DKA can result in death, especially in the elderly population when it's paired with other serious underlying diseases like heart disease, kidney disease, and infection. Over the age of 65, the death rate may be as high as 30 percent, but the overall death rate for DKA is less than 5 percent.

Considering some potential causes

About 30 percent of children and 20 percent of adults with T1DM have DKA as their initial presentation. They may have had T1DM for some time, but because they or their parents aren't aware of the signs and symptoms and because T1DM doesn't run in families, the illness progresses to the point that the individuals become severely sick.

DKA also occurs after the diagnosis of T1DM is known. The major reasons for this include:

- **Infections:** Usually the infection is pneumonia in the lungs or infection of the urine. Infection is the most common cause of DKA.

- **Interruption of insulin treatment:** Some children, particularly girls, recognize that not taking insulin shots results in weight loss. They may rapidly develop DKA hours after stopping insulin. Insulin treatment also may be interrupted in people using insulin pumps to deliver the insulin (see Chapter 11 for more about these pumps). Any cutoff of insulin from the pump may precipitate DKA. DKA occurs less frequently in pump users than in people who take shots of insulin and usually is most common at the start of pump usage. As patients become more familiar with the pump, it becomes rare.

- **Other acute conditions:** Conditions such as severe trauma, acute alcoholism, severe psychological stress, heart attack, stroke, and severe pancreatic inflammation can lead to DKA.

- **Certain drugs:** Drugs known to raise blood glucose, like cortisol and the thiazide class of drugs for high blood pressure, as well as certain drugs used to treat psychosis, like clozapine and olanzapine, contribute to DKA in people with T1DM.

- **Poor adherence to treatment, especially among people who can't afford their insulin:** Patients with financial difficulties may reduce the needed dose or stop taking insulin altogether. Some patients mistakenly think that if they're sick and can't eat, they don't need to take insulin.

Surveying the symptoms

Many signs and symptoms of DKA make the diagnosis obvious once it's considered. However, for the person who isn't known to have diabetes, DKA isn't always so clear. With or without an existing diabetes diagnosis, the major symptoms include the following:

- ✔ **Abdominal pain:** Especially frequent in children, abdominal pain occurs for unclear reasons but seems to be associated with the acid condition of the blood. With treatment, the pain disappears within hours.

- ✔ **Frequent urination and thirst:** As the blood glucose rises, it enters the urine, pulling water and other important nutrients along with it. The high glucose content of the urine prevents the kidneys from restoring the water to the body. The patient has to urinate a great deal, and the loss of water leads to dehydration and thirst.

- ✔ **Nausea and vomiting:** The acid condition of the blood along with failure of the normal movement of food and liquids down the gastrointestinal tract leads to nausea and vomiting.

- ✔ **Weakness:** Inability to get glucose into cells for energy, dehydration, and other factors lead to weakness.

- ✔ **Weight loss:** The lack of insulin means that glucose can't be stored in the liver, amino acids can't be turned into protein to produce muscle, and fat can't be stored when calories are excessive. In fact, fat breakdown takes place to provide the energy not available from glucose, further resulting in weight loss.

A strict diet doesn't lead to ketoacidosis. Diabetic or not, if you go on a strict diet to lose weight, your body burns its fat stores, producing ketones, in a way similar to how it burns fat when you lack insulin. But in the case of a strict diet, your glucose remains normal and enters cells, and (unless you have T1DM) you have sufficient insulin to prevent the excessive production of new glucose or the release of large amounts of glucose from your liver.

- ✔ **Smell of acetone on the breath:** This fruity smell is the smell of the ketone bodies, which are the products of fat breakdown that are excreted in the urine but can be exhaled as well.

- ✔ **Confusion or coma:** As the thickened, syrupy blood, which is very acid, circulates through the brain, brain cells are exposed to abnormal nutrients and miss other nutrients that have been lost in the urine.

- ✔ **Cold skin and body temperature:** Unless the cause is an infection, the skin is cold as the body's metabolism declines because cells don't get glucose for energy.

> ✔ **Rapid, shallow breathing followed by deep, labored breathing:** Called Kussmaul breathing after the German doctor who first described it, this unusual breathing pattern is an attempt to blow off some of the acid through the lungs.

If you suspect that your child has DKA, there are a couple of quick tests you can do at home to verify the diagnosis:

> ✔ Check the blood glucose with your home meter (see Chapter 7). With DKA, it will generally read greater than 250 mg/dl, but some cases of mild DKA may have a glucose under 250 mg/dl.
>
> ✔ Check the urine for ketones (see Chapter 7). With DKA, the reading will be high, as shown by a deep purple color when you immerse the test strip into a cup of urine.

After you verify DKA with a home test, or if you suspect that you or your child has DKA even without a diagnosis of type 1 diabetes, dial 911, and then call your doctor to tell him or her that you're on the way to the hospital.

Preventing and treating diabetic ketoacidosis

The basis of ketoacidosis treatment is to simultaneously

> ✔ Restore the proper amount of water to the body
>
> ✔ Reduce the acid condition of the blood by getting rid of the ketones
>
> ✔ Restore substances such as potassium that have been lost
>
> ✔ Return blood glucose to its normal level of around 80 to 120 mg/dl

The treatment of DKA is left in the hands of the experts, but you should know what's being done, in general, so that you understand what your child is going through. In the following sections, I explain what happens during treatment and give you a few pointers for preventing DKA entirely.

Although you can't take care of your child with diabetic ketoacidosis on your own, it's important that you recognize the signs and symptoms (see the previous section). Like most illnesses, the earlier you begin to reverse the abnormalities with treatment, the quicker the patient recovers and the lower the chance of further complications or death.

Taking measures to prevent DKA

Because infection is the major precipitating cause of DKA, prevention begins with the best possible sick-day care (see Chapter 15 for details). An important first step is realizing that just because your child's sick and not eating doesn't mean that he doesn't still need insulin — and perhaps needs more than usual. Performing more testing of glucose more frequently, especially on sick days, is another key step. It's also important to be very aware of the signs and symptoms of DKA.

Receiving treatment at the hospital

Traditionally, DKA has been treated in intensive care units, but there's no evidence that this setting has any benefit over the conventional medicine ward. Death rates, length of stay in the hospital, and rapidity of recovery are no lower in the intensive care unit, which is far more expensive. Ask the doctor if care in the intensive care unit is necessary before your child is admitted there.

In the hospital, your child's doctor sets up a flowchart to keep track of glucose, acid, potassium, and ketones. Although your child may have lost a lot of potassium, for example, the initial blood reading for potassium may be normal. As treatment progresses, potassium enters cells along with glucose to replenish the losses there, so his blood potassium may fall. Then the doctor administers potassium to fix the problem. As he does this, he looks for the underlying cause that may have set off the DKA, such as an infection, and treats it with antibiotics as necessary.

The first step in treatment is to begin replacing the large amounts of fluids that have been lost. At the same time, your child receives insulin to shut down fat metabolism and allow the large amount of glucose in the blood to enter cells. Traditionally, insulin is given as a constant intravenous (IV) drip, but if the hospital doesn't permit IV treatment outside the intensive care unit, injections of rapid-acting insulin every one to two hours are just as safe and effective. Injected insulin begins to work in ten minutes and continues for three to four hours, although it peaks in the first hour (see Chapter 10 for the basics of insulin use).

At some point, your child's blood glucose may fall towards hypoglycemia (which I discuss earlier in this chapter). When this begins to happen, the intravenous fluids that have contained no glucose up until then begin to contain glucose along with normal levels of sodium. Potassium is added in the IV if blood tests indicate that your child's potassium has fallen to low levels.

The doctor gives your child large volumes of a saltwater solution intravenously to replace the 6 or more liters of fluids lost during DKA. Replenishing body fluids relieves the nausea and vomiting that he's endured, and he should be able to eat and keep down liquid and solid food once again. Your child's normal mental function is returning as well. If you already were aware of your child's diabetes, you're ready to help him resume self-care. If not, you both have to begin the lifetime learning that diabetes requires (see Chapter 2 for an introduction).

Watching out for potential complications

Most cases of DKA respond to treatment, and the patient is able to resume daily life after a few days in the hospital. If the patient is being carefully monitored with frequent tests for blood glucose, potassium, and so forth, the most common complications can be avoided. Occasionally, a complication occurs; the major complications in order of frequency are

- **Hypoglycemia:** This usually happens because glucose hasn't been added to the intravenous fluids after the blood glucose reaches 250 mg/dl. Hypoglycemia also may result because the insulin being given isn't reduced sufficiently as the glucose falls. This complication is avoided by measuring the blood glucose every hour or two.

- **Low potassium:** A patient with DKA loses a lot of potassium from inside cells that have to regain their potassium in order to return to a normal state. Typically, glucose and potassium enter cells as insulin is given. However, prior to giving insulin, the blood potassium level can fall to dangerously low levels, which may result in serious abnormal heart rhythms. If the initial potassium measurement is low in the blood, it may be safer to replenish the potassium along with fluids before giving insulin to avoid this complication.

- **Relapse of DKA:** This may happen when there's a lack of insulin during the time between giving intravenous insulin for treatment of the DKA and giving subcutaneous insulin to return the patient to his usual program. To be safe, a long-acting subcutaneous insulin should be given two hours before the intravenous insulin is stopped. Or if only subcutaneous insulin is used, long-acting insulin may be given several hours before the frequent doses of subcutaneous insulin are stopped to provide some basal insulin until the next mealtime shot of insulin.

- **Cerebral edema:** This complication is a swelling of the brain that occurs less than 1 percent of the time, more often in children, and is associated with the rare deaths that occur in DKA. Symptoms include headaches, decreased consciousness, seizures, and urinary incontinence. The cause of cerebral edema is unknown. It begins about 12 hours after treatment begins for DKA, and drugs that are given to reduce the brain swelling are sometimes effective.

Chapter 5

Preventing Long-Term Complications

. . . .

. . . .

*T*his chapter is the bad news–good news chapter. The bad news is that if you don't manage your diabetes or your child's diabetes properly, you or your child will suffer one or several of the serious long-term complications that I discuss here. The good news is that everything is in place now to prevent this from ever happening; in Part III, I tell you what you need to know about controlling and treating type 1 diabetes.

The long-term complications in this chapter take between 10 and 20 years to develop. Long-term complications of type 1 diabetes (which I abbreviate T1DM) are divided into microvascular complications and macrovascular complications:

✔ **Microvascular complications** affect the tiny blood vessels that you wouldn't ordinarily see without magnification. They consist of

- Retinopathy, or eye damage

- Nephropathy, or kidney damage

- Neuropathy, or nerve damage

The abnormalities that cause eye disease, kidney disease, and nerve disease are similar. You can read more about them in the later sidebar "The potential causes of microvascular complications."

✔ **Macrovascular complications** affect the body's large blood vessels. They primarily consist of heart problems such as coronary artery disease and heart attacks.

The Diabetes Control and Complications Trial

The Diabetes Control and Complications Trial (DCCT) was published in *The New England Journal of Medicine* in September 1993. This study of patients with T1DM proved that control of the blood glucose would prevent complications from developing. Also, the study showed that the progression of complications that had already developed could be slowed.

Researchers divided patients involved in the study into two groups: 730 patients were treated with the usual treatment of the time, consisting of one or two insulin injections daily, and 711 patients were given intensive treatment with either three or more shots of insulin daily or an insulin pump. After six and a half years, the study was terminated because the results were so clear:

✔ It was possible even in 1993 to achieve a level of blood glucose control that would prevent long-term complications in T1DM.

✔ Intensive therapy reduced the risk of retinopathy (eye disease) by 76 percent compared to conventional therapy. In patients who already had retinopathy, intensive therapy reduced the risk that it would progress to a severe form by 47 percent and reduced the need for treatment by 56 percent.

✔ Intensive therapy reduced the risk of development of microalbuminuria, a early sign of diabetic kidney damage, by 43 percent.

✔ Intensive therapy reduced the risk of nerve damage due to diabetes by 69 percent.

After the DCCT, no one could doubt that persistently high blood glucose acts as a poison in the body. Furthermore, the patients in the DCCT continue to be followed. Fifteen years after the study, the group that had intensive therapy has a sustained benefit; they continue to have reduced eye damage, occurrence of kidney diseases, and nerve damage.

In this chapter, I discuss both microvascular and macrovascular long-term complications of T1DM as well as other diseases that occur more often in people with T1DM and complicate the treatment of T1DM because of the fact that autoimmune diseases tend to occur together.

Focusing on Eye Disease

The main eye complications of T1DM are cataracts and retinopathy.

✔ **Cataracts** are opaque areas of the lens. Cataracts occur in no more than 1 percent of children with T1DM. In both children and adults, if the cataract is blocking vision, the cataract is removed by surgery and a new lens is implanted, restoring vision.

✔ **Retinopathy** is considerably more common than cataracts, varying from 15 percent to 50 percent occurrence in patients with T1DM in different studies. It's considerably less common today than it was before the era of intensive diabetic treatment.

In order to understand retinopathy, you need to know the normal appearance of the eye and its structures. Figure 5-1 shows the structure of the eye.

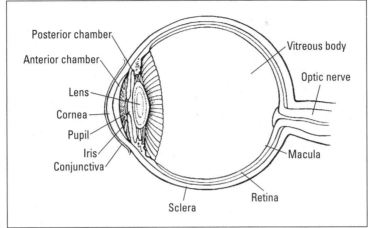

In a nutshell, vision works this way: Light enters the eye through the lens, where it's bent and focused upon the retina. The place in the retina where the lens focuses is called the *macula*. The retina collects the image and transfers it to the optic nerve, which carries it to the brain where the image is interpreted. Between the lens and the retina is a transparent material called the *vitreous body*. The eye muscles surround the eye on all sides and are attached to it, permitting you to look up, down, and sideways without moving your head. These eye muscles are important in the discussion of diabetic nerve damage called *neuropathy,* which I cover later in this chapter in the section "Knowing about Nerve Disease."

Retinopathy is broken down into two major forms depending upon the potential to cause vision loss: background retinopathy and proliferative retinopathy. In both forms, the major damage takes place on the retina. Figure 5-2 shows a normal retina, a retina with background retinopathy, and a retina with proliferative retinopathy. You can see that in Figure 5-2A, the normal retina shows a dark spot, the macula, which is the central spot that the image focuses upon. The light area is the optic nerve from which small blood vessels branch out, cascading toward the macula.

In the following sections, I explain the symptoms, prevention, and treatment of background retinopathy and proliferative retinopathy.

Because diabetic eye disease takes years to develop, the current recommendation is to have your or your child's eyes examined by an ophthalmologist or optometrist when T1DM is first detected, five years after T1DM is diagnosed, and once a year thereafter as long as the examination remains normal. See Chapter 7 for more about eye checks.

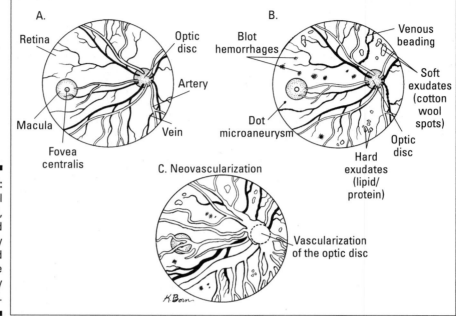

Adults in particular need to be aware of the following points about retinopathy, including behaviors and other conditions that are associated with it:

- Males and females develop retinopathy at about the same rate.

- The longer a person has diabetes, the more likely he or she is to develop diabetic retinopathy.

- High blood pressure worsens retinopathy.

- Smoking and heavy alcohol use worsen retinopathy.

- Persons with severe diabetic retinopathy are at increased risk for heart attacks.

Background retinopathy

Figure 5-2B shows the more benign form of diabetic retinopathy. The signs of background retinopathy, which are detected by an ophthalmologist or optometrist, include the following:

- *Retinal aneurysms* are the result of weakening of the capillaries of the eye, appearing like tiny balloons on the capillaries. This first symptom of the condition appears as small red dots on the retina. They usually disappear over time.

✔ Sometimes the weakened capillaries rupture and release blood, forming *retinal hemorrhages* and *hard exudates*. The hard exudates are yellowish and appear round and sharp. They're actually scars left from the hemorrhage. If they extend into the macular area, they reduce vision. If the capillaries in the retina allow fluid to flow into the macula, the patient gets macular edema, which also reduces vision. These exudates and hemorrhages can last for years.

✔ As the capillaries close, there's a decreased blood supply to the retina, and *cotton wool spots* or *soft exudates* appear. They appear as small areas of yellowish-white discoloration on the retina.

These changes usually don't cause complete loss of vision but may develop into the more serious proliferative retinopathy if the T1DM isn't brought under control by making the blood glucose as normal as possible.

Proliferative retinopathy

Figure 5-2C shows an eye that suffers from proliferative retinopathy. If untreated, this condition results in partial or complete loss of vision. Just as in many other parts of the body, when the blood supply in the eye is reduced, new vessels form to carry more blood to the retina. When this happens, the patient is entering the stage of proliferative retinopathy. The blood vessels grow into the vitreous body where they can hemorrhage and block vision. A hemorrhage forms a clot, which contracts, pulling up the retina to produce *retinal detachment*. The lens can no longer focus the light on the macula, resulting in complete loss of vision.

Many studies have aimed to develop drugs that may block proliferative retinopathy, but none has been successful so far. However, laser surgery may be used to reduce the damage caused by retinopathy and prevent blindness. Laser surgery causes burns in the retina that result in scars that prevent the retina from being pulled away by a hemorrhage in the vitreous body. Only 5 percent of diabetics with proliferative retinopathy who undergo laser treatment develop severe vision loss. However, there's some minor loss of vision at the sites where the retina is burned, and there's a decrease in night vision and the visual field (the area the eye can see at one time). Laser treatment can be used to treat macular edema that affects vision as well.

If a person with T1DM has already experienced retinal detachment, an operation called a *vitrectomy* is necessary. Under general anesthesia, the vitreous body is replaced with a sterile solution. Attachments to the retina are cut, and the retina falls back into place. Vitrectomy restores vision 80 to 90 percent of the time.

The potential causes of microvascular complications

The exact cause of microvascular complications isn't certain, but a number of different mechanisms have been proposed (persistent high blood glucose is the basis for all the mechanisms as shown by the DCCT study discussed in the earlier sidebar "The Diabetes Control and Complications Trial"):

✔ When glucose is elevated, some of it gets converted to another compound called sorbitol. Sorbitol accumulates in the lens of the eye, where it causes swelling and damage to the lens; the result is a cataract, an opaque area that you can't see through. Sorbitol also accumulates in the retina of the eye, the glomeruli in the kidneys, and the Schwann cells that provide insulation for nerve tissue. In each area, excess sorbitol causes damage.

✔ Protein kinase C consists of a group of chemicals in the body that help to control movement of substances in and out of cells and enlargement of blood vessels to improve flow. Persistent high blood glucose leads to increase in protein kinase C, especially in the retina and the glomeruli as well as in nerve tissue. At these high doses, the protein kinase C leads to reduced blood flow by promoting atherosclerosis in small vessels and therefore diminished oxygen to these tissues. The tissues then may die or fail to function normally.

✔ Elevated glucose causes advanced glycation end products (AGEs) to form in tissues. AGEs cause increased flow of damaging substances into cells and increased production of new cells, which block the tiny spaces needed for proper function in the kidneys and proper vision in the eyes.

✔ Vasoproliferative factors are compounds that cause increased production of small blood vessels in the retina of the eye that are very fragile and can bleed and block vision. In nerve tissue, new vessels may carry blood away from the nerves that need it.

Coping with Kidney Disease

Kidney disease due to diabetes is known as *diabetic nephropathy,* and it develops in less than half of the people at risk to get it. Some important factors contribute to kidney disease (some of which you can't change and some of which you can):

✔ Abnormal blood fats promote thickening in the kidneys. You can reduce this contributing factor.

✔ Certain ethnic groups, especially African Americans, Native Americans, and Mexican Americans, tend to have nephropathy more often. You can't change this.

✔ Elevated blood pressure damages the kidneys of a person with diabetes. Blood pressure should be measured at each doctor's visit and compared with the appropriate chart for age, height, and weight (Chapter 7 has more about measuring blood pressure). You can control blood pressure; for assistance, check out my book *High Blood Pressure For Dummies* (Wiley).

In the following sections, I explain the impact of uncontrolled diabetes on the kidneys and tell you how to prevent and treat kidney damage.

The effects of uncontrolled diabetes on the kidneys

Uncontrolled diabetes can affect the kidneys in many ways, depending on the stage of the disease. Luckily, with regular testing for an important indicator (microalbuminuria), anyone can lessen the impact of kidney disease before it progresses.

Early changes in the kidneys

Figure 5-3 shows the appearance of the normal *glomerulus* of the kidney, the structure that filters the blood. There are 2 million of these glomeruli in a person's kidneys, so loss of even a whole kidney isn't fatal.

Blood passes through the tiny glomerular capillaries, which are in intimate contact with tubules through which filtered blood travels. As the filtered blood passes through the tubules, most of the water and the normal contents of the blood are reabsorbed into the body while a small amount of water and waste passes from the kidneys into the ureter, into the bladder, and out the urethra (refer to Figure 5-3). The loops of capillaries are supported by a thin membrane called the *mesangium* and are surrounded by a sac called the *Bowman's capsule.* Between the capillaries and the mesangium is the *glomerular basement membrane,* the membrane through which filtration takes place.

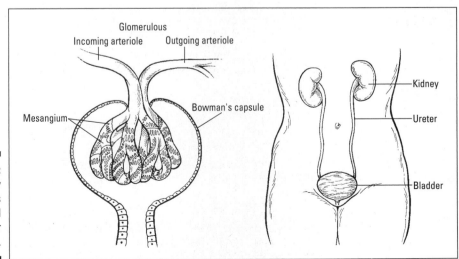

Figure 5-3:
The kidney and its normal glomerular structure.

As diabetes proceeds, if control of the blood glucose is poor, the glomerular basement membrane and other nearby structures begin to thicken and take up the space occupied by the capillaries (see Figure 5-4). The tight quarters mean that the capillaries can't filter as much blood as they should. The rate of filtration, or *glomerular filtration rate,* begins to fall.

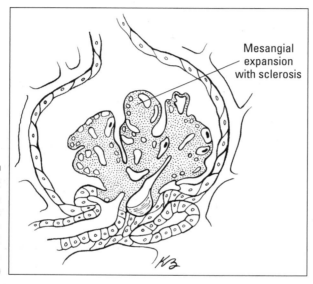

Mesangial expansion with sclerosis

Figure 5-4:
The glomerulus in un-controlled diabetes.

Microalbuminuria: An early indicator

As diabetes affects the kidneys, they begin to leak tiny amounts of protein. This indicator of kidney disease is called *microalbuminuria* and can be measured in a small sample of urine (see Chapter 7 for more about regularly testing for microalbuminuria).

Microalbuminuria should be measured on more than one occasion to confirm the elevation because many events can cause a falsely elevated reading, including the following:

- Blood in the urine
- Fever
- Heavy exercise
- Infection
- Menstruation
- Smoking
- Very high blood glucose

Microalbuminuria is rare in children before puberty, regardless of the duration of the diabetes and the level of control. Some specialists suggest, therefore, that it isn't necessary to screen prepubescent children for microalbuminuria. The American Diabetes Association recommends that all patients with T1DM be screened for microalbuminuria beginning at five years after the diagnosis and every year thereafter.

Microalbumin can be detected about five years before a urine dipstick (which tests for macroalbuminuria — greater than 300 mg/ml) would test positive for albumin, which is great news because treatment in this early stage can reverse the kidney disease. A study in *The New England Journal of Medicine* in June 2003 showed that lowering blood pressure, blood glucose, and abnormal blood fats decreased the microalbuminuria and the decline in kidney failure.

Progressive changes

If the blood glucose isn't kept down so that a test called the hemoglobin A1c (see Chapter 7) is less than 7 percent over 10 to 20 years, changes begin to occur in the kidneys. The earliest signs are enlarged kidneys that seem to be functioning abnormally well judging by how fast they clear wastes from the body. This over-functioning results from the large amount of glucose that the kidneys are filtering. The glucose draws a lot of water with it, causing an increase in the pressure in each glomerulus.

After about two years of poor glucose control, a biopsy of the kidney should indicate that the basement membrane and the mesangium are thickened.

The next 10 to 15 years is a silent period during which there are no clinical signs that the kidneys are failing. But after 15 years of poor control, there are measurable signs of kidney failure as waste products accumulate in the blood, especially blood urea nitrogen and creatinine. This is the stage of *azotemia,* significant reduction in kidney filtration but not complete cessation.

By 20 years of poor control, the patient either begins dialysis or has a kidney transplant in order to survive. At this stage, the patient has *uremia,* which is an inability to cleanse the blood at all.

Preventing kidney disease

The best treatment for kidney disease is preventative. If you can't prevent it with the following measures, you can at least slow it down if you

✔ Control your child's (or your) blood glucose. If you keep your child's blood glucose close to normal, he won't develop diabetic neuropathy. Part III is all about controlling blood glucose with testing, a healthy diet, regular exercise, and more.

✔ Keep your child's (or your) blood pressure below the 95th percentile for age and height. If you have microalbuminuria, you can use a class of drugs called *angiotensin converting enzyme inhibitors.* These drugs reverse microalbuminuria while lowering blood pressure.

✔ Control the blood fats by lowering total and bad cholesterol and triglycerides and increasing good cholesterol. The best way to do this is to take one of a class of drugs called *statins.*

✔ Avoid other kidney damage. People with diabetes tend to have urinary tract infections that can further damage the kidneys, so your child needs to drink plenty of fluids and acidify the urine with cranberry juice (the bugs don't like an acid urine) to avoid these infections. Nerve damage is also a risk, resulting in a neurogenic bladder with poor emptying of urine and a tendency to develop more urinary tract infections. (I discuss nerve damage later in this chapter.)

Treating kidney disease if prevention fails

When the kidneys reach the stage of uremia (see the earlier section "Progressive changes"), there's no alternative to *dialysis,* a mechanical cleansing of the blood, or transplantation of a healthy kidney. Two techniques are currently in use for dialysis:

✔ **Hemodialysis** requires that the patient's artery be hooked to a tube that runs through a filtering machine. This machine draws blood from the body, cleanses it, and sends it back into the patient's bloodstream. When the patient is moderately well, hemodialysis is done three times a week in a hospital-like setting. Hemodialysis can be associated with complications like infections and low blood pressure. The patient usually has to go to the center to have it done.

✔ **Peritoneal dialysis** may be done at home. A tube is inserted into the *peritoneal cavity,* the body cavity containing the stomach, liver, and intestines. A large quantity of fluid is dripped into the peritoneal cavity, and the body wastes are drawn out into the peritoneal cavity. After several hours, the fluid is drained out with its wastes. Glucose must be placed in the fluid, and this complicates control of the patient's diabetes. Peritoneal dialysis usually must be done daily, and it's possible to travel while undergoing this type of dialysis. Peritoneal dialysis may be associated with infection of the tube, just like hemodialysis.

There's little difference between these two forms of dialysis in terms of long-term survival. The decision to go with one over the other is based on convenience and whether your insurance has better coverage for one or the other.

For patients with diabetes, transplantation works better than dialysis, but healthy kidneys are difficult to come by in the United States, so 80 percent of all kidney failure patients use dialysis while 20 percent have kidney transplants. A transplanted kidney is foreign to the recipient, so his or her body tries to reject it. That's why the recipient receives antirejection drugs, which unfortunately complicate diabetes control, especially steroids. Transplantation works best if the kidney is from a donor closely related to the recipient; this arrangement reduces the chance of rejection. Control of the blood glucose is essential to prevent damage to the new kidney.

Knowing about Nerve Disease

The third kind of microvascular complication resulting from poor glucose control involves the nervous system and is called *diabetic neuropathy*. The tiny blood vessels supplying the nerve tissue are damaged by the mechanisms discussed in the earlier sidebar "The potential causes of microvascular complications." The result is loss of nerve conduction with numbness and tingling in some cases and pain in others.

Neuropathy becomes more severe the longer diabetes remains out of control. It usually takes ten years to develop, so it's not seen in young children who have had diabetes only a few years. Diabetic neuropathy occurs in some form or another in up to 75 percent of patients with T1DM, but this figure is falling. Neuropathy is made worse in adults by the following conditions:

- **Age:** It becomes more common with age.
- **Height:** It's most common in taller individuals who have longer nerve fibers to damage.
- **Alcohol consumption:** Even small quantities of alcohol can make neuropathy worse.

The speed with which a nervous impulse travels down a nerve is called the *nerve conduction velocity* (NCV). In diabetic neuropathy, the NCV is slowed. At first, the only symptom is an abnormal NCV, which is tested by using needles at the ends of a nerve and detecting how long a stimulus takes to travel from one end to the other. As early minor symptoms like mild loss of sensation develop, the only way to verify the result of any treatment, whether it's better glucose control or some medication, may be repeating the NCV. However, the degree of NCV slowing doesn't always correlate with the severity of symptoms.

Several different kinds of nerve fibers are responsible for different kinds of sensation such as vibration, light touch, and temperature. These fibers can be tested in the following ways:

✔ **Vibration testing:** A tuning fork discloses damage to vibration nerve fibers, which are large. A result of damage to these nerves may be that you have poor balance.

✔ **Temperature testing:** A hot or cold item discloses damage to temperature fibers, which are small and frequently damaged in people with diabetes. The result of damage may be that you get into a very hot bath without realizing that it may burn you.

✔ **Light touch testing:** A filament reflects the large fibers that sense anything that touches the skin. The amount of force needed to bend the filament to a point that you feel it is measured in grams (g). A person who can feel a 10 g filament is able to feel anything that may damage his foot. A person who can't feel a filament requiring 75 g of force is considered to have lost all sensation in the tested area. The consequence of such damage may be that you're unaware of stepping on a nail.

The various disorders of the nervous system in diabetes are broken down into the following categories:

✔ Disorders associated with loss of sensation, where the sensory nerves are damaged

✔ Disorders associated with loss of motor nerves, which carry impulses to muscles to make them move

✔ Disorders due to loss of automatic nerves (also known as *autonomic nerves*), which control muscles that you don't have to think about, such as the heart, the intestinal muscles, and the bladder muscles

The following sections describe the various conditions associated with these disorders.

Disorders of sensation

Disorders of sensation are the most common and bothersome nerve disorders associated with diabetes. A number of different conditions break down into diffuse neuropathies involving many nerves and focal neuropathies involving one or a few nerves.

Distal polyneuropathy

Distal polyneuropathy is the most frequently occurring form of diabetic neuropathy. "Distal" means "far away from the center of the body," like the feet and hands. "Poly" means "many," and neuropathy is disease in nerves. So this is a disease of many nerves noticed in the hands and feet.

The signs and symptoms of distal polyneuropathy include:

- ✔ Diminished ability to feel light touch (numbness) or feel the position of a foot, whether bent backward or forward, resulting from the loss of large fibers

- ✔ Diminished ability to feel pain and temperature, resulting from the loss of small fibers

- ✔ Minimal weakness

- ✔ Tingling and burning

- ✔ Extreme sensitivity to touch

- ✔ Loss of balance and coordination

- ✔ Worsening of symptoms at night

The danger of this kind of neuropathy is that the patient doesn't know, without looking, whether he has trauma to his feet, such as a burn or a puncture. When the small nerve fibers are lost, the symptoms aren't as serious. The majority of patients with distal polyneuropathy are unaware of the loss of nerve fibers, and the disease is detected by nerve conduction studies.

The most serious complication of loss of sensation in the feet is the neuro-pathic foot ulcer. A person with normal nerve function feels pain when pressure mounts on an area of the foot. However, a person with diabetic neu-ropathy doesn't feel this pressure. A callus forms, and with continued pressure, the callus softens and liquefies, finally falling off to leave an ulcer. This ulcer becomes infected. If it isn't promptly treated, it spreads, and amputation may be the only way to save the patient. In this situation, loss of blood supply to the feet isn't an important contributing factor to the ulceration; in fact, the blood supply may be good, but an ulcer still develops.

A less common complication in distal polyneuropathy is *neuroarthropathy,* or Charcot's joint. In this condition, trauma occurs to the joints of the foot and ankle without the patient feeling it. The bones in the foot go out of line, and many painless fractures occur. The patient has redness and painless swelling of the foot and ankle. The foot becomes unusable and is described as a "bag of bones."

Treatment of distal polyneuropathy starts with the best possible glucose con-trol and extremely good foot care. Your doctor should look at your feet during each visit, particularly if you have evidence of loss of feeling. Chapter 7 has more information on checking your feet.

Some drugs, such as the non-steroidal anti-inflammatory agents ibuprofen and sulindac, can reduce the inflammation associated with the unfelt trauma. Other drugs, such as the antidepressants amitryptiline or imipramine, reduce the pain and other discomfort that becomes worse as distal polyneuropathy continues. A drug called capsacin that's applied to the skin reduces pain as well. The results of these treatments are variable and seem to work only 60 percent of the time. However, the longer the pain has been present, and the worse the pain is, the less likely the drugs are to work.

Other drugs called gabapentin and pregabalin have been found to work more often than many of the older drugs in treating distal neuropathy, but they cause sleepiness and dizziness, which may make treatment more complicated. New drugs continue to be developed, but perhaps because so many factors cause the neuropathy, no one drug has proven to be successful all the time.

Polyradiculopathy-diabetic amyotrophy

Polyradiculopathy-diabetic amyotrophy is a mixture of pain and loss of muscle strength in the muscles of the upper leg so that the patient can't straighten the knee. Pain extends from the hip to the thigh. This is the second most common diabetic nerve condition after polyneuropathy. Time may heal the problem; it usually lasts weeks to months, but it may last years. Tight glucose control doesn't seem to have as much of an effect on this condition as it does on others. Painkillers may help.

Radiculopathy

Sometimes a severe pain along the location of a specific nerve suggests that the root of the nerve is damaged as it leaves the spinal column. The usual clinical picture for this condition known as *radiculopathy* is pain distributed in a horizontal line around one side of the chest or abdomen. The pain may be so severe that it's mistaken for an internal abdominal emergency. Fortunately, the pain goes away in 6 to 24 months. In the meantime, good glucose control and pain management with various painkillers are helpful.

Disorders of movement (mononeuropathy)

Diabetic neuropathy can affect nerves to individual muscles. The result is a sudden inability to move or use those muscles, called *mononeuropathy*. These disorders are believed to originate as a result of a sudden closing of a blood vessel supplying the nerve. The clinical picture depends on which nerve or nerves are affected. For example, if one of the nerves to the eyeball is damaged, the patient can't turn his eye to the side that nerve is on. If a nerve to the face is affected, the eyelid may droop or the smile on one side of the face may be flat. The patient with mononeuropathy can have trouble with vision or problems with hearing. Focusing the eye may not be possible. There's no specific treatment for mononeuropathy, but fortunately the disorder goes away on its own after several months.

Disorders of automatic (autonomic) nerves

Disorders of automatic (or autonomic) nerves often go unrecognized even though they may have a profound effect on the patient's quality of life and even survival.

As you're reading this page, many movements are going on in your body, but you're unaware of them. Your heart muscle is squeezing down and relaxing. Your diaphragm is rising up to empty the lungs of air and then relaxing to draw air in. Your esophagus is carrying saliva (or food, if you're a multitasker who's eating and reading) from your mouth to your stomach, and in turn, your stomach pushes it into the small intestine, which pushes it into the large intestine.

All these muscle functions are under the control of nerves from the brain, and diabetic neuropathy can affect them all. The nerves that perform these functions are called *autonomic nerves.* As many as 40 percent of people with T1DM have some form of autonomic neuropathy.

The clinical presentation of this type of neuropathy depends upon the involved nerve. Some possibilities include:

✔ Bladder abnormalities starting with a loss of the sensation of bladder fullness. The urine isn't eliminated, and urinary tract infections result. After a while, loss of bladder contraction occurs, and the patient has to strain to urinate and loses urine by dribbling. The diagnosis is made by determining how much urine is left in the bladder after urination has taken place. It's treated by remembering to urinate every four hours or by taking a drug to increase the force of bladder contraction.

✔ Sexual dysfunction, which occurs in as many as 60 percent of males and 30 percent of females with diabetes. Males can't sustain an erection, and females have trouble lubricating the vagina for intercourse. The drugs Viagra, Cialis, or Levitra are helpful for males with sexual dysfunction. For females, use of lubricating fluids may be helpful.

✔ Intestinal abnormalities of various kinds. The most common abnormality is constipation. In 25 percent of patients with autonomic neuropathy, nerves to the stomach are involved, so the stomach doesn't empty on time in a condition called *gastroparesis.* The precise timing of injected insulin and food intake (see Chapter 10 for the basics of using insulin) is thrown off; hypoglycemia occurs as the insulin finds no food, and hyper-glycemia occurs later as the food finds no insulin (see Chapter 4 for more about these conditions). Several drugs are helpful in treating intestinal abnormalities from autonomic nerve disorders, including metocloprimide and erythromycin. Some changes in eating habits are also helpful, including lowering fat intake and eating up to six small meals daily.

✔ Gallbladder involvement leading to gallstones. Normally the gallbladder empties each time you eat, especially if you eat a fatty meal, because the substances in the bile (which is in the gallbladder) help to break down fat. If disease to the nerve to the gallbladder prevents emptying, gallstones form, often requiring surgical removal of the gallbladder.

✔ Large intestinal involvement resulting in diabetic diarrhea and up to ten or more bowel movements per day. Accidental loss of bowel contents can also occur. Autonomic neuropathy may cause bacteria to grow abnormally in the intestine. The problem may respond to antibiotics, and diarrhea is treated with one of several drugs that quiet the large intestine.

✔ Heart abnormalities. If loss of nerves to the heart occurs, the heart may not respond to exercise by speeding up as it should. The pressure from the heart may not increase as the patient stands and he may become lightheaded. A very fast fixed heart rate also may occur, and patients experiencing this are at risk for sudden death. Autonomic neuropathy can also cause decreased perception of heart pain. Several drugs are available that may help.

✔ Sweating problems, especially in the feet. The body may try to compensate for the lack of sweating in the feet by sweating excessively on the face or trunk. Heavy sweating can occur when certain foods like cheese are eaten. There's no particular treatment other than avoidance of foods that set it off.

✔ Abnormalities of the pupil of the eye. Neuropathy may prevent the pupil from opening to let more light in when necessary. Reduced vision in low light means that the patient has to be much more careful about driving at night. There's no treatment other than better glucose control.

This long list can be a bit scary, but none of it need ever happen if you control your blood glucose.

Macrovascular Complications: Protecting Your Heart

Macrovascular complications are the complications involving the large blood vessels of the body, particularly the coronary arteries in the heart. In this section, I discuss how diabetes can lead to damage to the heart by causing blockage of these arteries.

Heart disease and heart attacks are the major macrovascular complications found in people with T1DM. How does heart disease lead to a heart attack? *Coronary artery disease* (CAD), which is also known as *atherosclerotic heart disease,* is the progressive closure of the arteries that supply blood to the heart muscle. (To understand how coronary artery disease develops, see the later sidebar "Picturing a plaque.") When one or more of your heart arteries close completely, the result is a heart attack (or *myocardial infarction*).

People with diabetes have more CAD than people without diabetes. When X-ray studies of the blood vessels of the heart are compared, people with diabetes have more arteries of the heart involved with CAD than non-diabetics. The incidence of CAD is increased even in young patients with T1DM. The duration of diabetes promotes CAD in type 1 patients, and CAD affects males and females with T1DM to the same extent.

People with diabetes often are unaware of heart pain because of cardiac neuropathy (I explain general neuropathy earlier in this chapter). Assuming that they don't have cardiac neuropathy, the symptoms are chest pain, pain down the left arm, and shortness of breath along with sweating. If a heart attack occurs, the risk of death is much greater for the person with diabetes. More than half of all people with diabetes die of heart attacks. Even if a person with T1DM survives a heart attack, he faces more complications, such as shock and heart failure, than the person without diabetes, and the outlook is much worse for him. A second heart attack occurs in 50 percent of diabetics compared with 25 percent of non-diabetics, and the death rate in five years is 80 percent compared with 25 percent for non-diabetics.

CAD is found in the arteries of people with T1DM who die of other causes as young as age 20 or even younger, and it's extensive in older people with T1DM who die of other causes. However, it's not found in everyone. Those folks with T1DM who don't have other risk factors, such as uncontrolled high blood pressure, cigarette smoking, a sedentary lifestyle, and high cholesterol levels, rarely have problems with coronary artery disease. A family history of coronary artery disease is another risk factor and one that you can do nothing about, but its effect is minimized when the other risk factors are avoided or controlled.

The picture is not a pretty one for the person with diabetes who has coronary artery disease. The treatment options are the same as for non-diabetics.

✔ Therapy to dissolve the blood clot obstructing the coronary artery (called *percutaneous transluminal coronary angioplasty,* or PTCA) can be used, but people with diabetes don't do as well with this form of treatment as non-diabetics because they may have many separate lesions in the artery. PTCA also can't be performed when an artery is completely closed.

✔ The other option is the use of a coronary artery bypass graft (CABG), in which a blood vessel is attached above and below the obstructed artery, thereby bypassing the obstruction. The long-term prognosis for keeping the graft open isn't as good in people with diabetes as in non-diabetics because the diabetes leads to increased promotion of atherosclerosis. The complications of CABG include an acute heart attack, stroke, infection in the area of the body that undergoes surgery, and even death on the operating table. The risk of complications is especially serious in older patients (more than 70 years old) and those patients with other diseases, such as kidney disease.

Although there's no data yet in T1DM, studies have shown that lowering the LDL cholesterol and raising the HDL cholesterol (see Chapter 7) will prevent first heart attacks and decrease the occurrence of second heart attacks in the general population. Hopefully, data will soon be available that will allow a recommendation for treatment of blood fats in T1DM.

For general information about heart health, check out *Heart Disease For Dummies* by James M. Rippe, MD (Wiley).

Considering Associated Diseases

Because T1DM is an autoimmune disease (a disease caused by the body inappropriately attacking itself), there's a greater tendency to develop other autoimmune diseases like celiac disease and hyperthyroidism. Non-autoimmune diseases also occur frequently in T1DM patients, however. The most important of these long-term complications are hyperthyroidism, hypothyroidism, skin disease, and celiac disease.

Hyperthyroidism and hypothyroidism

Thyroid disorders based on autoimmunity such as *hyperthyroidism* (an overactive thyroid) and *hypothyroidism* (an underactive thyroid) occur more frequently in people with T1DM. Both conditions are the result of autoimmune thyroiditis, which is usually missed because it causes no symptoms most of the time. In a study of 58 people enrolled in the Diabetes Control and Complications Trials published in *Diabetes Care* in April 2003, 18 patients had hypothyroidism and one had hyperthyroidism.

When symptoms are present, they alter metabolism. Hyperthyroidism and hypothyroidism affect diabetic control, and it's important to diagnose them by doing thyroid blood tests. Treatment for hypothyroidism is replacement of thyroid hormone. Treatment of hyperthyroidism is with antithyroid drugs, radioactive iodine, or surgery. The symptoms of the more common hypothyroidism are weight gain, slowness, dry skin, brittle nails, tiredness, and intolerance to cold. With hyperthyroidism, you get weight loss, palpitations, high body temperature, nervousness, and trouble sleeping.

Picturing a plaque

When diabetes, high blood pressure, smoking, and/or increased levels of cholesterol (especially low-density lipoprotein, or LDL cholesterol) damage the inner lining of the arteries, a plaque begins to form. The following figure shows the parts of a normal artery and the artery after a plaque has developed.

After damage has occurred, fat begins to accumulate within a part of the artery wall called the *intima.* In the intima, fat is protected from the chemicals in the blood that prevent changes in the fat because they can't reach the fat, and fat begins to take a more damaging form.

White blood cells, especially monocytes and lymphocytes that enter the intima from the blood, are transformed into other cells called *macrophages,*

and the macrophages begin gobbling up the changed fat to turn the cells into *foam cells.* Calcium also is deposited in the walls where the plaque is forming and is responsible for the calcification seen in X-rayed arteries.

The accumulation of foam cells and calcium is called *plaque.* It grows and begins to stick out into the *lumen,* the hollow part inside of the artery. After 80 percent of the lumen is blocked, blood flow to the heart muscle is reduced.

The irregular surface of a plaque can be the site of accumulation of blood platelets and the formation of a clot. The clot can go on and reduce the opening of the lumen even more, or it can break off and lodge in a smaller artery, completely closing off blood flow beyond it.

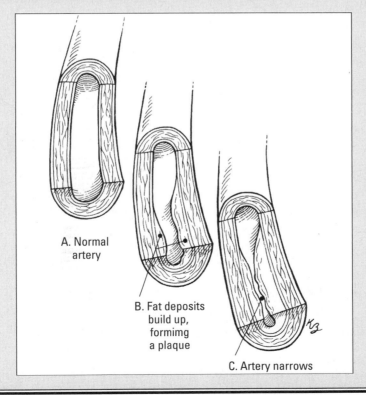

A. Normal artery

B. Fat deposits build up, formimg a plaque

C. Artery narrows

All people with T1DM should have routine thyroid function testing with a blood test that checks the level of thyroid-stimulating hormone on an annual basis.

See my book *Thyroid For Dummies,* 2nd Edition (Wiley), for general information about hyperthyroidism and hypothyroidism.

Skin disease

Many skin conditions are unique to the person with diabetes because of the treatment and complications of the disease. The most common and important skin complications include the following:

- Bruises occur because insulin needles cut blood vessels.

- *Vitiligo* (loss of skin pigmentation) is part of the autoimmune aspect of type 1 diabetes and can't be prevented.

- *Necrobiosis lipoidica,* which also affects people without diabetes, creates patches of reddish-brown skin on the shins or ankles, and the skin becomes thin and can ulcerate. Females tend to have this condition more often than males. Steroid injections are used to treat this condition, and the areas eventually become depressed and brown.

- *Xanthelasma,* which are small, yellow, flat areas called *plaques* on the eyelids, occur even when cholesterol isn't elevated. Treatment may not be necessary.

- *Alopecia,* or loss of hair, occurs in people with type 1 diabetes, but the cause is unknown.

- *Insulin hypertrophy* is the accumulation of fatty tissue where insulin is injected. This condition is prevented by changing the injection site (see Chapter 10 for more information on insulin injection).

- *Insulin lipoatrophy* is the loss of fat where the insulin is injected. Although the cause is unknown, this condition is rarely seen now that human insulin has replaced beef and pork insulin in diabetes treatment (see Chapter 10).

- Dry skin is a consequence of diabetic neuropathy, which leads to a lack of sweating (refer to the earlier section "Disorders of automatic (autonomic) nerves" for more on sweating). Treatment is with skin lubricants.

- Fungal infections occur under the nails or between the toes. Fungus likes moisture and elevated glucose, so lowering glucose and keeping the toes dry prevents these infections. Medications may cure this problem, but it recurs if glucose and moisture aren't managed.

- Diabetic thick skin, which is thicker than normal skin, occurs in people who have had diabetes for more than ten years. No treatment exists for this condition.

Celiac disease

Celiac disease is an inherited autoimmune disease present in as many as 2 to 3 percent of patients with T1DM. A person who has celiac disease, also known as *celiac sprue,* can't eat foods that contain gluten, including wheat, barley, and rye, because gluten damages the wall of the gastrointestinal tract. Patients with celiac disease (both adults and children) complain about these symptoms:

✔ Failure to gain weight

✔ Failure to thrive (a failure to grow and develop normally)

✔ Unexplained diarrhea

✔ Weight loss

Clearly, these kinds of symptoms make control of diabetes much more difficult because there's no dependable absorption of food. Hypoglycemia (which I discuss in Chapter 4) occurs much more often in patients suffering from T1DM and celiac disease, and it's difficult for them to choose a correct insulin dose.

A positive blood test for gastric parietal cell autoantibodies rules in the diagnosis of celiac disease. Confirmation comes from direct viewing of the stomach by gastroscopy.

When this diagnosis is made, it's time to consult with a dietitian, who can help identify safe foods. Foods that are safe for the type 1 patient with celiac disease include:

✔ Cereals made without wheat or barley malt

✔ Dairy products

✔ Fruits and vegetables

✔ Meat

✔ Potatoes, rice, corn, and beans

✔ Foods specially made with alternative grains and starches, like from rice, potato, and cornflower

All items made with flour, whether all-purpose, white, or wheat, are strictly prohibited in a gluten-free diet. For more on this topic, check out *Living Gluten-Free For Dummies,* by Danna Korn (Wiley).

Chapter 6

Handling Emotional Effects

Discovering that your little girl or little boy has a chronic disease called type 1 diabetes (or T1DM) that you know little about but have heard can cause premature death can be devastating, to say the least. I hope that in the course of reading this book you realize that much of what you've heard is myth. With the tools that are currently available, your child should be able to live a long, quality life, though it's true that he'll spend a lot of time doing things that his friends without diabetes won't have to do. On the other hand, the attention that your child will devote to taking care of himself will probably prolong his life beyond that of someone who isn't careful about eating, drinking, smoking, and exercise.

This chapter is about the emotional consequences of type 1 diabetes. They're not limited to the person with the disease but rather affect every family member. Having to deal with diabetes is a huge burden on a growing child, but the experience of numerous patients in the past shows that this burden is manageable.

Coming to Terms with the Diagnosis

When your child is diagnosed with type 1 diabetes, he may experience a wide range of emotions, such as shock, sadness, anger, and denial. Having these initial emotions is perfectly normal, but your child needs to accept the diagnosis eventually in order to take charge of his treatment and start living a healthy life. You can use the information in the following sections to show your child that he's not alone in dealing with type 1 diabetes and to help him develop positive coping skills.

Knowing that your child is in good company

So many people have T1DM that there are bound to be some really outstanding scholars, athletes, politicians, and leaders in all walks of life in the mix. They prove that there's no limit to what your child can do in his life with T1DM. In particular, they prove that T1DM doesn't make you uglier, dumber, slower, or weaker.

Your child is a person with T1DM. How he lets that fact affect his life will determine the shape of his life, not the diabetes. The people I describe in the following sections are able to live their lives to the fullest regardless of their diabetes. And your child can, too. Right now, your child can't be cured of T1DM, but he doesn't have to let it get in the way of whatever he wants to be and do.

World-class athletes

In 2007, a cycling team of 11 men with T1DM called Team Type 1 bicycled 3,043 miles across America in five days. This feat would have been impressive had it been accomplished by a group of completely well people; what makes it exceptional is that these cyclists had to test their blood glucose, give themselves continuous insulin with pumps, and make sure that their nutrition kept them fit for the many miles of biking each day. These men and the other athletes in this section show that your child can do anything even though he has T1DM.

Each of the people I describe in this section is at the top of his or her game, despite having to deal with T1DM. They represent a number of different sports, each doing what he or she loves the most:

- **Missy Foy** is an elite athlete who, in 2000, became the first athlete in history with T1DM to qualify for the Olympic Marathon Trials. In 2005, she broke the course record for the 50-mile Ultramarathon and was number one in the world for a woman at that distance.

- **Kris Freeman** is the top cross-country skier in the United States. He has won numerous cross-country championships and was preparing for the Olympics in 2000 when he developed T1DM. He competed anyway and remains a member of the US Ski Team.

- **Gary Hall, Jr.** won two gold medals in Olympic swimming (in 2000 and 2004). He also won silver and bronze medals in other swimming events.

- **Jonathan Hayes** was a star football player in college and then played tight end for the Cincinnati Bengals of the National Football League. He played in the NFL for 12 seasons and didn't miss a single game in his last six seasons.

✔ **Chris Jarvis** is a world champion Canadian rower who has won gold medals in several World Cup rowing events. He plans to compete in rowing at the Olympic Games in Beijing in 2008.

✔ **Adam Morrison,** a basketball player who developed T1DM in the eighth grade, entered the National Basketball Association after three years of college basketball and now plays for the Charlotte Bobcats of the NBA.

Entertainers and politicians

People with T1DM are unlimited in their physical and mental attributes, as the following individuals prove. They represent a large number of unique and successful entertainers and politicians with T1DM.

✔ **Halle Berry** is an Academy Award–winning actress who developed T1DM at age 23. The first African American woman to win an Academy Award, Berry has several high-profile endorsement deals and is one of the highest paid actresses in Hollywood.

✔ **Jim Turner** developed T1DM in high school and went on to become an actor, starring in numerous television shows. He's a strong advocate for the American Diabetes Association and gives many talks on how to live with diabetes.

✔ **Nicole Johnson** developed T1DM as a sophomore in college and went on to become the first woman with T1DM to win the Miss America crown (in 1999). She travels the world educating people about diabetes mellitus; her work has earned her numerous awards including the Koop Medal for Health Promotion and Awareness and the Victory Over Diabetes Medal of the Polish Diabetes Association. She also has written several books, including her autobiography, *Living With Diabetes*.

✔ **Charles (Buddy) Roemer** developed T1DM as an adult. Thereafter, he held numerous political offices, including four terms as Louisiana Congressman followed by one term as Governor of Louisiana.

Encouraging positive coping skills

What are some of the tools that your child can use to thrive with T1DM? They consist of the coping skills that he may or may not know he possesses. These are the traits that you want to promote by constantly emphasizing them. Praise the child when he does the right thing for his diabetes, whether it's eating properly, taking the injection correctly, or exercising. Also remember to limit the criticisms for mistakes.

To your child, you represent the chief "judge" in his life. If you constantly reinforce the positive qualities that he possesses, that's how he'll think of himself. On the other hand, if you dwell on his negative qualities, he'll see himself in that light.

Some of the key tools for helping your child deal with T1DM include the following:

- **Let him be the one in control of his diabetes.** As much as your child would like to have his parents, doctor, or diabetes educator handle things for him, he's the one constantly making the important decisions as to what to eat, how much to exercise, how much insulin to take, how much to rest, and so forth. (Of course, if your child is too young to make such decisions on his own, it's your job as parent or caretaker to step in.) It's important that an older child have the knowledge he needs to make the right decisions. This book is a great start to gaining that knowledge, but you can also help your child talk to his doctor, diabetes educator, pharmacist, and other helpful folks to find out the info he needs.

- **Focus on his successes.** When managing T1DM, you and your child know that there are times when things go better than other times. Try to figure out why that happens and use the knowledge to improve his diabetes management. For example, summer may be approaching and your child wants to be in good shape for summer sports, so he's willing to exercise more. When he increases his exercise level, he may find that he needs less insulin to get good control of his blood sugar and blood levels. You and your child can work together to develop an exercise program to maximize the benefits of exercise regardless of the time of year. (See Chapter 9 for full details on exercise.)

- **Get the family's help.** T1DM is a family disease, which means that a supportive family can really improve your child's control of his diabetes. For example, if family meals aren't consistent with your child's needs, it's harder for him to control his blood glucose. If a sibling encourages him to eat things that he knows are problematic, the sibling isn't doing him any favors. And things can be just as difficult if the sabotage is less direct, like if family members constantly complain about how he manages his diabetes. As the parent, you and your child can work together to let other family members know exactly the extent to which you want them to be involved in the diabetes. I say much more about this in the next section.

- **Develop a positive attitude.** A little optimism can go a long way. You will find as you read this book that there's an enormous amount of work going on to cure your child's diabetes. Some of the best brains in the world are concentrated on doing this. But even before "the cure" is found, your child should know that he's blessed by having the best set of tools that has ever existed to control his blood glucose.

In the decade and a half since researchers studied the benefit of glucose management in preventing or slowing complications from T1DM (see the sidebar "The Diabetes Control and Complications Trial" in Chapter 5), the knowledge of diabetes treatment has expanded with new tools and tests. Someone may announce the definitive cure tomorrow. In the meantime, a positive attitude helps your child keep his diabetes in the best possible control so that he's ready when the cure is available. Pessimism only leads to an "I don't care" attitude that doesn't motivate him to do all the things he needs to do with regard to his T1DM.

✔ **Help your child identify the most difficult issues and figure out how to overcome them.** Remember that every problem has a solution. For instance: Does your child have trouble remembering to take his insulin or do his blood glucose tests? Meters are now available with alarms that he can set to remind him (see Chapter 7). Because he generally tests just before he takes his insulin, one alarm may solve both problems.

Is he having trouble figuring the correct insulin dose, perhaps? His doctor and dietitian can be of help. Learning how much insulin he needs for the glucose in his blood (see Chapter 10) as well as the carbohydrate he's about to eat (see Chapter 8) will solve this problem.

✔ **Don't expect perfection.** Although things need to go right most of the time, there will be times when they don't. So many different inputs determine the result of your child's blood glucose that even if he eats the same food, exercises the same amount, and takes the same amount of insulin each day, his next glucose level may be very different from what he expects. If this happens consistently, a change may correct the problem. But if a surprise is a rare event, encourage your child to forget about it. One or even several bad blood glucoses won't damage him in the long run.

Realizing that Type 1 Diabetes Is a Family Disease

Both the patient and the patient's family have to deal with the emotional impact of T1DM. If the patient is a small child, Mom and Dad may have to take care of everything for a number of years, and siblings may feel ignored as all the attention goes to the patient. How the whole family copes with all the challenges of T1DM may make a huge difference in the future of the patient. If the gang can keep things in good control until he takes over, he has a great start in preventing future complications.

In the following sections, I provide some helpful general tips for parents of children with T1DM and explain how diabetes care changes at different stages of a child's growth. I also help siblings develop an understanding of T1DM.

Getting a grip on general guidelines for parents

Parents commonly feel fear when they discover that their child has T1DM. The first step in overcoming the fear is to become knowledgeable about the diabetes. You can do that by attending a course on T1DM available in most local hospitals. Also find a diabetes educator and a dietitian with whom you feel comfortable (see Chapter 2 for tips on finding these folks). When you know that there are ways to prevent the complications of T1DM (covered in Chapters 4 and 5) and a broad range of treatments should the complications occur, you'll feel much more able to handle the challenges that come your way.

As a parent, you can do a number of things to ease yourself through the experience of having a child with diabetes.

- ✔ **Try to maintain a balance between good diabetes care of your child and overbearing control.** If you try to control every blood glucose result in an attempt to achieve perfection, you'll rapidly find that your child rebels. He'll refuse his insulin, eat foods that aren't appropriate, and refuse to exercise.

- ✔ **Understand that anger is a natural response to the limitations that a child feels when he has diabetes.** Discover the source of his anger by asking questions like "What makes you angriest about having diabetes?" and try to find a compromise that addresses his anger without sacrificing diabetic control. Sometimes it's even okay to sacrifice control for a short while in order to gain the child's support. For example, allowing him a small piece of cake on his birthday is a small price to pay to maintain his cooperation.

- ✔ **Be aware that neither you nor your child is to blame for the fact that he has diabetes.** T1DM doesn't result from consuming too much sugar, failing to exercise sufficiently, or any other failure that you may imagine. (Turn to Chapter 2 to find out how T1DM actually develops.)

- ✔ **Don't overreact to a temporary loss of control over your child's glucose level.** Control of the blood glucose may be lost temporarily when your child gets sick with a virus or encounters one of many other problems. When it happens, move on and try to restore the control as soon as possible without being judgmental and implying that the child was bad or did the wrong thing. A child who's really trying but gets blamed when things go wrong will quickly lose interest in trying.

- ✔ **Recognize that depression can occur in patients with diabetes.** If your child's sleep is disturbed, if he doesn't want to eat, if his usual positive outlook changes to sadness and unhappiness, it may be the time to talk to his doctor about getting help. Maintaining good diabetic control in the face of depression is very difficult. Even if the child isn't depressed, a visit to a psychologist may be a valuable baseline to establish in case things go wrong later on; you can obtain a referral for a psychologist from your diabetes specialist.

- ✔ **Know when to begin turning over control of the day-to-day management of diabetes to the child.** Previously it was thought that this should be done as early as possible. Now, doctors and other people in the know feel that the child shouldn't have control of daily diabetes management until he clearly understands how his lifestyle, eating, exercise, rest, insulin, emotional state, and more affect his diabetes. For example, when the child knows how a level of blood sugar combined with the amount of carbohydrate about to be eaten and with the kind and amount of insulin previously taken all play a role in the next insulin shot — and he can calculate the amount correctly — he's ready to assume more responsibility. When a child gets more involved in his T1DM control, he and his parents need to work out who's responsible for what part of diabetes management so that poor diabetic control doesn't result from confusion. The age at which you hand over some control is entirely dependent on your child and what he's ready for.

✔ **Make it clear that the limitations on food, exercise, and so forth are associated with living, not necessarily diabetes.** Whether diabetes is present or not, you don't want your child to be obese, and you do want your child to be physically fit. By framing responsibilities as part of a healthy lifestyle rather than a diabetes lifestyle, your child will be much more receptive to eating right and keeping fit just like his siblings and friends who don't have diabetes. If he associates every limitation in his life with diabetes, he'll hate his disease and either ignore it or not do the things that are critical to good diabetes control.

✔ **Make sure that your children without diabetes know about the disease.** This is a great opportunity to find out what the "patient" knows by having him explain his disease to his siblings. (You can correct any mistakes.)

Caring for children of all ages

Your growing child will have different reactions to diabetes at different ages. Young children passively but not happily accept the insulin shots, whereas young adults want to take charge of their condition. The following sections describe what you can expect from children with T1DM at different ages.

Infants up to 18 months

Missing the initial diagnosis of T1DM in an infant up to 18 months of age is easy to do because the child can't tell you what's wrong. You may not notice that diapers have to be changed more often because of excessive urination, and the baby's nausea and vomiting may be ascribed to a stomach problem. Call your doctor immediately to get a diagnosis if you suspect that your baby has T1DM; Chapter 2 has more information on typical symptoms.

The infant up to 18 months of age with T1DM is completely under the care of his parent (usually the mother). He'll resist his shots and his glucose tests but must clearly understand that they're essential. This is something you have to insist upon even though the child can't understand the reason.

It's better for the baby's neurological system to allow his blood glucose to be a little higher. A blood glucose between 150 and 200 mg/dl (8.3 to 11.1 mmol/L) is a good target to shoot for. Chapter 7 has full details on measuring and monitoring blood glucose.

Toddlers between 18 months and 3 years

The toddler who is 18 months to 3 years old is at the stage of beginning to test his parents, establishing himself as a separate human being. He's starting to learn to control his environment (by toilet training, for example). With diabetes, he may refuse shots, refuse to eat enough and at the right time, and generally make it difficult for you to manage the disease. You have to set limits and be firm, know when to insist when the item is essential (like taking insulin) and when to give in so that the child can have some victories as well (like allowing the child a piece of birthday cake).

Use of very short-acting insulin like lispro (see Chapter 10) is very helpful in toddlers because the child's eating habits tend to be irregular and you can give the insulin just as the child begins to eat.

Children between 3 and 6 years

The child between ages 3 and 6 is still home and tests your limitations even more than a toddler. But at last he can tell you when he has symptoms of hypoglycemia (see Chapter 4). At this age, the child is wondering what he did to deserve diabetes when all his friends don't have it. Get the child involved with food preparation so that he feels he plays a part in his care.

As your child gets closer to 6 years old, think about enrolling him in a diabetes camp or a children's diabetes group. There he'll be surrounded by kids like him and will realize that everyone has similar concerns and limitations. It turns out that diabetes isn't a punishment after all but something to be managed. (For information on camps for children with T1DM go to the Web site of the American Diabetes Association at www.diabetes.org/community programs-and-localevents/diabetescamps.jsp.)

Don't try to teach your young child about the complications of diabetes yet. He doesn't possess the skills or knowledge to manage his disease and will simply be frightened.

Children between 6 and 12 years

As the child begins school between 6 and 12 years of age, he wants to know more. This is the time for you and the child to go to a diabetes education program and to sit down together with a dietitian to work out the best diet to promote continued growth and good diabetic control. It's also the time to hand over some of the control (don't give up control of the insulin just yet), especially because you're not at school to monitor the child all the time. Establish that the school has food that's healthy for your child and also has a program where knowledgeable people are available to help him in the event of hypoglycemia. This is mandated by law. Your child should have access to immediate sources of glucose and permission to take them if necessary as well as the right to go to the bathroom when required. You also want to be sure that one parent is always available and reachable in case of an emergency. (Check out Chapter 14 for more information about adjusting to school with type 1 diabetes.)

Diabetes camp is a valuable place for your child to go at this age because he can make friends with other children with diabetes and also can learn more about his condition. In addition, nutrition is especially important as the child is growing rapidly (see Chapter 8). Snacks between meals will smooth out the glucose control.

Teens between 13 and 15 years

When the child reaches age 13 to 15 and officially becomes a teenager, he's extremely curious and wants to know about everything, including his diabetes. Another trip together to a diabetes education program and the dietitian isn't overdoing it at all. He's probably forgotten a lot of information since his last visit, and there's usually some new and hopeful information that you can both learn from the program. At this age, involving both parents in diabetes education and treatment is even better than just one parent.

It's time to give up more and more control while still overseeing the way your child is managing his diabetes. Continuing attendance at diabetes camp confirms that he's doing the right things and reinforces the notion that diabetes can be associated with fun.

This and the following stage may be a very difficult time in terms of trying to keep good glucose control because of the production of large amounts of growth hormone, which tends to raise blood glucose. Don't expect perfection, and make sure your child doesn't either! Maintaining reasonable good diabetic control, allowing the average blood glucose to be a little higher (to avoid hypoglycemia), and knowing that after your child grows out of the teen years he can achieve tighter control will get you through these stages with your sanity intact.

Teens between 15 and 19

The stage of puberty, from age 15 to 19, with all the new and powerful hormones (especially the sex hormones) may prove to be the most difficult time of all to manage T1DM. All the problems of attraction to and being attractive for a significant other seem to get in the way. Who wants his girlfriend to know that he has a chronic disease? Your child also has a lot of buddies of the same sex that he wants to impress. Telling them he can't eat this or that or that he has to take a shot several times a day or must leave for a regular doctor's appointment hardly makes a good impression.

In this age range, teenagers want to see the doctor on their own. They want to know that their diabetes won't prevent them from doing whatever they want in life. Teenagers also need their friends to know about diabetes and to help them when needed. This may be difficult for the teenager who really doesn't want anyone to know about his disease, but it's essential.

This is the stage when girls, especially, are highly conscious of their weight and may skip insulin shots in order to lose weight. Skipping insulin will show up in the hemoglobin A1c (see Chapter 7). If this level starts to rise as the child is losing weight, you need to step in to deal with the problem; see Chapter 8 for details.

Despite the difficulty of achieving excellent glucose control, this also is the point at which you really need to emphasize the importance of tight blood glucose control for two reasons: Tight control beginning now will help to prevent diabetic complications later on; and your young adult is preparing to go off to ·college, where you'll have little or no control over what happens. If he has developed good habits of eating, insulin administration, and so forth, these habits are likely to continue when he's on his own.

Be sure to discuss alcohol use and sexual activity before your teenager leaves the nest. Make sure he understands that overdoing it with alcohol provides many empty calories and can lead to hypoglycemia (see Chapter 12). In addition, be certain that your daughter is aware of the danger of pregnancy when diabetes isn't well-controlled (see Chapter 16) and that children of either sex are aware of sexually transmitted diseases. You may not be comfortable talking about these subjects with your child, but think how you'll feel if they suffer the consequences of ignorance.

Helping siblings be understanding

Being the brother or sister of someone with T1DM is a tough assignment. On the one hand, your other children envy all the time and attention that your child with diabetes gets from you (the parent). On the other hand, they may be fearful of getting it themselves. They also may witness a severe hypoglycemic episode, which can be very scary. It's a good idea to educate your other children so that they know something about diabetes, especially how to manage hypoglycemia. You can certainly take non-diabetic children to diabetes education sessions.

It's important that all your children share things as kids together, playing together, going to movies together, and so forth. Their relationship should be based on the fact that they're members of the same family, not a sibling and a child with diabetes. The sibling with T1DM is first of all a person, and the fact that your children share the same parents creates a special bond that lasts a lifetime.

Handling Issues of Self-Esteem

Children with T1DM face many issues of self-esteem, even after they've been treating their T1DM for a while. Among the reasons are

✔ The feeling that you must be a bad person or have done something wrong to have been stuck with such a bad disease

✔ The idea that diabetes makes you less handsome or pretty than your friends

✔ The notion that you're mentally inferior, particularly when you've had hypoglycemia and think that it has damaged your brain

✔ The fear that you may someday give this disease to your child

✔ The fear of the complications of T1DM that will make you less of a human being

✔ The fact that you must constantly plan when to eat, what to eat, when to take your medication, when to test, and so forth unlike your friends without diabetes

✔ The reliance that you have on others, including parents and doctors

These are realistic fears, although most of them are based upon myth and not fact. I address them in the following sections.

Busting myths about having a chronic disease

Neither you nor your child or anyone else is to blame for your child's diabetes. As I explain in Chapter 2, T1DM occurs in a susceptible individual who comes in contact with a virus that shares tissue similarities with the person's beta cells. As your child's body attempts to reject the virus, it destroys his beta cells, the ones that make insulin. As a parent, you're not responsible if your child gets diabetes; you certainly had nothing to do with that villainous virus.

Help your child remember that he's first a person and then a person with diabetes. As a person, a nice haircut, nice clothes, and so forth make him indistinguishable from any other good-looking person. There is no big D printed on his forehead.

It's also true that your child is just as intelligent as any other person with or without diabetes. Although there's some suggestive evidence that severe hypoglycemic reactions under the age of 3 may decrease a child's intelligence quotient (IQ), hypoglycemia after that has been shown to have no harmful long-term effect on the mind.

Clearing up fears about having special needs

Managing your child's diabetes requires many products, including the following:

- He uses needles, syringes, and insulin (see Chapter 10).
- He has a glucose meter and test strips to test his blood glucose (see Chapter 7).
- He may have an insulin pump (see Chapter 11) to slowly administer insulin over 24 hours and a continuous glucose monitor to take glucose levels at five-minute intervals throughout the day.

He also needs a variety of people to help him, including:

- A diabetes doctor for overall health
- A dietitian to help choose the right foods
- An eye doctor to check his vision regularly
- A diabetes educator to teach him about diabetes
- A psychologist or social worker to get him through the stressful occasions that accompany any chronic disease
- A pharmacist for the right medication
- Family and friends to give support all the time

Type 1 diabetes certainly puts strains on your child that a person without diabetes doesn't have, especially when it comes to planning meals, taking medications, and monitoring blood glucose. But as I point out in the earlier section "Knowing that your child is in good company," it also molds character. If your child can overcome the limitations of T1DM, he can overcome many other of the challenges that he'll face in his lifetime. Like Frank Sinatra said, if you can make it there, you'll make it anywhere.

While it's true that your child with T1DM has a lot more special needs than the average person, he's a unique individual with a special role to play in the world. He may become an entertainer bringing joy to many people he'll never know, or he may be a writer teaching people about subjects they want to know more about. He may be an inventor, creating a product that improves the lives of many other people, or he may be a teacher, helping others to learn how they can thrive in the world. Sit down with your child and help him understand that his special needs are the foundation that makes it possible for him to make his contribution to the world. And remember that at one time or another, everyone has to draw on society to help them along. In a real way, everyone is interdependent.

Maintaining a High Quality of Life

Again and again it has been shown that the people with T1DM who feel that they have the highest quality of life are those who have the best control of their diabetes. And having control of diabetes means controlling the blood glucose especially for the young person and later, controlling the blood pressure and the blood cholesterol.

The keys to your child maintaining a high quality of life with T1DM are

- ✔ Regularly measuring his blood glucose and knowing how to respond to highs and low (see Chapter 7).

- ✔ Getting all the important examinations at regular intervals (see Chapter 7).

- ✔ Knowing how to count carbohydrates so that he can estimate insulin needs (see Chapter 8).

- ✔ Enjoying good food that's also nutritious (see Chapter 8).

- ✔ Developing a program of aerobic and anaerobic exercise to keep his muscles in excellent shape thereby helping to keep his metabolism functioning well (see Chapter 9).

- ✔ Taking insulin in appropriate amounts and at appropriate times (see Chapter 10).

- ✔ Making sure he gets sufficient rest so that he's alert and able to respond to the challenges of T1DM.

- ✔ Maintaining a positive attitude as he recognizes that he can control his diabetes and avoid complications.

- ✔ Keeping himself aware of the most current treatments.

- ✔ Making full use of all the resources available to him, including tools and people.

- ✔ Avoiding blaming himself or others when things don't go exactly according to plan. Help him just pick himself up and move on.

Part III
Treating Type 1 Diabetes

The 5th Wave   By Rich Tennant

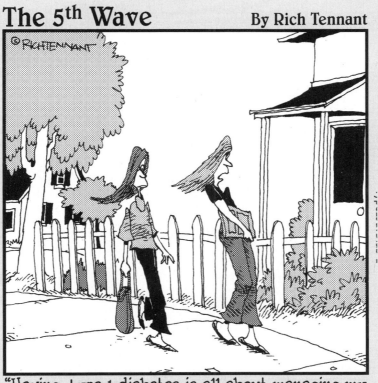

"Having type 1 diabetes is all about managing my insulin. Like, if I see this real nice jacket, but my mom won't buy it for me, but I know if I get all on her about it she will, but that takes up a lot of my blood sugar? Then I adjust my insulin that day."

In this part . . .

If you live in the United States in the 21st century, you're blessed with everything you need to become and remain healthy. This holds true for people diagnosed with type 1 diabetes. Whether it's equipment for monitoring the disease or tools for treating the disease, the problem is selecting from the abundance available. In this part, I guide you through the choices involved in treating this disease, pointing out the best options and how to use them not just to survive but to thrive with type 1 diabetes.

Chapter 7

Undergoing Essential Tests and Monitoring Blood Glucose

In This Chapter

▶ Doing essential tests at the doctor's office regularly

▶ Checking your child's blood glucose several times daily

▶ Picking a home blood glucose meter

*A*s the parent of a child with diabetes, I have no doubt that you want to use every available method to keep your child healthy and prolong his life. Doing the tests in this chapter will make the difference between a long life and a shorter one. Most of them are designed to discover diabetic complications early in their development, when you can use all the great tools available to slow or reverse them. Some tests are part of the doctor's physical exam each time your child visits him. Most of the tests should be performed at least annually, but certain tests must be done quarterly. Others, like self-monitoring of blood glucose, are done several times a day. Taken together, these tests provide information that you and your doctor can use to make the adjustments in your child's treatment plan necessary to ensure not just a long life but a high quality one.

Twenty-five years ago, many of the tests I discuss in this chapter didn't exist. Self-monitoring of blood glucose, the biggest advance since the isolation of insulin in 1921, only began to become available in 1980. Unfortunately, people who developed T1DM before then didn't have the benefit of these tests and often developed diabetic complications. *This should not happen to your child (or to you, if you're the patient).* Getting all these tests done may be inconvenient and expensive, but it's worth your time and money. The things you *won't* have to worry about happening to your child if you follow my recommendations carefully include:

✔ Blindness

✔ Kidney failure

✔ Amputations

✔ Painful nerve disease

✔ Strokes

I'm reminded of the story of the wonderful violinist Midori, when she performed for the first time with the New York Philharmonic under Leonard Bernstein. In the middle of the violin concerto, one of her strings suddenly broke. She put down her violin, walked over to the first violinist, borrowed his violin, and continued playing. Moments later, a string broke on this violin. She put that one down, walked over to the second violinist and borrowed his violin to complete the concerto to one of the biggest ovations ever heard at Tanglewood, where the concert was taking place. Asked later how she maintained her calm under such adversity, she said, "What could I do? My strings broke and I didn't want to stop the music."

If you think of your child's life as a beautiful song and diabetes as a broken string, you want to continue and complete the music. In this chapter, you find all the keys you need to make that happen.

Doing Key Tests at the Doctor's Office

Treating your child's type 1 diabetes (or T1DM for short) means that his doctor must order many tests, but as a responsible parent, you shouldn't depend on the doctor's memory to make sure the tests are done. After all, he's a busy guy with hundreds of patients to worry about. Instead, keep a flow chart for your child's tests and fill in the blanks as time goes by. I've created such a chart for you on the Cheat Sheet at the front of this book. Copy it and use it to make sure that your child's tests get done at the appropriate times.

Following are the tests that must be done on a regular basis to evaluate the status of your child's diabetes (I go into detail on them in the following sections):

✔ The doctor should download your child's blood glucose results from the home glucose meter at every office visit into a computer program that he can use to adjust treatment. (I discuss home meters later in this chapter in the section "Selecting a Home Blood Glucose Meter.")

✔ You should examine your child's feet daily; the doctor should examine your child's feet at every office visit.

✔ The doctor should measure the blood pressure at each visit.

✔ Your child's height and weight should be measured at each visit.

✔ The doctor should send your child to the laboratory for a hemoglobin A1c test every three months. You can also do this test at home and give the results to the doctor.

- ✓ The doctor should do an ankle-brachial index study every five years.

- ✓ The doctor should check the thyroid function with a TSH at the beginning of treatment and every five years thereafter.

- ✓ The doctor should order an annual microalbuminuria test to look for early kidney damage.

- ✓ The doctor should send your child to an ophthalmologist or optometrist for an annual dilated eye examination.

- ✓ The doctor should order an annual lipid panel on your child.

If any abnormalities are found in these tests, the frequency of testing is increased and steps are taken to reverse the abnormalities.

If you want more information on every aspect of proper diabetes care for your child, go to the Web site of the National Diabetes Education Program at ndep. nih.gov. There you can find information for parents and children including standards of care. Another great resource for parents is the Web site Better Diabetes Care at betterdiabetescare.nih.gov/MAINintroduction. htm. Although this is a site for professionals, it tells you what your child's doctor should be doing for your child to provide the best diabetes care possible.

Foot problems

Just like eye problems associated with diabetes, foot problems take more than ten years to develop and are preventable by good diabetes care. Although amputations are rare in children, the damage that leads to an amputation can start at a young age.

Make sure that your child has full sensation in his feet. It's up to you as the parent to check the young child if there's any question of loss of sensation. Here's what you must do:

- ✓ Examine his feet with your eyes and hands daily. If you notice redness, swelling, or a cut, be sure to call your doctor.

- ✓ Test the heat of water that he's about to enter for a bath to make sure that it isn't burning hot.

- ✓ Check his shoes for stones or other objects that he may not feel but that could cause damage.

- ✓ Make sure that he wears foot protection, like good sturdy shoes. (Flip-flops aren't a good idea!)

- ✓ Keep his feet clean and moisturized.

The doctor should examine your child's feet at each visit, although you'll probably pick up any abnormality long before he does because you examine your child daily. Doctors usually have a 10-gram filament as well as a tuning fork that they use to detect loss of sensation in the feet.

You also want the doctor to do an ankle-brachial index test on your child every five years. This is done by measuring the systolic blood pressure at the ankle and in the arm (see the later sidebar "The meaning of blood pressure numbers" for an explanation of systolic blood pressure). The ankle reading is divided by the arm reading. A normal result is greater than 0.9, meaning the two readings are very close. A result of 0.4 to 0.8 means that the blood pressure is much lower in the leg than in the arm, suggesting a blockage somewhere in the leg. Below 0.4 indicates a severe blockage. If necessary, surgery can be done to open the artery. If severe obstruction is present, it may be treated by *angioplasty*, a procedure in which a balloon is inserted in the artery to open it up, or *bypass surgery*, in which the obstruction is bypassed with a piece of the patient's vein or a synthetic tube.

The ankle-brachial index is much worse in older people with T1DM if they're smokers, have high cholesterol, or have high blood pressure.

Blood pressure

There's no question that blood pressure plays a key role in the development of complications of diabetes. Your child's blood pressure should be measured each time he sees the doctor. An increase in the average blood pressure of children is especially harmful for the child with T1DM. Here are just some of the reasons for the increase:

- Children are getting fatter.

- Children are more sedentary than before.

- Children with diabetes may have increased sensitivity to salt, which raises blood pressure.

- Children with diabetes may lack the nighttime fall in blood pressure that normally occurs in people without diabetes.

In order to tell if your child with T1DM has high blood pressure, you have to know the normal levels of blood pressure for his age and height. (See the nearby sidebar "The meaning of blood pressure numbers" for more detailed explanations of each type of blood pressure.) Table 7-1 shows the highest normal blood pressure at each age.

Table 7-1	Maximum Normal Blood Pressure at Different Ages
Age	*Maximum Blood Pressure*
Newborn	70/45 mm Hg
5	115/75 mm Hg
6–12	125/80 mm Hg
13–15	126/78 mm Hg
16–18	132/82 mm Hg
Over 18	139/89 mm Hg

To compare your child's blood pressure with other children his age and height, go to www.nhlbi.nih.gov/health/prof/heart/hbp/hbp_ped.pdf. This takes you to The Fourth Report on the Diagnosis, Evaluation, and Treatment of High Blood Pressure in Children and Adolescents. Scroll through the document to find Blood Pressure Levels for Boys (Table 3) and Girls (Table 4) by Age and Height Percentile. Check the tables to see if your child is above the 90th percentile, which is considered too high.

High blood pressure worsens all the complications of diabetes, and controlling blood pressure slows or reverses the progression of the complications. Blood pressure is treated with lifestyle changes like exercise and weight loss and medications if needed.

You can check your child's blood pressure (and your own) using one of the home blood pressure monitors that you can buy in pharmacies. The Panasonic and Omron models are reliable, accurate, and not very expensive.

For much more information on every aspect of high blood pressure, check out my book *High Blood Pressure For Dummies,* 2nd Edition (Wiley).

Weight and height

A child's height and weight is such an easy measurement to make, and it tells so much about whether he's growing normally that there's absolutely no reason for the doctor not to make this measurement at every visit. Your child with T1DM should be compared to the height and weight charts for children without diabetes of the same age in order to determine if he's growing normally and is underweight or overweight.

The meaning of blood pressure numbers

How do you interpret a blood pressure reading? Suppose you see something like 125/75; it consists of a top reading and a bottom reading.

✔ The **top reading** is the *systolic blood pressure* (SBP) — the amount of pressure in your arteries as the heart pumps. *Systole* is the rhythmic contraction of your heart muscle when it's expelling blood from your left ventricle (the large chamber on the left side of your heart). The aortic valve sits between that chamber and your *aorta,* the large artery that takes blood away from the heart to the rest of the body. During systole, the aortic valve is open and blood flows freely to the rest of your body.

✔ The **bottom reading** is the *diastolic blood pressure* (DBP). After your heart empties the blood from the ventricle, the aortic valve shuts to prevent blood from returning into the heart from the rest of your body. Your heart muscle relaxes, and the ventricle expands as blood fills it up from the left atrium, which has received it from the lungs. Within your arteries, the blood pressure rapidly falls until it reaches its lowest point. The diastolic blood pressure reflects this lowest point of blood pressure. Before the pressure falls further, the ventricle contracts again and the blood pressure starts to rise back up to the systolic level.

If you're an adult with T1DM, you can use one of the following formulas to calculate your ideal weight depending upon your sex:

✔ A woman should weigh 100 pounds for 5 feet of height plus 5 pounds for every inch over 5 feet. Therefore, a 5-foot, 4-inch woman is ideally 120 pounds. That's the center of the range. Normal weight may be plus or minus 10 percent, so this woman is considered normal in weight if she weighs between 108 and 132 pounds.

✔ A man should weigh 106 pounds for 5 feet of height plus 6 pounds for every inch over 5 feet. For example, a 5-foot, 4-inch man should weigh 130 pounds with a normal range of 117 to 143 pounds.

Another way to determine whether an adult with T1DM is the proper weight is to figure out his body mass index (BMI). This is a very useful measurement because it takes the height into account in deciding whether the weight is appropriate. To calculate BMI, follow this formula:

$$[\text{Weight (lb)} \div \text{Height (in)} \div \text{Height (in)}] \times 703 = \text{BMI (kg/m}^2)$$

The final result is interpreted as follows:

✔ **Normal weight for height:** BMI from 22 to 24.9

✔ **Overweight for height:** BMI from 25 to 29.9

✔ **Obese for height:** BMI from 30

Hemoglobin A1c

A single blood glucose measurement is necessary to tell you how much insulin to give for the next meal and whether the insulin you gave your child previously was sufficient. However, it doesn't give you the big picture. Even four blood glucose measurements a day say little about overall diabetic control because blood glucose can and does change within minutes; you're looking at four points in time, but the blood glucose may be very different the rest of the time, especially during the long period of sleep when no measurements are made at all. The test that gives you the big picture is called the *hemoglobin A1c test*. It looks at the last three months and gives you an average of all the ups and downs in blood glucose levels. (To understand how it does this, see the nearby sidebar, "What the hemoglobin A1c test measures.")

At the beginning, the hemoglobin A1c tells you just how out-of-control your child's glucose was when the disease began. Every three months after that, it tells you how close he's coming to a level of control associated with avoiding the complications of diabetes that I discuss in Chapters 4 and 5.

Targeting certain levels

Figure 7-1 compares the hemoglobin A1c with the whole blood glucose and the plasma glucose (which is important to know because the plasma glucose is what you're measuring multiple times a day, not the hemoglobin A1c).

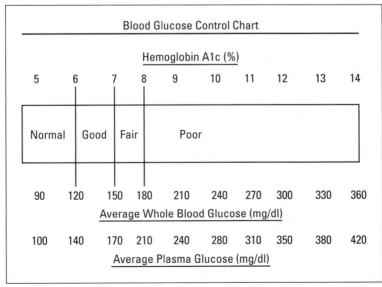

Figure 7-1: Hemoglobin A1c compared to whole blood glucose and plasma glucose.

Blood Glucose Control Chart

Hemoglobin A1c (%)

| 5 | 6 | 7 | 8 | 9 | 10 | 11 | 12 | 13 | 14 |

| Normal | Good | Fair | Poor |

| 90 | 120 | 150 | 180 | 210 | 240 | 270 | 300 | 330 | 360 |

Average Whole Blood Glucose (mg/dl)

| 100 | 140 | 170 | 210 | 240 | 280 | 310 | 350 | 380 | 420 |

Average Plasma Glucose (mg/dl)

What the hemoglobin A1c test measures

Hemoglobin A1c is the largest of three subfractions of the protein *hemoglobin,* the carrier of oxygen in the bloodstream. As hemoglobin is being formed, it binds to glucose to form glycohemoglobin. Glycohemoglobin ordinarily makes up 6 percent of the total hemoglobin in the blood. The glycohemoglobin takes three forms: hemoglobin A1a, A1b, and A1c. Because hemoglobin A1c is the largest subfraction of the three, it's the easiest to measure. The more glucose there is in the blood, the more glycohemoglobin will be formed. As it's formed, hemoglobin is transferred into red blood cells where it remains for 60 to 90 days. So by measuring the hemoglobin A1c in a sample of red blood cells, you can determine how much glucose was circulating in the blood over the last two to three months.

A hemoglobin A1c of 6 percent, considered normal, corresponds to an average whole blood glucose of under 120 mg/dl. A good hemoglobin A1c reading of 7 percent corresponds to an average whole blood glucose of 150 mg/dl. A reading of 8 percent, corresponding to an average whole blood glucose level of 180 mg/dl, is considered fair; anything above that figure is considered to be poor. In terms of plasma glucose, a good hemoglobin A1c of 7 percent corresponds to a plasma glucose of 170 mg/dl. A reading of 8 percent means the plasma glucose is 210 mg/dl.

For very young children, whose brain cells are still developing, it's advisable that the hemoglobin A1c be kept a little higher, perhaps up to 8 percent, until they've reached the age of 2. That's when low blood glucose levels will no longer damage their brains.

During puberty, as a result of the brain's increased production of growth hormone, it's extremely difficult to keep the hemoglobin A1c below 8 percent. Your teenager is considered to have poor control of his glucose if his hemoglobin A1c is 9 percent or higher.

The American Diabetes Association recommends that the goal of therapy for adults and adolescents with diabetes should be a hemoglobin A1c of 7 percent or less. This was the goal of the Diabetes Control and Complications Trial that was associated with a tremendous decrease in microvascular complications like eye disease, kidney disease, and nerve disease (see Chapter 5). However, for long-term prevention of macrovascular complications including heart attacks and strokes, a hemoglobin A1c of 6.5 percent is recommended.

Using test results

When working with people with T1DM, I use the hemoglobin A1c test for many purposes.

✔ It gives me a first indication of how well or poorly controlled a person's T1DM is when I first see her.

✔ It motivates the patient to try harder when the hemoglobin A1c is higher than the goal of 7 percent.

The difficulty with achieving a hemoglobin A1c of 7 percent or even 6.5 percent is the occurrence of hypoglycemia (see Chapter 4). The good news is that the longer the hemoglobin A1c is maintained at a normal value, the less hypoglycemia seems to be a problem.

✔ It clarifies the diabetic control when blood glucose measurements are up and down. A hemoglobin A1c of 7 percent, for example, means that most of the glucoses are in a satisfactory range, whereas a hemoglobin A1c of 8 percent means that they aren't. And if the glucoses aren't in a satisfactory range, the treatment should be revised.

✔ It permits me to encourage a woman with T1DM who wants to get pregnant to go ahead if the value is satisfactory or to tell her to wait if the level isn't right.

If a pregnant woman's hemoglobin A1c is high (over 8 percent for example), it mean's that her blood glucose was high on average at the time of conception of the baby. As a result, she's at high risk of delivering a baby with a congenital malformation. If she isn't yet pregnant, a measurement of the hemoglobin A1c tells her whether she can become pregnant now or should wait until her glucose is under better control. (See Chapter 16 for details on T1DM during pregnancy.)

Surveying potential issues with the test

One problem with the hemoglobin A1c test is the slowness with which it changes when major changes are occurring in treatment. Despite marked improvement in the blood glucose levels, the hemoglobin A1c changes slowly. Obtaining a hemoglobin A1c more often than every three months is of little value in showing improved glucose control.

Another problem with the hemoglobin A1c measurement is the difference in how the test is performed in different labs. Because each insurance company mandates it, I send my patients to three different labs to have the test done. The normal values in one lab aren't the same as in the other labs. Recently, the significance of this problem became clear when an insurance company changed the lab to which I could sent its patients. The change left me unable to compare the old test results to the new test results because of different normal values. Fortunately, there's an ongoing effort to standardize the method of performing the hemoglobin A1c test; the movement is based on the method used in the Diabetes Control and Complications Trial, where the normal level was 6.05 percent or less.

Testing at home

You can also do the hemoglobin A1c at home every three months. A test called A1c Now can be performed with a finger stick, similar to a blood glucose measurement (see the later section "The Basics of Testing Blood Glucose at Home"). You mix a large drop of blood with a solution and put it in the testing device. It takes eight minutes to get the result of the hemoglobin A1c. The test is accurate, and you can bring the result to your child's doctor so he can act on it immediately. The A1c Now test is available without a prescription at pharmacies.

You can also obtain the materials to collect a drop of your child's blood and send it to one of the following testing laboratories. This approach to A1c testing takes a little longer than a home test (a few days rather than eight minutes), but you can still get the result to pass along to your child's doctor.

- **AccuBase A1c Glycohemoglobin:** Each test costs $26.95 and includes lab analysis and reporting.

    Diabetes Technologies, Inc
    P.O. Box 1954
    Thomasville, GA 31799
    Phone 888-872-2443
    Fax 229-227-1752
    Web site www.diabetestechnologies.com

- **A1c at Home:** Each test costs $19.95 and includes lab analysis and reporting.

    Flexsite Diagnostics, Inc.
    3543 SW Corporate Pkwy.
    Palm City, FL 34990
    Phone 772-221-8893
    Fax 772-221-9671
    Web site www.flexsite.com

- **BioSafe A1c Hemoglobin Test Kit:** Each test costs $24.95 and includes lab analysis and reporting.

    Lab 123, Inc
    100 Field Drive, Suite 240
    Lake Forest, IL 60045
    Phone 888-700-8378
    Web site www.ebiosafe.com

GlycoMark

In contrast to the traditional hemoglobin A1c test, changes occur rapidly in the GlycoMark test. Like the hemoglobin A1c, it's a blood test, but a better result in the GlycoMark test is a higher value, not a lower one.

The GlycoMark test takes advantage of the fact that the compound 1,5-anhydroglucitol (or 1,5 AG) is normally found in healthy people. It's filtered by the kidneys and reabsorbed into the blood. However, when a lot of glucose is present in the urine, reabsorption is blocked, and the level of 1,5 AG in the blood falls. As glucose is reduced by treatment, blood levels of 1,5 AG rise.

Table 7-2 shows the values for GlycoMark found in people without and with diabetes.

Table 7-2	GlycoMark Test Results	
GlycoMark (ug/ml)	*Diabetes Control*	*Glucose (mg/dl)*
14.0 or higher	Normal (no diabetes)	Under 160
10–13.9	Well-controlled	Under 200
6–9.9	Moderate control	200–300
2–5.9	Poor control	
Less than 2	Very poor control	

Large changes in GlycoMark results occur in just two weeks, so you can use the test to detect early improvement or deterioration in your child's glucose control. In addition, the glucose after eating (called *postprandial glucose*) seems to have a big effect on the result of the GlycoMark test. Many specialists believe that the postprandial glucose has a greater effect on diabetic complications than glucose at other times. I expect the GlycoMark test to find a more prominent role in following diabetes care in years to come.

Thyroid functions

Increased and decreased thyroid function affect metabolism, and diseases that result in abnormal thyroid function are generally autoimmune, similar to T1DM. For these reasons it's important to verify that thyroid function is normal in your child with type 1 diabetes.

Too much thyroid hormone leads to insulin resistance, making diabetes worse. Too little thyroid hormone increases insulin sensitivity, so people with low thyroid function have reduced levels of blood glucose.

All children born in the United States are tested at birth with a *thyroid-stimulating hormone* (TSH) blood test because low thyroid function during development of the brain may lead to reduced intelligence. The TSH is the most sensitive test of thyroid function.

TSH is produced by the pituitary gland in the brain. When the thyroid gland makes the right amount of thyroid hormone, the pituitary produces the right amount of TSH to keep it working properly. The normal TSH level in the blood is 0.5 to 2.5 microunits per milliliter (mU/ml).

When the thyroid makes inadequate amounts of thyroid hormone, the pituitary increases its production of TSH to stimulate the thyroid, and values of 10 mU/ml or more aren't uncommon. On the flip side, when the thyroid makes too much thyroid hormone, the pituitary turns down its production of TSH, and values less than 0.5 mU/ml are found.

TSH should be measured when a person develops T1DM. The other test that should be done is a blood test for thyroid autoantibodies. If the TSH is normal and antibodies are present, TSH is tested every year. If the TSH is normal and antibodies are absent, TSH should be retested at least every five years.

Treatment for low thyroid function *(hypothyroidism)* is with replacement thyroid hormone. Treatment for increased thyroid function *(hyperthyroidism)* is with antithyroid drugs, radioactive iodine, or surgery. See my book *Thyroid For Dummies* (Wiley) for much more on this topic.

Microalbuminuria

A *microalbuminuria test,* a measurement of tiny amounts of protein in a urine specimen, indicates if T1DM is affecting your child's kidneys. Finding excessive levels of microalbumin is a very early and reversible sign of kidney damage due to diabetes. If the test finds abnormal amounts of microalbumin, there's plenty of time and opportunity to do something about this complication (see Chapter 5). The usual test for albumin, which involves a test stick put into a urine specimen, is only positive if there are large amounts of protein in the urine — greater than 300 mg per day. The microalbumin test is positive if the amount of protein in the urine is greater than 30 mg per day. A finding of small but abnormal amounts of protein (albumin) indicates the earliest evidence that diabetes is damaging the kidneys.

This test is first done about five years after your child has a diagnosis of T1DM. A negative test should be repeated annually. A positive test should be rechecked at the next appointment because the test can be falsely positive after strenuous exercise or if the patient is dehydrated. If your child has several positive microalbumin tests, the following actions are taken:

   ✔ **The doctor puts your child on a drug called an ACE inhibitor.** The microalbumin test can become negative after several months of taking the ACE inhibitor, and it may be possible to stop the drug after a while.

✔ **You take steps to get your child's blood glucose as normal as possible.** The Diabetes Control and Complications Trial showed that normal blood glucose can reverse early kidney damage. Chapters 7, 8, and 9 help you get going on tightening control of your child's glucose.

✔ **The doctor checks your child's blood pressure and treats it if it's not normal.** I discuss blood pressure later in this chapter.

✔ **The doctor checks your child's blood fats.** High cholesterol can damage the kidneys. I discuss checking cholesterol later in this chapter.

FlexSite Diagnostics, Inc., offers KidneyScreen At Home, a urine-collection kit that you use to send a sample to a lab to test for microalbuminuria (it costs $19.95). The lab sends the result to you and your child's doctor. You can find more information about this kit at www.flexsite.com. The company's other contact information is listed in the earlier section "Testing at home."

Eye problems

Fortunately, it takes 15 to 20 years of poor diabetic control for your child to develop eye problems. Unfortunately, that means that he may be only 30 years old when his vision begins to deteriorate. This can be prevented by keeping his hemoglobin A1c at 7 percent or below as much as possible (I discuss hemoglobin A1c earlier in this chapter).

An eye examination must be done annually to check for diabetic eye disease called *retinopathy* (see Chapter 5). An ophthalmologist or an optometrist can perform the exam; as a side note, it has been shown that no other doctor does as good a job with the exam as these two professionals. Make sure you insist that your doctor arrange for your child to have this examination annually.

During the exam, your child's eye is treated with drops to enlarge the pupils so that the doctor can see most of the back of the eye. He also measures the pressure in the eye and the appearance of the lens of the eye.

Fortunately, excellent treatments are available for diabetic eye disease, as you find out in Chapter 5. If it's discovered early by this examination, blindness is usually prevented in patients with T1DM.

Cholesterol

You may think that your child doesn't have to worry about cholesterol and other fats, but with T1DM, you have to pay attention to elevated cholesterol, excessive bad cholesterol, and too little good cholesterol; all can be major problems. In the following sections, I define cholesterol and describe a test that measures it.

Breaking down types of fat particles

Cholesterol circulates in the blood in the form of small particles called *lipoproteins*. Because cholesterol (the "lipo" part of "lipoprotein") doesn't dissolve in water, it has to be surrounded by proteins so it can remain suspended in blood. Otherwise it would separate just like oil separates from water.

Most of the fat your child eats is in a form called *triglyceride*. For example, the fat you see surrounding a piece of steak is triglyceride.

The different fats are neatly packaged into four particles in the blood. To treat high cholesterol properly, you need to know the levels of these different particles:

- ✔ **Chylomicrons,** the biggest fat particles, carry the fat from the meal your child just ate. They don't remain in the blood and don't cause *arteriosclerosis* (the hardening of the arteries). They disappear rapidly from the blood and usually aren't measured in a lipid panel.

- ✔ **High Density Lipoprotein (HDL)** is the particle that carries cholesterol back to the liver where it's broken down. HDL is known as "good" cholesterol because it reduces the danger of arteriosclerosis. The size of HDL particles is between the size of LDL and VLDL particles.

- ✔ **Low Density Lipoprotein (LDL),** known as "bad" cholesterol, is the smallest in size. It's bad because it's the particle that carries cholesterol to the arteries in which it's deposited, leading to arteriosclerosis.

- ✔ **Very Low Density Lipoprotein (VLDL)** particles contain mostly triglyceride as the fat. These are smaller than chylomicrons.

Deciphering lipid panel results

If your doctor wants to know the levels of all the fat particles in your child's bloodstream, your child has to fast for 12 hours before undergoing a test known as a *lipid panel*, but if he is satisfied with the results of a total cholesterol and the good cholesterol, no fasting is required before the test. Make sure that the doctor performs a lipid panel on your child once a year (or more often if the results aren't normal). A lipid panel is done with a blood specimen in which the various types of fat particles are measured.

Table 7-3 lists the current recommendations for everyone for the levels of fats in terms of the risk for coronary artery disease.

Your child's risk for coronary artery disease is greater if his HDL cholesterol is low and LDL is high. The famous Framingham study has shown that if you measure the total cholesterol and the HDL cholesterol and divide the total by the HDL, patients who have a ratio of 4.5 or less have a low incidence of heart attacks. Patients with ratios of greater than 4.5 are at higher risk, and the higher the ratio, the worse the risk.

Table 7-3	Levels of Fat and the Risk for Coronary Artery Disease		
Risk for Coronary Artery Disease	**LDL Cholesterol Level**	**HDL Cholesterol Level**	**Triglycerides Level**
Higher	Greater than 130	Less than 35	Greater than 400
Borderline	100–129	35–45	200–399
Lower	Less than 100	Greater than 45	Less than 150

A study in *The New England Journal of Medicine* in March 2004 indicated that the LDL level is also very important. In the study, a drug called atorvastatin was used to lower the HDL cholesterol of more than 4,000 men who had just had heart attacks. Those who received the maximum dose (so their LDL was reduced to a mean of 62) had a much lower incidence of subsequent heart attacks, heart pain, and strokes than the group whose LDL was lowered to a mean of 97; although Table 7-3 says that the risk is lower when the LDL is below 100, it may be that the best LDL is simply the lowest LDL.

The treatment of abnormal fat levels depends upon the type of fat that's not normal. For example, if the patient has too much LDL cholesterol, the statin group of drugs is used. If the patient doesn't have enough HDL cholesterol, niacin is taken and the patient is encouraged to exercise more.

The Basics of Testing Blood Glucose at Home

When self-testing of blood glucose was developed around 1980, it was the first huge advance in T1DM treatment since the isolation of insulin. Previously, glucose testing was done with urine specimens, but this method didn't produce accurate or helpful results because glucose generally doesn't enter the urine until the blood glucose is over 180 mg/dl. By that standard, a patient with T1DM may never show glucose in the urine and still suffer complications of diabetes!

All the thousands of research papers in the medical literature before 1980 that used urine testing for glucose are of no value and should be burned. (However, testing the urine for other things, such as ketones and protein, can be of value. See the earlier section microalbuminuria and the nearby sidebar on ketones for more information.)

The new method of testing blood glucose revealed some valuable information. Following is just a sampling:

✔ Under what seem like the exact same conditions, the blood glucose may be very different from time to time. It's impossible to control many of the variables involved in testing, like the depth of the insulin injection or the emotional state of the patient at the time. Little differences in carbohydrate intake, taking fiber with food, and so forth also can make a big difference in the reading. *It isn't an exact science.* Because it isn't an exact science, blaming a child for poor blood glucose levels is ridiculous.

✔ When blood glucose levels could be downloaded to a computer, it was seen that, for the most part, patients had been reporting them honestly in their logbooks. You see, many doctors thought that their patients weren't recording their results honestly, causing them (the docs) to pay less attention to patient logbooks of glucose results.

✔ The approximate response of blood glucose to exercise and to food can be gauged.

✔ It's possible to see if a child's blood glucose is going too low (or too high) in the middle of the night.

In the following sections, I explain how often to test blood glucose and walk you through the testing process. See the later section "Selecting a Home Blood Glucose Meter" for details on a variety of meters available.

Deciding on the frequency of testing

The minimum frequency to test your child is before each meal and at bedtime. You can test his glucose more frequently depending upon the situation. The minimum testing frequency must be met because you're constantly using this information to make adjustments in his insulin dose. No matter how good you think his control is, he can't feel the level of the blood glucose without testing unless he's hypoglycemic (see Chapter 4). And even then, he knows the glucose is low but doesn't know just how low it is.

On numerous occasions, I've asked my patients to guess their blood glucose and then test it. Their guesses are close to the actual number less than 50 percent of the time. That degree of accuracy isn't good enough for good glucose control!

You should occasionally test your child one hour after a meal and in the middle of the night to see just how high his glucose goes after eating and whether it drops too low in the middle of the night. These results guide you and his doctor to make the changes your child needs. Just be sure not to make more than one change at a time and to give it a couple of weeks to make a difference.

Blood glucose test results can be useful many other times of day, such as during intense exercise, during illness, and after eating food with unknown amounts of carbohydrate.

Performing the test

You get blood for testing glucose, which usually requires no more than a drop, by sticking your child's finger with a sharp device called a *lancet.* Most meters come with a spring-loaded holder that permits you to penetrate the skin quickly and usually without much pain.

The SoftClix lancet and the BD Genie lancet are both in the low-pain category. Let your child try out many different lancets and select the one that causes him the least pain.

Here are some standard rules for using the lancet:

- The finger being pricked should be clean, but wiping it with alcohol isn't necessary.
- Use the side of the finger, where there's less sensation.
- Change fingers every time.
- *Never* use your child's lancet on someone else or use someone else's lancet on your child.

Ready to test? Put the strip into the appropriate opening in the meter unless you're using a meter that holds the strips and ejects them. Inserting the strip usually turns on the meter and prepares it for a test. Place a drop of blood from the lancet on a specific part of a test strip. The result will appear on the meter screen in 5 to 40 seconds, depending upon the meter. Also, depending upon the strip, you may have 30 seconds to add more blood if you didn't have enough; you can twist a rubber band at the base of the finger if you're having trouble getting enough blood for the strip.

Test strips left loose in a tube of strips rapidly become worthless if exposed to air; just two hours of exposure is enough to ruin them. That's why I like the test strips in a drum, like AccuChek Compact Plus strips (see the later section "Surveying standard blood glucose meters"), that are protected within the drum until they're used.

I tell you how to use glucose test results to manage diabetes in the section "Using a typical data management system" later in this chapter.

In order to interpret your child's glucose reading, you need to know whether his meter gives a reading for whole blood or for plasma. The whole blood glucose is 11 percent less than the plasma glucose. Charts that tell you what his blood glucose should be use plasma glucose levels. Most meters give a plasma reading, but you should check the instruction booklet to be sure.

Testing away from the finger

Some glucose meters can perform the test away from the fingers. This gives the fingers a rest and offers a huge number of other sites for testing, such as the forearm and the thigh. If you want to test your child away from his finger, there are a few things to consider:

✔ Blood glucose changes rapidly right after a meal. There may be a large difference in glucose results between the finger and another site, as much as 50 to 100 mg/dl, but the finger is giving the correct result (the higher one).

✔ During and after exercise, glucose also changes rapidly, so use the finger to test.

✔ After an insulin shot, there may be a large difference between the finger and an alternate site. Again, the finger is the correct site.

The difference in glucose readings results from the fact that the finger gets much more blood flow than other sites.

If there's any question of your child having hypoglycemia, the finger should be used. It reflects the true blood glucose much more rapidly than other sites in the body.

Selecting a Home Blood Glucose Meter

All home meters now on the market are accurate enough to measure your child's glucose correctly. They're generally plus or minus 10 percent of the reading done in a laboratory. For example, a lab reading of 100 mg/dl may be anywhere from 90 to 110 mg/dl on your child's meter. This is sufficiently accurate to help you decide on treatment and evaluate the results of treatment.

Meters that measure the blood glucose use one of two methods, both of which are highly accurate (Figure 7-2 shows a typical meter):

✔ The first method depends on the production of a color when the glucose reacts with a chemical in the strip. The meter reads the darkness of the color to produce a blood glucose reading.

✔ The second method uses a strip that produces electrons when the glucose reacts with the chemical in the strip. The meter measures the amount of electrons produced to give a glucose reading.

In the following sections, I give you some factors to consider as you select a home glucose meter, and I explain how a data management system works. I also provide details on a wide variety of meters.

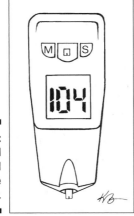

Figure 7-2:
A typical home blood glucose meter.

Get a new meter for your child every two years at the very least. They're like cars in that a new model with new features is available practically every year. With each new meter, the batteries last longer, and the testing procedure becomes simpler. With recent meter developments, manufacturers have been trying to do away with coding the meter each time you use new test strips.

Considering a few factors when choosing a meter

Here are some practical tips to consider when purchasing a glucose meter for your child:

✔ The meter companies are happy to give away most of their meters. What they want you to buy are the test strips, which are different for each meter. Even within one manufacturer the test strips may differ for the different meters the company makes.

The strips tend to cost about the same for each meter. If you find strips that cost significantly less per test, you may want to go with them. A meter should cost no more than $25 to $50, and test strips are about $1 per test.

✔ Make sure that you can download your child's meter information to a data management program. (Some doctors have a preference for a particular meter that can be downloaded to a computer because the glucose results can be viewed in a way that's especially useful for that doctor.) Trying to determine trends in the blood glucose is next to impossible simply by looking at results in a logbook. The computer can do so much with the results that your brain can't, like putting results from different days into the same time slots or putting entire days into separate slots so you can see if your child's T1DM is managed the same on different days. For example, many patients do better Monday through Friday and loosen up on the weekend. This trend is obvious with a data management program. (See the next section for more about these programs.)

Don't buy a meter that doesn't have a memory for at least 100 test results. If you test your child four times a day, a 100-result memory allows you up to 25 days of results, enough to give you and your doctor a good overall picture of the trend of the glucose.

✔ If your insurance company will only pay for one particular kind of meter or strips, you may have to go with that meter. But if you and your doctor are willing to go through the hassle of contacting the insurance company and requesting authorization, you still may be able to use the meter of your choice.

✔ If you want your child to learn to test himself, make sure that he can use the meter easily.

Using a typical data management system

You can use a data management system on just about any home blood glucose meter to plot your child's blood glucose and determine where changes need to be made. Figure 7-3 plots the results before changes were made in the treatment, and Figure 7-4 shows the results after those changes. You can see the difference very clearly. Here are the elements of each figure:

✔ The Trendgraph at the top of each page shows the individual blood glucose values. The horizontal or x-axis represents the days, and the vertical or y-axis represents the blood glucose values shown by a X. Underneath the Trendgraph, the program has figured out the MBG, the mean blood glucose, 159 mg/dl on the before page and 119 mg/dl on the after page. The program also shows the percentage of readings in three categories: less than 80 mg/dl (low), 80 to 180 mg/dl (normal), and over 180 mg/dl (high).

Comparing the two graphs, the percentage of normal readings in the after page is much greater (63.4 percent before, 77.4 percent after), whereas the percentage of high readings is substantially lower (31.7 percent before, 6.5 percent after). The thick black line averages out the glucose values for each day. You can see that it hovers around 150 mg/dl before and 110 mg/dl after treatment.

✔ Below the Trendgraph, the Standard Day puts all the blood glucoses from a specific range of time into the same area of the graph. Night is midnight to 5:30 a.m., before breakfast is 5:30 to 8:30 a.m., and so forth. It's easy to see by the position of the large X (the average for that time range) that the blood glucose is around 150 mg/dl throughout the day before treatment and is usually at 100 mg/dl after treatment.

> ✔ The Pie Chart graphically shows that the control is much better after treatment than it before, although there are more low readings (less than 80 mg/dl) after treatment.

You can also use the data management software to show every permutation of the blood glucose values. For example, it's easy to produce a graph that shows the average blood glucose for each day of the week. From such a graph, your child's doctor can see what time of day requires more or less insulin, more or less food, and more or less exercise to improve control.

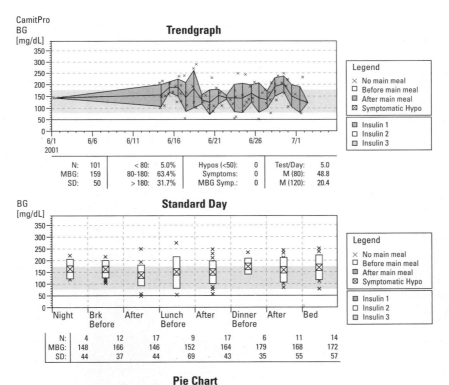

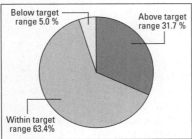

Figure 7-3:
Test results
before
therapy.

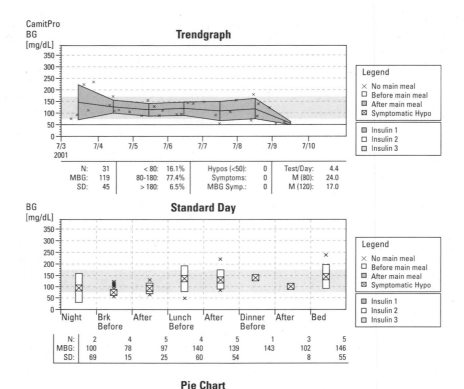

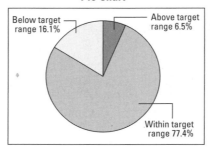

Figure 7-4:
Test results
after
therapy.

Surveying standard blood glucose meters

More than a dozen companies currently manufacture blood glucose meters. However, in the following sections I discuss the meters of the four major players in the field. Among them, they have every new feature you may want or need. The meters generally have warranties longer than you'll keep the meter. They also have 24/7 backup by calling a toll-free phone number (and you won't be speaking to someone in Zamboanga).

I'm sure that you want to know the name of the meter that I prefer. It's the AccuChek Compact Plus meter. The Compact Plus uses whole blood, not plasma. The features that I like about this meter are the drum with 17 strips wrapped up until they're used, the ability to add blood if there isn't enough on the strip, and the fact that it's very fast and accurate. I also like its data management system, and my patients have been very happy with the help they get from the company when anything goes wrong.

One limitation of this meter is that you have to put the date and time back into the meter each time you change the batteries, which is after about 500 tests. Despite the fact that it's simple to do, many patients forget to do it, and all the results that don't have date and time stamps can't be used by the data management system.

Abbott Laboratories

Abbott Laboratories has one of the longest warranties in the industry at four years, but you'll probably replace your child's meter long before that anyway. The batteries are built in, so after 4,000 tests or about three years you need to send the meter back for new batteries. The manufacturer is likely to give you a new meter at that point.

- **Freestyle Flash:** Abbott considers this the smallest meter available in the industry. It requires very little blood and allows the addition of blood within 60 seconds if necessary. You can get a 14-day average of readings on the meter, and the Freestyle Flash works with diabetes management software (DMS) called the *Precision Link Direct Diabetes Data Management System* through a data port and has a result memory of 250 tests. It allows alternate site testing, away from the fingers, and it has programmable alarms to prompt you to test. Coding for the test strips is done with the keys on the meter.

- **Freestyle Freedom:** This meter is basically identical to the Freestyle Flash, but the display screen is much larger for people with vision trouble.

- **Freestyle Lite:** This meter uses different tests strips from the other two Freestyle meters that don't require coding the meter each time a new bottle of strips is used. It has a memory for 400 tests. Otherwise, its features are like the other Freestyle meters.

- **Precision Xtra:** This meter requires a code key with each new bottle of test strips to code the meter. It remembers 450 tests. It's also able to test for ketones in the blood with the appropriate test strips. The Precision Xtra can test at multiple sites, has a rapid test time, and doesn't start the test until enough blood is on the strip.

Bayer Healthcare LLC

Bayer Healthcare LLC, which is a branch of Bayer Group, sells the following two meters in the United States but continues to support several of its old meters (like the Elite models) with test strips. You can replace the batteries for these meters at home. The meters are descendants of some of the first meters available. They both allow testing away from your fingers and don't require coding each time you use new strips. These meters use *GLUCOFACTS Diabetes Management Software* for data management.

- **Breeze 2:** The Breeze 2 uses a ten-test cartridge that calibrates the meter and requires no coding. It remembers 420 tests. It can provide 1-, 7-, 14-, and 30-day averages. It was the first meter to receive the "Ease of Use" commendation from the Arthritis Foundation.

- **Contour:** This meter uses individual test strips that require no coding. Tests may be done at sites away from the finger. It can remember up to 480 tests.

LifeScan

Johnson & Johnson owns LifeScan, which is one of the older meter companies. The company makes good, reliable meters that compete with one another. You can replace the batteries in LifeScan meters at home, and all the meters are coded with keys on the meter itself. LifeScan meters use *One Touch Diabetes Management Software*.

- **One Touch Ultra 2:** This system uses a tiny sample and therefore can work with LifeScan's ultrafine lancets, which are included with the blood glucose meters and can be ordered when needed. The blood is drawn up by capillary action, and the result is displayed in five seconds. This meter allows testing away from the fingers. It has a 500-test memory that allows averaging on the screen and connects to a data port. You can get averages for 7, 14, and 30 days.

- **One Touch UltraSmart:** This meter is like the One Touch Ultra 2 with the addition of other features, including 60- and 90-day averages. You can enter information about your child's exercise, health, medication, and food. The meter prompts you to comment on out-of-range results. You can view charts and graphs that help to analyze your child's blood glucose on the meter's screen. The meter remembers 3,000 tests.

- **One Touch Ultra Mini:** This meter is very small and portable, and the company promotes it for travel. It uses a tiny sample of blood and remembers 50 tests, but it doesn't permit downloading results or data management. For this reason, I can't recommend it.

Roche Diagnostics

Roche Diagnostics sells the meters of Boehringer Mannheim. The batteries in these meters are replaceable at home, and the meters may be used away from the fingers. All the meters come with Spanish language instruction and a

---

Ketones: Testing at home

The breakdown of fat produces ketones (a type of chemical compound), which can be measured easily by putting a ketone strip into a tube of urine. If your child's blood glucose is above 250 mg/dl, or if you have diabetes and are pregnant and your blood glucose is below 60 mg/dl, it's time to test for ketones. The test is usually done at home.

To perform the test, you place a ketone strip into urine and observe the purple color. Comparing it to a color chart tells you whether your child's ketones are negative, low, medium, or high. A finding of high ketones with high blood glucose

means that your child (or you) may be on the way to ketoacidosis (see Chapter 4). A finding of high ketones with low blood glucose means that your child (or you) isn't getting enough carbohydrates. and his body is turning to fat for energy. (This happens during a pregnancy because of the demands of the growing fetus.)

If you find that your child has high ketones, high blood glucose (over 250 mg/dl), and can't keep liquids down, it's definitely time to call the doctor.

If you find high ketones with a low blood glucose, it's time to feed your child more carbohydrates.

---

phone number for a Spanish-speaking representative. Roche promotes this feature, but all the major manufacturers offer it.

- **Accu-Chek Aviva:** This meter works with diabetes management software (DMS). It has a very large memory, storing up to 500 blood glucose values, and can also record other information such as insulin dosages and carbohydrate intake. It requires a tiny sample of blood and can produce on-screen graphs and statistics. It has a code key with each new bottle of test strips.

- **Accu-Chek Advantage:** This meter also works with DMS and stores 350 blood glucose values. It uses a test strip that takes 27 seconds to produce results but doesn't require cleaning or wiping. This meter requires a snap-in code key.

- **Accu-Chek Compact Plus:** This meter uses a 17-test drum that requires no test strip handling or calibration. It has a lancing device attached to it, which can be removed for separate use. The results are displayed in five seconds, and it has a 350-test memory that's downloadable to a DMS. It allows testing away from the fingers. You can see a 7-, 14-, and 30-day average on the screen.

- **Accu-Chek Active:** This meter uses a tiny sample of blood and gives a result in five seconds. It can be used at alternate sites besides the fingers. It has a 200-value memory that's downloadable to a DMS, and it needs a snap-in code key.

- **Accu-Chek Voicemate:** This meter is designed for the visually impaired. A new version of this meter is being prepared as of this writing; the main difference is that it reports the blood glucose result audibly. Otherwise, it's similar to the other meters in this list.

Roche's Data Management System is called *AccuChek Compass*. You need the right hardware and software to download the glucose values, but you can get it from the company.

Checking out meters for continuous glucose monitoring

Continuous glucose meters obtain glucose readings from a needle placed under the skin into the interstitial fluid (the fluid that bathes the tissues). You can see a typical continuous monitoring meter in Figure 7-5. The needle is usually changed every three days. The meter still has to be calibrated with finger-stick blood glucose tests several times a day. The results of a continuous glucose meter can lag behind changes in the blood glucose, especially when the blood glucose falls rapidly. The interstitial glucose may not fall to the same extent for 30 minutes. The GlucoWatch G2 Biographer that I describe later doesn't use a needle under the skin.

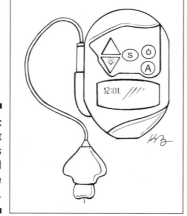

Figure 7-5:
A meter that monitors blood glucose continuously.

Several companies are making this product, and with improvements, it may replace individual blood glucose monitoring because it provides so much more information. When continuous meters no longer require calibration by finger-stick testing, one insertion of the needle will replace 12 finger-sticks for patients with T1DM.

The main advantage of these meters is the huge amount of data they provide — blood glucose values every five minutes throughout the day compared with four readings in 24 hours for traditional meters. The main disadvantages are that they still need calibration by doing a finger stick blood glucose several times a day, and they tend to lag behind the blood glucose when conditions are changing rapidly, such as after exercise and after eating. Also, the huge amount of information that these devices provide can only be understood with the data management software provided for each one.

Continuous meters are being used for children and in patients in whom the traditional four glucose readings daily don't correlate with the hemoglobin A1c test.

By knowing the direction of the blood glucose over 24 hours (see Figure 7-6 for an example), the doctor can adjust the rapid-acting and long-acting insulins or the insulin pump to provide tight control of the blood glucose without causing hypoglycemia.

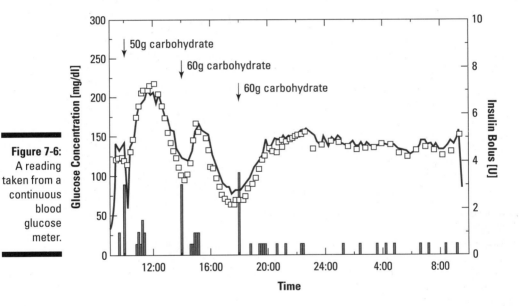

Figure 7-6:
A reading taken from a continuous blood glucose meter.

Dexcom STS Continuous Blood Glucose Monitor

This unit has a small sensor that transmits glucose values wirelessly to the STS receiver. The receiver displays glucose readings averaged over five minutes as well as one-, three-, and nine-hour trends. It alerts you to high or low levels. It has to be calibrated with LifeScan's One Touch Ultra 2 blood glucose meter, and it must be recalibrated with a finger-stick glucose test at least every 12 hours.

The meter is meant to detect trends and track patterns in adults 18 or older. It hasn't been tested in children, adolescents, or pregnant women.

GlucoWatch G2 Biographer

This device is worn on the forearm. Readings are taken through the skin, so there's no insertion of a needle. Readings are provided every ten minutes for up to 13 hours. Low and high blood glucose readings are marked by alarms. This meter is meant to detect trends and track patterns but not replace finger-stick testing. After a two-hour warm-up period, you calibrate the meter, which sounds an alarm if the reading is below a low-alert level or above a high-alert level set by the doctor. This meter stores more than 8,500 individual readings. Perspiration interferes with the readings. Redness, itching, and blisters may appear at the site of the device.

Guardian RT Glucose Monitoring System

This device has a sensor inserted into the skin; a wireless transmitter connects the sensor to a receiver. It takes readings every ten seconds and averages them every five minutes. You can see the readings by pushing a button. The meter holds 21 days of data, which may be downloaded to a computer. It sounds an alarm or vibrates to alert you of low and high glucose levels. However, any significant abnormalities should be verified by a finger stick. Also, you must calibrate the meter daily with at least two finger sticks.

Chapter 8

Eating a Healthy Diet

- -

- -

*I*f your child has type 1 diabetes (T1DM for short), what he eats will play a large role in his health. This doesn't mean that he has to follow a boring and unpalatable diet. It means that you have to be more aware of what he eats, especially how it contributes to his blood glucose, blood cholesterol, and blood pressure. (He should be aware of all this too, if you think he's old enough to understand and contribute to this aspect of his diabetes management.)

A healthy diet accomplishes a number of things for the person with T1DM. Here are some of the more important benefits:

- ✔ **It makes controlling blood glucose much easier.** When you're aware of the amounts of fat, protein, and especially carbohydrate in your child's diet, it's easier to keep the blood glucose in a range that keeps the hemoglobin A1c at 7 percent or less, thereby preventing complications like eye, kidney, and nerve disease. (See Chapter 7 for more about hemoglobin A1c.)

- ✔ **It makes it easier to help your child maintain a normal weight.** With a healthy diet, you have a better grasp of your child's total calorie intake. Therefore, you avoid adding insulin resistance to lack of insulin as the cause of high blood glucose.

- ✔ **It helps you keep your child's total cholesterol and bad cholesterol low while increasing his good cholesterol.** A healthy diet involves reducing the fats that are bad for him and substituting fats that are healthy. The effect on cholesterol reduces the risk of the heart disease complication of diabetes.

✔ **It keeps you aware of your child's salt intake, allowing you to control that contribution to his blood pressure.** High blood pressure is an important factor that leads to diabetic kidney disease. (Another important factor is high blood glucose.)

✔ **It improves your child's energy level.** Eating the right foods in the right amounts means that your child's getting the vitamins, minerals, and other nutrients that his body requires for peak performance.

In this chapter, you find out all you need to know to help your child (or yourself, if you're the patient) enjoy food while maintaining a balanced blood glucose.

Be sure to consult a dietitian for help with calorie intake and meal planning (see Chapter 2 for info on adding a dietitian to a diabetes care team).

Carbohydrates: The Energy Source with the Biggest Impact on Blood Glucose

When you eat, you take energy into your body from three different sources: carbohydrate, protein, and fat. Each source is important to your body, and you can't live without the contribution of all three. However, when it comes to T1DM, the energy source that's directly responsible for the level of your blood glucose is carbohydrate. Protein and fat play a role but only indirectly and to a much lesser extent (I discuss protein and fat later in this chapter).

Most people who think of carbohydrate think of sugar, but there are many forms of carbohydrate. The following simple carbohydrates can be digested by enzymes in the stomach and intestine:

✔ **Glucose** is the sugar that circulates in the bloodstream and provides energy for movement and for all the chemical reactions taking place in the body. It's a *monosaccharide* because it contains only one molecule of sugar, as do fructose and galactose.

✔ **Sucrose** is a *disaccharide* because it has two sugar molecules. You may know it as the sugar in sugar cane and beets or as simple table sugar. Other disaccharides are lactose (milk sugar) and maltose (malt sugar).

✔ **Starches** are made up of large numbers of sugar molecules.

Other types of carbohydrate are complex carbohydrates including cellulose, the carbohydrate that forms the walls of plant cells; and fiber. Neither of these complex carbohydrates can be digested, which means that they provide no calories.

These are the important functions of all carbohydrates in the body:

- ✔ They're the major source of energy for muscles.
- ✔ The carbohydrate glucose stimulates the pancreas to release insulin, if the pancreas can. In the absence of effective insulin in the body, glucose can rise to very high levels.
- ✔ They raise the level of the blood fat called *triglyceride.*

In the following sections, I explain what you need to know about the use of carbohydrates in the diet of a person with type 1 diabetes, including some smart food choices and the relationship between carbohydrate amounts and insulin intake.

Americans are eating less fat yet continue to get fatter. Analysis of the American diet shows that people haven't increased their protein intake, so they must be eating more carbohydrates. Carbohydrates can be turned into fat in the body, so if you consume excessive amounts, you'll gain weight. This ancient characteristic of mammals was fine when humans could only find food in the summer and had to live on body fat in the winter. Today, the conversion of carbohydrates into fat causes all kinds of disturbances like heart attacks and strokes. Experts recommend that 40 to 50 percent of a person's daily calorie intake should be from carbohydrates (1 gram of carbohydrate contains 4 kilocalories). And yes, people with diabetes can eat real carbohydrates rather than artificial sweeteners so long as they don't eat too many total calories. (I discuss sweeteners in detail later in this chapter.)

Getting a grip on the glycemic index

The *glycemic index* (GI) of a carbohydrate is the effect that a particular carbohydrate has on the blood glucose. Here's how it works: Glucose itself is assigned a GI of 100. A food with the same number of grams of carbohydrate as glucose (usually 50 grams) is eaten, and the blood glucose is measured two hours later. If the food raises the blood glucose as rapidly and as high as glucose does, it too has a GI of 100. If it raises the blood glucose half as much, its GI is 50. If it raises it one and a half times more, its GI is 150.

The GI isn't used as much as it could be in nutritional planning for T1DM for several reasons, including the following:

- ✔ GI values are for isolated foods. The values change when the carbohydrate is part of a mixed meal.
- ✔ GI is dependent on the way food is cooked; for instance, the GI of a baked potato is different from that of a boiled potato.
- ✔ Just because the GI is low doesn't mean that the food is good for your child with diabetes if it contains a lot of fat. Chocolate is one example.

✔ Some diabetes educators feel that the concept is too confusing for people with diabetes to understand. I think that if you're smart enough to read this book, you're smart enough to understand the GI. You need to use every available tool to keep your child's blood glucose level under control, and the GI can be a valuable tool for people with T1DM. It has been shown that people whose overall food history incorporates more foods with low GI have lower incidences of diabetic complications.

In the following sections, I give you the GI values of a few common foods and show you how to swap out high-GI foods for healthier, low-GI versions.

The best source for more information on the glycemic index is www.glycemic index.com, a site maintained by the University of Sydney in Australia. The site offers two valuable books: *The New Glucose Revolution,* 3rd Edition, which offers a complete explanation of the concept plus a list of the GI values of most foods; and *The New Glucose Revolution, Shopper's Guide to GI Values, 2007,* which contains only the list of GI values.

Comparing the GI values of a few common foods

Table 8-1 shows the GI values of several common foods. A high GI is in the range of 65 to 100, a medium GI is the range of 45 to 64, and a low GI is in the range of 0 to 44. You can see that plenty of good choices are in the medium- and low-GI categories. With the exception of milk, you could say that you should avoid the white foods: potatoes, white rice, and white bread.

Table 8-1	Glycemic Index Values of Several Common Foods	
High GI	*Medium GI*	*Low GI*
Glucose: 100	Rice, long grain: 58	Banana, yellow-green: 42
Potato, baked: 85	Honey: 55	Orange: 42
Waffles: 76	Banana, all yellow: 51	Ice cream: 37
Potato, boiled: 74	Pasta: 48	Kidney beans: 28
White bread: 70	Lactose: 46	Milk (2%): 21
Table sugar: 68	Grapes: 46	Fructose: 19
White rice: 64	Rye bread: 46	Peanuts: 14

Some foods can't be given a GI value because they have so little carbohydrate. Examples are beef, chicken, fish, vegetables, and alcohol. They don't affect blood glucose immediately, but the fat in beef and the empty calories in alcohol make them poor food choices anyway. (See Chapter 12 for information on alcohol use.)

Replacing high-GI foods with low-GI foods

Table 8-2 shows some simple substitutions you can make in your child's diet (or your own) to emphasize low-GI foods. If you do this consistently, you'll find the result in terms of blood glucose levels and hemoglobin A1c very gratifying.

Table 8-2	Simple Diet Substitutions
High-GI Food	*Low-GI Food*
Whole-meal or white bread	Whole-grain bread
Processed breakfast cereal	Unrefined cereals like oats or processed low-GI cereals (such as Kellogg's All-Bran Complete Oat or Wheat Flakes)
Plain cookies and crackers	Cookies made with dried fruits or whole grains like oats
Cakes and muffins	Cakes and muffins made with fruit, oats, and whole grains
Potatoes	Pasta or legumes
White rice	Basmati or brown rice

Table 8-2 confirms that it's relatively easy to make a switch from high- to low-GI foods. Just choose grainier foods and foods that are less processed. If possible, rather than switching, feed your child low-GI foods from the start. It will make the task of controlling his blood glucose that much easier.

Low-GI foods aren't a good choice when you're treating hypoglycemia. In that situation, you want to give your child foods that provide a glucose load as quickly as possible. See Chapter 4 for more about hypoglycemia.

Understanding the glycemic load

In addition to glycemic index, you may want to consider the *glycemic load*. The glycemic load of a food is based on the glycemic index but also takes into account the amount of carbohydrate in a portion. A food that has a high glycemic index may not be that bad for your child if the portion is so small that the total grams of carbohydrate don't raise his glucose that much. An example is pumpkin, which has a high GI of 75 but few grams of carbohydrate in the small portion that's usually consumed. Another example is cantaloupe, which has a glycemic index of 65 but a low glycemic load in the typical portion size. Many foods that have low glycemic loads aren't necessarily good for your child, like ice cream and beef, so you should emphasize glycemic index rather than glycemic load in making food choices for your child.

Filling up with fiber

Although fiber is a carbohydrate, the digestive enzymes in the stomach and intestine can't break it down, so it can't be used for energy and isn't counted as calories. It plays an important role in the diet in its two forms:

- **Soluble fiber:** Dissolves in water and forms a jelly-like material that blocks the digestive enzymes from getting to food, thereby slowing the uptake of carbohydrate from the intestine.

- **Insoluble fiber:** Doesn't dissolve in water but can be processed so much when it's milled that it doesn't prevent digestive enzymes from getting to food. Insoluble fiber is the *roughage* in the intestine that prevents constipation and colon cancer.

It seems that people prefer "smooth" foods — foods with few whole grains that can give the food a chunky, grainy taste. But it's the grainy, unrefined foods that are full of fiber and much better for the health of your child with T1DM because they help keep the blood glucose at the right level. Foods with lots of fiber (especially insoluble fiber) include fruits and vegetables, multigrain bread, and legumes like peas and beans.

Although the recommendation for adults is 20 to 30 grams of fiber daily, children can't comfortably consume that much. For children, the daily fiber intake should be their age plus 5, so a 5-year-old should have 10 grams of fiber a day.

Don't suddenly introduce a lot of fiber into your child's diet. Add it slowly (1 to 2 grams a week) so that he doesn't complain of a lot of gas. (The gas occurs when the carbohydrate in the fiber reaches the bacteria in the large intestine that break it down.)

Carbohydrate counting

Using the amount of carbohydrates in a meal to determine your child's insulin dose is called *carbohydrate counting.* The key to this system is knowing the carbohydrate in your child's food. Here's where you make use of your friendly dietitian, who can go over his food preferences and tell you how many grams of carbohydrate are in them. The dietitian also can show you where to find carbohydrate counts for any other foods that your child may eat.

For carbohydrate counting, you also need to know how many grams of carbohydrate are controlled by each unit of insulin your child takes. This is determined by checking his blood glucose one hour after eating a known amount of carbohydrate. For example, one person may need 1 unit of rapid-acting insulin to control 20 grams of carbohydrate, whereas another person needs

1 unit of rapid-acting insulin to control 15 grams of carbohydrate. If both people eat a breakfast of 75 grams of carbohydrate, the first person may take 4 units of insulin, whereas the second person takes 5 units of insulin. Then they add units to the base number for the amount that the blood glucose needs to be lowered. A typical insulin schedule involves taking 1 unit of insulin for every 50 mg/dl that the blood glucose is above 100 mg/dl. You also can subtract insulin if the blood glucose is too low. For every 50 mg/dl that the glucose is below 100, subtract 1 unit. (To see how carbohydrate counting works in practice, see the sidebar "A true-to-life example of carbohydrate counting.")

By measuring your child's blood glucose frequently, you find out how different carbohydrates affect his blood glucose. He needs less insulin to control the carbohydrate sources that have a low glycemic index (I discuss the GI earlier in this chapter).

Another great advantage of carbohydrate counting is that your child can eat a variety of foods as long as you know the carbohydrate count of what he's eating. Children who are allowed this variety are much happier with their food, and their hemoglobin A1cs are significantly lower.

A true-to-life example of carbohydrate counting

To find out how you can accomplish carbohydrate counting in everyday life, take a typical type 1 patient. Salvatore is a 41-year-old who has had type 1 diabetes for 31 years. His diabetes has been well controlled because he follows a good diet, gets lots of exercise, and takes his insulin appropriately. He takes 30 units of insulin glargine (see Chapter 10 for details on this and other types of insulin) at bedtime.

Salvatore has a list of dosages of lispro insulin that tells him to take 1 unit of insulin for each 20 grams of carbohydrate he eats. He's about to have breakfast and knows that it will contain 80 grams of carbohydrate. Therefore, he needs 4 units of lispro insulin. He measures his blood glucose before breakfast and finds it at 202 mg/dl. His doctor has told him to take an extra unit of lispro insulin for each 50 mg/dl above 100 mg/dl. He adds two more units for a total of 6 units of insulin taken just before breakfast.

At lunch, his blood glucose measures 58. He's about to have a lunch of 120 grams of carbohydrate, so he needs 6 units. However, he reduces it by 1 unit because the glucose measurement is approximately 50 mg/dl lower than 100, so his final dose is 5 units.

Before supper, Salvatore's blood glucose measures 120. His supper contains only 60 grams of carbohydrate, so he needs 3 units. He doesn't have to adjust the dose because the glucose is close to 100, so he takes only 3 units.

At bedtime, his blood glucose is 108, so he's doing very well. Unless the blood glucose is 200 or greater, he doesn't need to take any bedtime lispro because he's taking insulin glargine to control his glucose overnight.

Other tips for managing carbohydrate intake

There's a lot to know about the way that carbohydrates affect blood glucose in addition to the grams of carbohydrates eaten (see the previous section). Carbohydrates aren't usually eaten alone, and as I mention earlier in the chapter, the other foods eaten with them play a role in how rapidly the carbohydrates are absorbed and raise blood glucose. Check out these facts about how carbohydrates work with other foods:

✔ When your child eats carbohydrates that tend to be swallowed in larger pieces like rice and pasta, absorption is slowed by the need to break down those pieces in the intestine. His blood glucose rises more slowly.

✔ When your child eats carbohydrates with fat, the fat slows down the movement of food through the intestine, so the blood glucose rises more slowly.

✔ Chewing food thoroughly means that food is broken down into small pieces; therefore, the carbohydrate is absorbed more rapidly.

✔ Whole fruit, like an orange, requires breakdown of cell walls in the intestine, but that breakdown has already occurred in orange juice. The carbohydrate in orange juice is absorbed more rapidly than the carbohydrate in a whole orange. The same is true of finely ground flour, as found in white bread compared with whole-grain bread.

✔ Drinking a beverage with a meal makes the food pass more rapidly into the intestine where it's absorbed, so blood glucose rises more rapidly.

✔ Light exercise like walking speeds up the absorption of glucose, whereas heavy exercise like running slows it down.

✔ Very cold or hot food slows down the emptying of the stomach, thus slowing the absorption of glucose.

✔ A high blood glucose slows the emptying of the stomach, whereas a low blood glucose speeds it up.

✔ Smaller meals with snacks in between result in a more consistent level of blood glucose.

These effects help to explain why the blood glucose rises as much as it does after some meals and rises very slowly after others. Being aware of them allows you to adjust the timing of your child's insulin to match the absorption of the glucose. For example, if he takes rapid-acting insulin and you know that a particular meal will result in slower absorption of glucose because it's high in fat, you may want to give his insulin after the meal rather than before. That way the insulin is active when the food is being absorbed. Flip to Chapter 10 for full details on using insulin properly.

Looking at Other Sources of Energy

Even though carbohydrates are the most important source of energy for everyone (especially folks with T1DM), you can't forget about protein and fat. In the following sections, I explain the effects of protein and fat on blood glucose and provide examples of good (and bad) foods that contain them.

Protein

Protein, the second major source of calories in your child's diet, is found in the muscles of animals (beef, poultry, and fish), cheese, eggs, and milk. It's usually accompanied by more or less fat, depending upon the source.

Protein in a meal doesn't contribute to the blood glucose immediately. It takes several hours for protein to be converted into sugar in the body unless the blood glucose is low, in which case the conversion happens much more rapidly.

You should be selecting low-fat sources of protein for your child, developing his palate so that he enjoys food without fat. Following are some fast facts about sources of protein:

- The protein sources with the least amount of fat (only 1 gram per ounce of protein) are very lean meat or fish and fat-free cheese. Shellfish like lobster and shrimp are included in this category.

- Lean protein with 3 grams of fat per ounce includes lean beef and pork, dark meat chicken, oily fish like salmon, and some cheese. These sources of protein are still a good choice for your child, especially oily fish because the fat in it is omega-3 fatty acid, which has beneficial effects on the heart. Omega-3 fatty acid has been shown to:

  - Decrease abnormalities of the heart rhythm
  - Reduce triglyceride levels
  - Slow the growth of arteriosclerosis
  - Slightly reduce blood pressure

  Serve your family a minimum of two meals of oily fish per week so that everyone gets enough omega-3 fatty acid.

- The categories of medium-fat proteins with 5 grams of fat per ounce and high-fat proteins with 8 grams of fat per ounce include foods that should be limited in your child's diet (because of the very high fat content, of course). Fried foods, processed sandwich meats, regular fat meats, and very fatty meats like bacon and pork are in these categories.

Fat has more than twice as many calories per gram as carbohydrate and protein. Eating a lot of protein in the medium- to high-fat category will cause weight gain, and the fat in these foods is the kind that raises cholesterol and worsens arteriosclerosis (hardening of the arteries).

Another factor to consider when selecting protein sources (besides fat content) is the amount of mercury in certain fish. Regularly eating fish with high levels of mercury can lead to mercury poisoning and is especially bad for young children and pregnant and nursing mothers. The fish with the most mercury that you should avoid are shark, swordfish, mackerel, and tilefish.

For several reasons, experts feel strongly about limiting protein in the diet to 20 percent of calories (a gram of protein contains 4 kilocalories). One reason is the fat that's consumed with the protein, although choosing low-fat sources of protein reduces this problem. Another reason is that although higher levels of protein haven't been shown to hurt normal kidneys, they do seem to worsen the damage in kidneys that are failing. A study in *The Journal of Renal Nutrition* in May 2007 showed that a diet very low in protein could postpone the need for dialysis in all patients with chronic kidney disease.

Fat

Fat doesn't have a direct immediate effect on the blood glucose level. Consumed to excess, it causes weight gain, and increased weight results in resistance to insulin. In fact, as I mention earlier, fat in a meal may lower blood glucose by slowing the absorption of the glucose.

Children need a lot of fat in their diet up until the age of 5. Breast milk is 50 percent fat, for example. After the age of 5, children should begin eating a diet of less fat, with the emphasis on types of fat that decrease the development of arteriosclerosis rather than increase it. The fats to avoid are saturated fats and trans fats.

When a child is a little older (over age 5), the recommended daily intake of fat is 30 percent of kilocalories and no more than 300 mg of cholesterol (which is one type of fat) in the diet. That much cholesterol is found in an egg yolk. An ounce of hard cheese like cheddar has 28 mg of cholesterol, and a glass of whole milk has 35 mg of cholesterol. Switch your child to skim milk and you drop to just 5 mg of cholesterol.

In addition to cholesterol, fat comes as several forms of triglyceride.

  ✔ **Saturated fat** raises a person's cholesterol level and worsens arteriosclerosis. It's the main fat in meat, but it's also present in certain vegetable oils, especially coconut oil, palm oil, and palm kernel oil. If your child must have that occasional steak, encourage him to cut off all visible fat.

✔ **Trans fatty acid,** though present in nature, is mostly added to foods by food manufacturers looking to replace butter. The trouble is that trans fatty acids not only raise LDL (bad) cholesterol, but they lower HDL (good) cholesterol at the same time, so they are even worse than butter! (See Chapter 7 for an introduction to good and bad types of cholesterol.)

✔ **Unsaturated fat** is a much better choice than saturated fat and trans fatty acids because it doesn't raise bad cholesterol. It can be either of the following:

- **Monounsaturated fat,** which is in avocado, olive oil, canola oil, and nuts like almonds and peanuts.

- **Polyunsaturated fat,** which is in soft fats and oils such as corn oil, mayonnaise, and margarine. Polyunsaturated fat lowers good cholesterol, however.

Fat should make up 30 percent of your child's daily caloric intake, and most of that 30 percent should be from the unsaturated fat group.

What do you feed your child with T1DM to improve his cholesterol level without damaging his blood glucose? Here are some suggestions:

✔ Oatmeal lowers the bad cholesterol but also contains soluble fiber, so it slows the absorption of glucose. Apples and pears make good snacks because they also provide soluble fiber (which I discuss earlier in this chapter).

✔ A handful of walnuts or almonds is a great snack that reduces bad cholesterol. But don't overdo the nuts — the "good" fat in them is still fat and has 9 kilocalories per gram.

✔ Delicious salmon provides the omega-3 fatty acids described in the previous section on protein to lower triglycerides. Walnuts, canola oil, and soybean oil have omega-3s that do the same.

Soy protein, once thought to have cholesterol-lowering power, has now been shown to have little effect on the cholesterol.

Getting Enough Vitamins, Minerals, and Water

In addition to carbohydrate, protein, and fat, people with type 1 diabetes need vitamins, minerals, and plenty of water in their diets. I explain the basics of these nutrients in the following sections.

Vitamins

Vitamins and minerals are food substances that the body needs in minute quantities. Luckily, a balanced diet usually provides all these in sufficient amounts. Table 8-3 shows the various food sources that you need to provide for your child to make sure he gets enough vitamins.

Table 8-3	Essential Vitamins and Where to Find Them	
Vitamin	*Function*	*Food Sources*
Vitamin A	Needed for healthy skin and bones	Milk and green vegetables
Vitamin B1 (thiamin)	Converts carbohydrates into energy	Meat and whole-grain cereals
Vitamin B2 (riboflavin)	Needed to use food properly	Milk, cheese, fish, and green vegetables
Vitamin B6 (pyridoxine), pantothenic acid, and biotin	Needed for growth	Liver, yeast, potatoes, bananas, and chicken breasts
Vitamin B12	Keeps the red blood cells and the nervous system healthy	Animal foods, such as meat, dairy products, and eggs
Folic acid	Keeps the red blood cells and the nervous system healthy	Green vegetables
Niacin	Helps release energy	Lean meat, fish, nuts, and legumes
Vitamin C	Helps maintain supportive tissues	Fruit and potatoes
Vitamin D	Helps with absorption of calcium	Dairy products
Vitamin E	Helps maintain cells	Vegetable oils and whole-grain cereals
Vitamin K	Needed for proper clotting of the blood	Leafy vegetables

Kids don't need vitamin pills (nor do most adults) if they eat a healthy diet. Only in cases in which the body rapidly uses food and vitamins, as in pregnancy, is there a possibility that the person doesn't get enough of these vitamins. Then a supplemental vitamin pill makes sense. Otherwise, it's just a waste of money.

Minerals

Minerals provide structure in your child's body, and he may need extra amounts of them to ensure that he gets enough. This is true for any child, not just one with T1DM. Here are a few important minerals for both children and adults:

- ✔ **Calcium, phosphorus, and magnesium:** These minerals build bones and teeth. Fortunately, children get enough of them from milk and other dairy products. Adults, especially women, usually need to supplement their calcium intake by taking calcium tablets.

- ✔ **Iron:** This mineral is a major component of hemoglobin in red blood cells. Thanks to Popeye, spinach is considered a good source of iron, as are other leafy green vegetables. Other good sources are meat, beans, and seafood.

  As your daughter with T1DM begins to menstruate, she loses iron each time she bleeds. It's important to make sure she gets foods with extra iron.

- ✔ **Sodium:** This mineral helps to regulate body water. It seems like everything has salt in it naturally, and it's pretty difficult to avoid consuming too much, especially if you ever take your child to a fast-food place. Teach your child to enjoy the taste of food without added salt. His blood pressure will benefit. Don't put salt on the table at mealtimes, and don't use it in cooking.

- ✔ **Chromium:** This mineral, which is found in whole grains, bran cereals, and potatoes, is often claimed to be missing in people with diabetes. This claim is one of the myths you're likely to come across when looking on the Internet for treatments for diabetes. Scientific literature still hasn't proven this point.

- ✔ **Iodine:** This mineral is a critical part of the thyroid hormones. If your child eats any kind of bread, he gets enough iodine because the bread is fortified with iodized salt.

- ✔ **Various other minerals, like chlorine, cobalt, tin, and zinc:** These minerals are found in many foods. There is very little likelihood that a child will be deficient in any of them, which generally are required in very small amounts.

Water

The last nutrient in this section by no means is the least important. The human body is 50 to 70 percent water. A child needs to drink a minimum of 5 cups, or 1¼ quarts, of water a day; adults need a minimum of 8 cups. Most children drink exactly what they need according to how thirsty they feel. Keep fresh, cool water available for your child so that he doesn't turn to fruit juice or soda when he's thirsty. Water comes from many sources in addition to a glass of water; for example, all foods contain some water.

Understanding Diet Challenges at Every Age

Children with T1DM should follow the nutritional guidelines that I provide earlier in this chapter, but as with all children, diet challenges can arise. Here are some issues that you may face as your child grows (for any serious diet issues, be sure to consult a dietitian):

- ✔ **The newborn:** Hopefully, the newborn is breast-feeding, but if breast-feeding isn't possible, formula may be used for a baby with T1DM. It's unusual for a newborn to develop T1DM, but should it occur, the high fat content of breast milk (50 percent fat) will result in very slow absorption of the sugar in milk. Short-acting insulin should be given before each breast or formula feeding. Very small amounts of insulin are required, sometimes measured in half units.

- ✔ **The toddler:** A child at this age may be a picky eater, but he'll probably eat enough to grow normally. It may be necessary to determine the dose and give insulin after the child has eaten so that you know how many grams of carbohydrate have been consumed. Toddlers often don't feel hungry early in the morning, so breakfast may be missed. If glucose is needed for low blood glucose, giving it in a gel form may be better than a tablet because the gel doesn't have to be chewed.

- ✔ **Preschooler:** A child at this age is beginning a growth spurt that will last the next 15 years. A preschooler's activity level and food intake is very erratic, so it's hard to predict the correct insulin dosage. Therefore, attempting to control the blood glucose in a child this age is difficult.

  Preschoolers obtain a large amount of their energy from fat rather than carbohydrates. They don't do well on high-fiber foods, which upset their stomachs. They may use food as a way of gaining some control, which makes feeding them even more difficult. Try to give your preschooler with T1DM a choice in what he eats, and praise him for good eating behavior. Never force-feed your child if you think he isn't getting enough calories. It's usually best to give a preschooler insulin after eating because you know how much carbohydrate he has eaten.

✔ **Primary school and prepuberty:** For children who are at the age of entering school, diet challenges shift from the home environment to the school because the children spend so much time at school and eat at least one meal there. It's necessary to work with the school dietitian to set up a good meal program. (Of course, the child may not follow it anyway.) One thing that may make control easier is the regimentation of the school environment and the tendency to serve the same thing on a regular basis.

Someone at the school has to be able to determine how much insulin should be given and give it (see Chapter 14 for more on handling diabetes at school). It's better to err on the side of too little than too much insulin. At this age, your child is increasingly active, and this has to be taken into account when determining the insulin dose. It may be easier to control his diabetes if the meals are smaller and the snacks more numerous, thus reducing the amount of insulin needed at any one time.

✔ **Puberty from 13 to 19 years of age:** Children at this age are much more capable of understanding the importance of good control of the blood glucose and, hopefully, will adopt the eating habits that make control easier. At this age, your child is under the influence of many hormones that tend to raise the blood glucose, especially growth hormone, so insulin needs may be higher. At the same time, he's doing his best not to stick out, so if the group goes for candy, he will too. Lapses like this will certainly make glucose control more difficult.

Children with T1DM generally know what they need to eat to grow normally and stop eating when they're no longer hungry. You can always check that this is the case for your child by comparing him with the standard height and weight tables for his age. You can find these charts at `pediatrics.about.com/cs/growthcharts2/l/bl_growthcharts.htm`. Your pediatrician should also have them, and you can check at a routine visit (see Chapter 7 for details about doctor visits).

Focusing on Other Food Factors

If only eating were just as simple as getting the right amount of nutrients! Folks with T1DM have to deal with a variety of factors that affect their basic diets, such as sugar substitutes, fast food, and vegetarianism. I delve into the details of these factors in the following sections.

Using sugar substitutes

Before the isolation of insulin in 1921, sugar was thought to be extremely dangerous for the person with T1DM. With nothing available to lower the blood sugar, consuming sugar actually was pretty dangerous. By completely cutting sugar from the diet of these patients, they survived a little longer (although most died in childhood soon after the diagnosis was made).

Old habits take a long time to die, and there are still plenty of people, even doctors, who think that people with diabetes must avoid sugar at all costs. Most physicians no longer believe this and permit some sugar in the diet of patients with T1DM, but the wish to avoid sugar has created an industry of products with fewer or no calories yet great sweetening power.

You can use sweeteners for your child with T1DM by substituting one for sugar in a recipe, but you need to know their sweetening power to use them correctly. I give you the scoop in the following sections.

Sugar-free food can still have plenty of fat and protein calories. Because total calories are what counts in the diet, there's no great advantage to eating sugar-free products when the result may be that your child's getting as many or more total calories.

Calorie-containing sweeteners

This group consists of a sugar similar to glucose and the so-called sugar alcohols, the names of which end in *–ol*. Fructose has the same number of kilocalories per gram as glucose (4), but the sugar alcohols have half as many (2). Food manufacturers like to use the sugar alcohols in all kinds of products that they call "sugarless," but it's important to remember that the sugar alcohols aren't calorie-free. Here's a rundown of fructose and sugar alcohols:

- **Fructose is fruit sugar found in fruits and berries.** Its great advantage it that it's absorbed much more slowly than glucose although it has about the same sweetening power as table sugar, which is sucrose.

- **Xylitol is a sugar alcohol found in strawberries and raspberries.** Xylitol has the sweetening power of sucrose. It's taken up slowly from the intestine, so it causes little change in blood glucose. Xylitol doesn't cause cavities of the teeth as often as the other sweeteners containing calories, so it's commonly used in chewing gum, hard candy, and some drugs.

- **Sorbitol and mannitol are sugar alcohols occurring in plants.** Sorbitol and mannitol are half as sweet as table sugar and have little effect on blood glucose. They change to fructose in the body. (I mention sorbitol in Chapter 5. When taken as a food, sorbitol doesn't accumulate and damage tissues.) Sorbitol is used in candies, chewing gum, jams and jellies, and baked goods. Mannitol is used in chewing gum, candies, jams and jellies, and frostings.

Non-nutritive or artificial sweeteners

These sweeteners contain no calories yet are much sweeter than sucrose by weight. Several of them have been very controversial as far as the possibility that they cause cancer. As a result, the Food and Drug Administration (FDA) has developed the concept of *acceptable daily intake,* or ADI. This is the maximum daily intake that's safe to consume each day over a lifetime. ADI is listed in the form that the sweetener usually appears or the food that it's usually added to. For example, saccharin's ADI is expressed in packets because it's used that way.

The ADIs in the following list are for adults. The ADI for a child is based on the size of a child compared to an average adult. For example, if the average adult is 150 pounds, the ADI for a 75-pound child is half the adult value.

- ✔ **Aspartame:** It's 150 to 200 times sweeter than sucrose. Many people seem to prefer the taste of aspartame, which is sold under the brand name Equal. It has an ADI of 18 to 19 cans of diet soda. It's not useful for cooking.

- ✔ **Acesulfame:** This sweetener is 200 times sweeter than sucrose and doesn't leave an aftertaste. Sold under the brand names Sunett and Sweet One, it can be used in cooking and is found in numerous foods and beverages as well as a tabletop sweetener. It has an ADI of 30 to 32 cans of diet soda.

- ✔ **Saccharin:** This sweetener is 300 to 400 times sweeter than sucrose. Brand names include Sweet'N Low and Sugar Twin. The ADI for saccharin is 9 to 12 packets per day.

- ✔ **Sucralose:** This sweetener is obtained from sugar and is 600 times sweeter. Sold under the name Splenda, it's very stable and can be used in place of sugar in any food. It leaves no unpleasant aftertaste. Its ADI is six cans of diet soda.

- ✔ **Neotame:** Authorized by the FDA in July 2000, neotame has 7,000 to 13,000 times the sweetening power of sucrose. It isn't used in commercial products yet, but food manufacturers are working with it because cooking it doesn't reduce its sweetening power. Because it isn't available in foods, there's no ADI for neotame and the brand name is not yet determined.

Considering fast food

Is it even important to include fast-food restaurants in a discussion of type 1 diabetes? McDonald's claims to serve 26 million customers every day in the United States. That's almost one in ten of all Americans. It has 13,700 restaurants, compared with 7,600 for Burger King, 5,900 for Wendy's, and 3,300 for Arby's. You bet these restaurants have a huge impact on eating in America.

People used to say that at fast-food restaurants, you could get more nourishment from biting your lip than from eating the food. This is definitely no longer the case. Because everyone is conscious of good nutrition these days, you can find something healthful to eat in any fast-food restaurant. In the following sections, I explain the benefits of being prepared before walking into a fast-food joint and recommend a few dishes at popular restaurants.

Knowing what you're getting into

The reason these establishments are called fast-food restaurants is that they've mastered food preparation, ordering, and serving so that they take the least amount of time possible. Because people are in a hurry when they're out and about, they don't want to stop for a long time. There's nothing wrong with enjoying that convenience, but you need to make sure that the food you choose is right for your child with T1DM.

Of course, it's possible to sit down and take your time eating at some of these places, but the food is still standardized and prepared pretty fast, so the result is about the same.

One advantage of franchise restaurants is that a hamburger in a Denny's in California is almost exactly the same as a hamburger in a Denny's in New Mexico or Oregon. You know exactly what your child is getting, which makes the meal easier to fit into your child's diet. On the other hand, the quick serving and eating often doesn't allow the brain enough time to recognize that the body has eaten enough calories, and you may be tempted to order more food. Don't.

A study published in *The Lancet* in December 2004 that followed 3,000 people over 15 years showed that those who ate at fast-food restaurants regularly gained 10 pounds more than those who didn't, and the fast-food eaters also were much more likely to develop diabetes.

Food that's fried in a fast-food restaurant may be fried in trans fats. These fats, also called *hydrogenated* or *partially hydrogenated oils,* not only increase hardening of the arteries like saturated fats and cholesterol do, but they also reduce the levels of good cholesterol. Since 2006, food labels have been required to include the amount of trans fats, and the better fast-food places are trying to eliminate them from their cooking processes. Trans fats are still present in large amounts, however, especially in foods like French fries, batter-dipped onion rings, fried mozzarella sticks, and buffalo wings. The best way to avoid trans fats is to order food that's low in all fats.

No one should say that a person with T1DM can't go to a fast-food restaurant and remain on his or her nutritional plan. But these places do offer many seductive and unhealthy choices. You need to plan in advance what you're going to choose for your child (or yourself, if you're the patient). If you want to be sure of the nutritional content of various fast foods, pick up a copy of the *Guide to Healthy Restaurant Eating* by Hope S. Warshaw and published by the American Diabetes Association; to order, call 800-232-6733 or check your local bookstore. This book covers a lot of the available restaurant chains (but definitely not all of them). You also can find a great deal of information about fast-food offerings on the Web. Enter the name of a specific franchise into your favorite search engine, and visit the homepage. Most of the franchises have links to the nutritional content of their foods. You can see the amount of carbohydrate, protein, and fat in your child's favorite foods as well as the total calories.

Some specific fast-food recommendations

Here are a few suggestions for decent food choices at some very popular fast-food restaurants:

- ✔ A hamburger at Burger King isn't a bad choice for lunch. It contains 330 kcalories (kilocalories is the correct measurement, not calories, which is a much smaller number) and about 30 grams of carbohydrate, 20 grams of protein, and 12 grams of fat. The Burger King hamburger contains 530 milligrams of sodium. If your child goes up to the bacon double cheeseburger, he consumes 640 kcalories with 1,240 milligrams of sodium, so keep him away from those.

- ✔ Denny's menu offers some healthy choices, such as the Grilled Chicken Dinner. It has about 200 kilocalories, 25 percent of which are fat calories, 25 percent carbohydrate calories, and 50 percent protein calories, which isn't a good balance. But your child can have some carrots and a baked potato to add carbohydrates. Without any extras, the Grilled Chicken Dinner contains about 824 milligrams of sodium, so the dish is not ideal as far as sodium is concerned. This dinner choice also contains 30 grams of carbohydrate.

- ✔ At Domino's Pizza, your child may have two slices of medium cheese, deep-dish pizza with peppers and mushrooms as the toppings. Peppers and mushrooms add very little to the calorie count, so you don't need to consider them in his food plan. Two slices of the pizza provides about 375 kilocalories with 10 grams of fat and about 500 milligrams of sodium. The carbohydrate count is 45 grams. A small green salad with fat-free dressing provides a satisfying, low-calorie addition.

- ✔ McDonald's has all kinds of choices for breakfast, some good and some not so good. The Egg McMuffin is a good choice at only 290 kcalories and 30 grams of carbohydrate. If your child orders the scrambled eggs, he still gets eggs but loses the carbs and a lot of sodium. That's the only suitable breakfast option at McDonald's for your child with T1DM, however.

Avoid McDonald's hotcakes at 600 kcalories; the biscuit with sausage, mostly made of fat and a gram of salt; and particularly the biscuit with bacon, egg, and cheese, which has 480 kcalories and 1.4 grams of salt with too much fat.

> ✔ Arby's roast beef sandwich looks good, but should your child get the junior, regular, or super size? It's not that hard a choice: The junior has 324 kcalories with about 22 grams of carbohydrate, not too bad. But the regular goes up to 388 kcalories, and the super tops out at 523 kcalories. The sodium content likewise climbs from 779 to 1009 to 1189 milligrams of salt. So the junior size is clearly the best choice for your child.

Choosing a vegetarian diet

Children need a lot of calories, particularly fat calories, and it may be difficult to provide enough calories with a vegetarian diet. Although it's possible to provide all the nutrients necessary for a healthy diet by eating vegetarian, it's wise to avoid this kind of diet with young children because their eating habits tend to be so erratic.

Your child with T1DM may decide that he wants to follow a vegetarian diet when he reaches his teens. At this point, I recommend that you meet with a dietitian to work out a program that provides the essential nutrients while avoiding meat. The fact that there are so many vegetarians who are doing so well and outliving many meat eaters suggests that the diet is a viable option, even for the person with T1DM who needs a specific balance of carbohydrate, protein, and fat.

Handling Eating Disorders

Children, especially girls, are often convinced that they're too fat, even when there's little or no evidence to support it. When the attempt to lose weight becomes dangerous to the health of the patient, it's an eating disorder.

Eating disorders take two different forms: anorexia nervosa and bulimia. I describe the differences in the context of someone with T1DM and provide sources of help in the following sections.

An eating disorder is particularly dangerous in a child with T1DM because she tends to reduce or stop her insulin, knowing that insulin is required to store fat. She can rapidly get into ketoacidosis (see Chapter 4). If you suspect that your child has an eating disorder, take her to her endocrinologist for a discussion, and get a recommendation for a therapist who handles eating disorders. They can be very complicated and very dangerous.

Different types of disorders

Both anorexia and bulimia are eating disorders, but they have some differences. For instance, anorexia involves starvation, and bulimia involves bingeing and purging. I explain the signs, complications, and treatment of both disorders in the following sections.

If you think you or your child has an eating disorder, try answering the questions at www.dartmouth.edu/~chd/resources/eating/risk.html. You can quickly rule it in or out with this questionnaire.

Anorexia nervosa

Anorexia nervosa is the form of eating disorder in which the patient starves herself. Her weight is at least 15 percent lower than the appropriate weight for her height and age either as a result of starvation from a normal weight or from never allowing herself to reach a normal weight. She looks in the mirror and sees fat where others see thin or even starvation.

Anorexia is more common in girls than boys. These girls often get their erroneous ideas about body weight from their mothers who are preoccupied with staying thin. Patients tend to come from middle-class or upper-class families. They often love to cook, but only for others; they won't taste the food themselves.

One clue that anorexia is present in someone with T1DM is that the person requires very little insulin because she's taking in so little food, especially carbohydrates. In fact, it's difficult to calculate her insulin needs at all. Other findings that suggest anorexia are low body temperature and low blood pressure as well as extremely low levels of cholesterol. Girls with anorexia usually miss several menstrual periods in a row or stop menstruating, and boys with this disease lose interest in sex.

Anorexia can be fatal. Some of the serious complications include

- ✔ Heart failure
- ✔ Abnormal heart rhythms
- ✔ Fainting
- ✔ Bone loss
- ✔ Hair loss
- ✔ Kidney stones and kidney failure
- ✔ Infertility and miscarriages

Patients with anorexia demonstrate some peculiar eating behaviors. They may

- Eat more rapidly than others do
- Skip many meals and make excuses for doing so
- Eat until uncomfortably full
- Eat very few foods and stick to foods that are low in calories
- Weigh themselves often and obsess about tiny changes
- Avoid going to parties where there's food and avoid buffets
- Eat by themselves because they're embarrassed
- Feel guilty or disgusted after overeating

First and foremost, treatment for anorexia involves restoring the body weight to avoid the medical dangers. This sometimes requires hospitalization. Then there's a long period of therapy during which the patient restores a healthy mental picture of her weight. No particular medications are effective, but antidepressants may be necessary.

Bulimia

Patients with *bulimia* eat large amounts of food but then induce vomiting and take enemas to purge the food and lower their weight. Their condition is a little milder than that of the patient with anorexia; those with bulimia aren't as thin as those with anorexia and don't tend to lose their menstrual periods.

Patients with bulimia also may do excessive amounts of exercise to burn up all the calories they're consuming. They're more likely than anorexic patients to become obese as adults. Also, they don't seem to respond to psychological therapy as well as those patients either.

Some signs of bulimia include

- Tooth decay from the stomach acids that enter the mouth when the patient induces vomiting
- Scarring of the hands from putting them in the mouth and rubbing against the teeth to induce vomiting
- Eating large amounts of food without weight gain
- Dehydration with light-headedness or fainting from the loss of fluids from inducing vomiting or diarrhea

Otherwise, the signs of bulimia are similar to those of anorexia. The child with T1DM and bulimia has poor control of the blood glucose as a result of the irregularity of food intake.

Treatment of bulimia requires psychotherapy as well as drugs such as antidepressants to manage the depression that's often present in the patient.

Sources of help

If you think that your child with T1DM may have an eating disorder and would like to know more about anorexia and bulimia, check out the following resources:

- **The Weight-Control Information Network:** Find information on binge eating online at win.niddk.nih.gov/publications/binge.htm. You can also contact the organization at 1 Win Way, Bethesda, MD 20892-3665; or call 202-828-1025.

- **The Eating Disorder Referral and Information Center:** Find information and treatment centers online at www.edreferral.com. You can also contact the center at 2923 Sandy Pointe, Suite 6, Del Mar, CA 92014-2052; or call 858-792-7463.

- **The National Eating Disorders Association:** You can find information online at www.nationaleatingdisorders.org. You can also contact the association at 603 Stewart Street, Suite 803, Seattle, WA 98101; or call 800-931-2237.

- **The National Association of Anorexia Nervosa and Associated Disorders:** Find information online, including referrals to support groups, therapists, and treatment centers, at www.anad.org. You can also contact the association at P.O. Box 7, Highland Park, IL 60035; or call 847-831-3438.

Chapter 9

Exercising to Improve Control of Type 1 Diabetes

....

In This Chapter

▶ Getting a grip on the role of exercise in type 1 diabetes

▶ Planning for safe exercise

▶ Sticking to the program

....

*T*he fact that your child has type 1 diabetes (also known as T1DM) just makes it more important that he develops a fitness program that's part of his everyday activities, like eating and sleeping. Chapter 6 draws your attention to world-class athletes who have T1DM, and although the average child with T1DM isn't likely to become a world-class athlete, he can certainly use physical activity not only to help to control diabetes but also to help to live a long and full life.

The Joslin Diabetes Center has been studying patients with T1DM who have been taking insulin for 50 years or more. In an article in the August 2007 issue of *Diabetes Care,* the center looked at the "clinical factors associated with resistance to microvascular (eyes, kidneys, nervous system) complications in diabetic patients of extreme duration." They concluded that "exercise was associated with reduced microvascular complications" and "exercise may be an important protective factor." In other words, despite 50 years of taking insulin for T1DM, these people don't have those complications.

Everyone should exercise regularly, not just people with diabetes. In this chapter, you find out why exercise is important in T1DM, how you can get started and get your child started, and what exercise may be best for you both. Stop finding excuses and begin enjoying the body that carries around your brain and heart!

The Diabetes Exercise and Sports Association is an organization that you can turn to for help, instruction, and friendship as you add exercise to your child's good diabetes care. Check out the organization's Web site at `www.diabetes-exercise.org/index.asp` or call 800-898-4322. They know all about diabetes and sports and are eager to share the information with you.

The skinny on how exercise affects glucose

In order for muscles to have energy for either moderate or vigorous exercise, they have to store glucose that's ready for use. As vigorous exercise like heavy weight lifting begins, the muscles rapidly use up their stored glucose. Then the liver is turned on to release its stores of glucose and to produce large amounts by converting protein into glucose. The liver can sometimes make so much glucose that the blood glucose is temporarily higher after exercise than before. This extra glucose is quickly taken up by the depleted muscles to restore their glucose.

In the case of moderate exercise, however, after the glucose in muscles is used up, the muscles begin to use fat for energy. This arrangement works well because there are more kilocalories of energy in fat than in glucose (a carbohydrate) and because fat turns into energy much more slowly than does glucose. As fat is burned up for energy, there's less fat available to cause arteriosclerosis. More HDL (good) cholesterol is formed to reduce the risk of a heart attack.

The Benefits of Exercise for People with Type 1 Diabetes

Although it doesn't normalize the blood glucose or lower the hemoglobin A1c in T1DM, exercise has several very important functions that are essential to a healthy body. They include:

- **Preventing heart attacks, strokes, and peripheral vascular disease:** People with T1DM usually die of cardiovascular disease due to arteriosclerosis (narrowing of the arteries). Exercise reduces the frequency of all forms of arteriosclerosis by increasing good cholesterol (HDL), decreasing bad cholesterol (LDL), making the heart more efficient, and improving lung function.

- **Controlling the blood glucose more easily:** When a person with T1DM exercises, his insulin sensitivity increases. This means that less insulin is needed to handle the carbohydrates he consumes. This increased sensitivity can last for 24 hours after exercise. In my practice, the people who take the least total daily insulin are the heavy exercisers. They also tend to be in excellent diabetic control with low hemoglobin A1c levels.

Increased insulin sensitivity means that a person with T1DM may be prone to nighttime hypoglycemia if he doesn't eat a bedtime snack after exercise and doesn't reduce his pre-exercise insulin. See Chapter 4 for more about hypoglycemia.

Some additional benefits of exercise for patients with T1DM include

- Lower blood pressure
- Easier loss of weight and weight maintenance

✔ Stronger bones

✔ Lower rates of heart disease and cancer

✔ More energy

✔ Greater libido

✔ Increased mental ability

You may think that kids with T1DM don't have to worry about blood pressure, weight maintenance, strong bones, and heart disease, but the earlier they develop good exercise habits, the greater the chances that they'll stick with their routine for the long haul and live full, healthy lives.

Taking Care Before Starting an Exercise Program

You should do a few things to prepare your child for an exercise program. Obviously, having the right clothes and sneakers is important. If your child is newly diagnosed with T1DM, there's no concern about making complications worse with exercise, but if the diabetes has been present for more than five years, make sure that his eyes are in good shape by having an eye examination. Other than that, you're both ready to get moving.

Talking to the doctor

Your child with T1DM can do any exercise he prefers (as you find out later in this chapter). As an adult with T1DM, though, you should probably see your doctor before beginning a vigorous exercise program, especially if T1DM has been present ten years or more. You also should schedule a doctor's visit before starting vigorous exercise

✔ If you already have a complication of diabetes (like those in Chapter 5)

✔ If you're obese with a body mass index (BMI) of 30 or more

✔ If you have a physical limitation

✔ If you already have coronary artery disease or elevated blood pressure

✔ If you use medications daily

You may also want to talk to a dietitian about getting good nutrition before and during exercise to avoid hypoglycemia.

Deciding to devote an hour each day

The amount of aerobic exercise that you do depends upon your goal.

> ✓ **For very good physical fitness and stamina,** 30 minutes of daily aerobic exercise such as walking, jogging, tennis, squash, swimming, and cycling does the job.
>
> ✓ **For weight maintenance,** one hour of exercise a day takes care of you.
>
> ✓ **For actual weight loss,** 90 minutes a day is necessary.

In 2002, the Institute of Medicine recommended at least one hour of exercise daily for good health and weight. This was based on numerous studies of the effects of exercise on health. This amount shouldn't be taken as an upper limit, though. If you want to do more, that's fine, but don't do less. An hour (not an apple) a day keeps the doctor away!

When I ask patients to do an hour of exercise a day, one of the most common replies that I get is, "I can't find the time." One way to find time is to keep a log of how you spend your time every day. When I ask my patients to do that, they're amazed at how much time is actually available. You may have to give up a little television viewing or shorten your lunch and walk instead. If you like to read, consider picking up audio books that let you get out and walk as you "read."

Determining how hard to exercise

Simple exercise for one person may be very hard exercise for another person. When I first ask patients to consider walking 10,000 steps a day (I recommend this exercise later in this chapter), most of them look at me as though I'm crazy. Yet when they get up to that level, they realize that it isn't nearly as difficult as they imagined. Push yourself to the place where you're about to be out of breath, and you'll be doing moderate exercise.

The Perceived Exertion Scale is very useful in determining whether an activity is making a difference in your fitness (or your child's). To use the scale, you rate the degree of your exertion while performing a certain activity from extremely light to extremely hard, according to your personal physical ability level. Here's the scale:

> ✓ **Extremely light exercise** is very easy to do and requires little or no exertion.
>
> ✓ **Very light exercise** is like walking slowly for several minutes.
>
> ✓ **Light exercise** is like walking faster but at a pace you can continue without effort.

- ✔ **Somewhat hard exercise** is getting a little difficult but still feels okay to continue.

- ✔ **Very hard exercise** is difficult to continue. You have to push yourself, and you're very tired. At this level, you have trouble talking. The very hard level of exercise is most beneficial.

- ✔ **Extremely hard exercise** is the most difficult exercise you've ever done.

To find out more about the Perceived Exertion Scale, go to `www.cdc.gov/nccdphp/dnpa/physical/measuring/perceived_exertion.htm`.

Adjusting insulin usage and following other precautions

Exercising when you have T1DM requires a lot more careful thought than exercising when you have type 2 diabetes (T2DM). The reason is, of course, that in T2DM you have insulin in your body that can rise and fall according to the needs of your cells, especially your muscles. In T1DM, however, the only insulin you have is what you take by injection or by inhalation. There are a number of things you must consider when exercising with T1DM:

- ✔ **Where you inject the insulin:** Insulin taken in the thigh just before a run is absorbed much more quickly than if it were injected in the stomach, for example. Avoid the thigh just before exercise so that you don't become hypoglycemic early in the exercise.

- ✔ **How much insulin you take:** There has to be some insulin in your body for your muscle cells to take up glucose, but if there's too much, you may become hypoglycemic during the exercise and be unable to continue. If there's too little insulin in your system, your muscles may not get enough glucose, and you'll rapidly become fatigued.

- ✔ **When you take the insulin in relation to the time of the exercise and the time of the last meal:** You can usually begin exercising starting one hour after taking rapid-acting, pre-meal insulin.

- ✔ **The type of insulin you take:** If you take short-acting insulin called regular insulin, it doesn't lower the blood glucose as much or as rapidly as rapid-acting insulin called Apidra, Humalog, or Novolog (see Chapter 10). For this reason, you may want to use regular insulin before strenuous exercise rather than the rapid-acting form.

Make sure your child with T1DM (or you) follows these additional precautions when he (or you) actually exercises:

- ✔ Wears a bracelet or necklace identifying himself as a person with T1DM

- ✔ Checks his blood glucose frequently (every hour) if the exercise lasts more than two hours

✔ Chooses proper socks and shoes

✔ Drinks plenty of water as he feels thirsty

✔ Has a source of rapid-acting glucose available for hypoglycemia

✔ Exercises with a friend

Developing (And Sticking to) an Exercise Plan

People with T1DM should do two types of exercise, aerobic and anaerobic exercise.

✔ **Aerobic exercise** is moderate exercise done for a long duration; it improves heart and lung function and strengthens your muscles. *Aerobic* refers to the fact that the body has time during the exercise to combine oxygen with glucose to produce energy.

✔ **Anaerobic exercise** is a short burst of exercise during which glucose is used without oxygen. It's much less efficient and is too intense to be sustained. Anaerobic exercise increases muscle strength and stamina. Whereas running is aerobic exercise, sprinting is anaerobic exercise. Lifting 10 pounds repeatedly is aerobic exercise, and lifting 125 pounds once is anaerobic exercise.

In the following sections, I explain how to incorporate both of these types of exercise into your child's (or your own) program; I start with aerobic activity and finish with a great method for anaerobic exercise: weight training.

You probably wonder how long you can go without exercise before you begin to lose all the conditioning you've accomplished. The answer is only two to three weeks. That's a good reason to continue to do something every day.

Encouraging exercise at all ages

You'll probably be surprised to hear that exercise should begin with your newborn. Although T1DM doesn't usually begin at this age, starting a child's exercise at such a young age makes it easier to progress his exercise regimen throughout childhood, adding more time and new tasks, than to suddenly impose an exercise regimen at some later stage. In the following sections, you discover what you and your child should do at each stage to make (and keep) exercise a priority.

Check out these great resources for more info on children and exercise:

✔ The National Association for Sport and Physical Education, made up of more than 25,000 professionals in the fitness and physical activity fields, offers excellent resources at www.aahperd.org/naspe. Here you find National Standards for Physical Education, the Shape of the Nation Report on the status of physical education in the United States, and Tools for Observing Your Children's Physical Education.

✔ The President's Council on Physical Fitness and Sports has a Web site at www.fitness.gov where you can find out about its work to improve physical fitness and connect to a large number of other resources on the Internet. The site also has a page of Physical Activity Facts. Among them are the following:

- Children and teens need 60 minutes of activity a day for their health.

- Physically inactive people are twice as likely to develop coronary heart disease as regularly active people.

- Only three in ten adults get the recommended amount of physical activity, which is at least 30 minutes of activity five or more days a week.

- One-quarter of children in the U.S. spend four hours or more a day watching television.

Newborns and toddlers

Infants go through great physical changes in the first year of life, tripling their birth weight and gaining about 9 inches in length. They're born with undeveloped muscles and spend the first year building up their muscle mass so that they can grasp objects and ultimately stand up and walk.

During this first year, infants also are building up the neurological connections that allow them to move their muscles in a coordinated fashion. For example, you can stimulate your infant to turn over or to move by putting objects just out of reach. You also can stimulate him to reach out by hanging a mobile over his crib.

To make sure that your infant develops strong muscles to hold up that head and build up those arms, you can

✔ Take time to play with your infant every day for 30 minutes to one hour.

✔ Encourage siblings and grandparents (as if they needed it) to play with your baby.

✔ Provide safe objects and toys for the baby to play with.

✔ Let the baby watch as you exercise to encourage imitation.

✔ See if your local sports club has a parent-infant program. If not, tell them to start one.

Preschoolers

By 2 years of age, a child weighs four times his birth weight and grows 2½ to 3½ inches per year from age 2 to 5. The preschooler's muscles and nervous system are growing and developing. His vision is improving, but his eye movements limit his ability to follow moving objects. The child's balance is improving, and he's learning all the time. From age 1 to 2, he's running; by 3, he's jumping; and by 5, he can skip.

There's much you can do to encourage daily exercise for your youngster (and keep it safe). Here are a few suggestions:

- ✔ Play simple games like Hide and Seek or Simon Says with him.
- ✔ Supervise the child during play.
- ✔ Make sure he uses safety equipment, like a helmet.
- ✔ Provide balls for him to throw, kick, and catch.
- ✔ Provide a tricycle so that he can start to learn to ride a bike.
- ✔ Provide devices to improve balance and climbing, like playground equipment.
- ✔ Sign him up for classes in tumbling, dancing, or gymnastics.
- ✔ Protect his skin from sun exposure.

Primary school children and preteens

Young children and preteens gain 7 pounds of weight and 2½ inches of height per year. There's significant increase in motor skills, strength, and stamina, so the child can begin to participate in competitive sports. This is a very important time in the development of a lifelong interest in physical activity.

Exercise with your child regularly and also on your own. Your child will follow your example, especially when he's young. The best way to share your exercise time is to select an activity that you can both enjoy together. Begin at the earliest age possible by pushing him for a good long walk in his stroller. As he begins to walk, let him hold onto the stroller as you walk together. When he has his balance, walk together with him. Keep emphasizing that exercise is for a lifetime.

Fortunately, most small children love to run around; you may be hard-pressed to keep up with your youngster after a while. However, there will come a time when television and the Internet become very attractive distractions for him. It's important that you continue to set an example by exercising yourself, but you also have to place limits on the amount of time your child spends in such sedentary inactivity. The American Academy of Pediatrics recommends no more than one to two hours a day of quality programming.

You can really emphasize the importance of exercise to your child while getting more of it for yourself and your child. Here are a few tricks to sneak in more exercise:

- ✔ Walk to shops and markets whenever possible. If it's too far to walk all the way, drive partway, park, and then walk to your destination.
- ✔ When you go to a store, park at the farthest end of a parking lot from the door.
- ✔ If you travel by public transportation, walk to and from the station if possible.
- ✔ When you travel, look into walking tours available at your destination. (You can usually find books or Web sites with such information.) Take the tours, and you're sure to see much more.
- ✔ Take the stairs.
- ✔ Get pedometers for you and your child, and see who can record more steps in a day. Be sure to reward your child for winning. (See the section "A good pick for everyone: Walking 10,000 steps a day.")

In addition, you can really help your child by doing some or all of the following:

- ✔ Make sure that his school has a daily break for physical education.
- ✔ Introduce him to a variety of physical activities, and encourage him to join teams (see the later section "Competing against others").
- ✔ Provide positive roles models for sports.
- ✔ Introduce the idea of weight or strength training with light weights.

Adolescents

Puberty is a time of peak growth similar to the first year of life. The adolescent gains the last fifth of his height and 50 percent of his adult weight. Strength greatly increases, especially if he does strength-training exercises. Girls have their pubertal growth spurt earlier than boys, but boys experience a longer growth period and are taller on average at the end of growth. The percentage of body fat in boys remains about the same but significantly increases in girls, sometimes leading to the eating disorders described in Chapter 8.

Adolescents are much more able to think logically. They're more aware of the future and the consequences of their behavior, so they can understand the importance of physical activity to a much greater degree.

This is a time of continued promotion of exercise not just by parents but by many others in the adolescent's environment.

✔ If the child is willing, you should continue to exercise with him, especially if you can make it fun and even competitive. For example, this may be the time when your child beats you in tennis for the first time, an important milestone.

✔ School physical exercise programs should be available to every student, not just the ones who want to participate in after-school competitive sports.

✔ Physical activities that include socialization, like dancing, encourage your child to want to participate.

✔ Vacations with lots of physical activity such as biking or walking continue the active tradition.

✔ It may be more difficult to limit your child's sedentary activities, but you must give it all you've got. After all, it's what's best for your child.

If you want to see how your child stacks up against many others, have him perform the President's Challenge Physical Fitness Test, which you can find online at www.presidentschallenge.org/educators/program_details/physical_fitness/events.aspx. For the test, your child performs five exercises, and you compare his results with the results accomplished by a large school population (last measured, unfortunately, in 1985). Your child receives a Presidential Physical Fitness Award if he scores in the 85th percentile compared to the national standard. Perform the test every six months to best track your child's physical fitness progress.

As your child gets older and takes more control over his physical activity, he may develop some behaviors that complicate his T1DM. Minimize the risk of dangerous behavior by

✔ Discussing the negative effects of substance abuse on the child's physical state as well as his diabetes

✔ Discouraging the use of performance-enhancing drugs

Choosing an activity

Choosing a specific activity for exercise requires some thought. It's best to do several different activities that use different muscles, and it can get boring doing the same thing day after day. Here are some points to keep in mind when choosing a physical activity, either for yourself or your child:

✔ Some people prefer a team sport, whereas others prefer a solitary sport.

✔ Some people like competition, and others just like to improve their own performance.

✔ Some people like to be very tired at the end of a workout, whereas others like to take it a little easier.

✔ Climate is a factor in the choice of physical activities. If you live in a climate that's warm year-round, you can pretty much do anything outdoors at any time. In contrast, winter weather may send you indoors and help determine what activities you can do. You may want to do one sport during the warm summer months and another when you have to be inside.

✔ Decide what you want to get out of the exercise: fitness, flexibility, or weight loss (or all three).

Table 9-1 shows you how each exercise can improve the body. Choose the one that accomplishes what you (or your child) need from physical activity.

Table 9-1	Match Your Activity to the Results You Want
If You Want to . . .	*Then Consider . . .*
Build up cardiovascular condition	Vigorous basketball, racquetball, squash, cross-country skiing, handball
Strengthen your body	Weight lifting (low weight and high repetition), gymnastics, mountain climbing, cross-country skiing
Build up muscular endurance	Gymnastics, rowing, cross-country skiing, vigorous basketball
Increase flexibility	Gymnastics, judo, karate, soccer, surfing
Control body fat	Handball, racquetball, squash, cross-country skiing, vigorous basketball, singles tennis

You and your child can choose any one or more of the activities in Table 9-1 that meets your goals. Unless you have an illness or have never exercised before, or your child has a complication of diabetes, feel free to do what you and your child enjoy.

If you're an adult patient, consider your current physical state when you choose your exercise. Here are some complications (which I describe in Chapter 5) and how they limit may your choices:

✔ Diabetic retinopathy should prevent you from doing exercises that increase your blood pressure. Anaerobic weight lifting is in that category. Bouncing exercises also aren't good for damaged eyes, and you should avoid underwater diving like scuba, which increases the pressure in your eyes.

✔ Nephropathy (kidney damage) is made worse by uncontrolled high blood pressure, which can accompany any prolonged, high-intensity exercise, such as a triathlon or marathon. You can find out if such activities put you at risk by measuring your blood pressure several times during the exercise. Trying something once doesn't damage you more, particularly if you check to see if the exercise causes an increase in BP, which it may not.

✔ Chest pain at rest certainly prevents you from doing any exercise because it gets worse with exertion and you run the risk of a heart attack. Get it cleared up with your doctor before you undertake any form of exercise, or you may be meeting with the undertaker next.

Competing against others

If your child with T1DM wants to compete against others (or if you're an adult interested in competitive sports), he should be permitted to do so. Chapter 6 shows you that there are many world-class athletes who have T1DM. So if it's your child's goal to join in on competitive sports, you and he need to make several important changes to his diet and insulin program. Here are some suggestions for making his competition not only fun but safe:

✔ Check with his doctor before he starts playing, and work with a dietitian and sports physiologist who know how people with T1DM can compete successfully.

✔ Make sure he's well prepared as far as training is concerned.

✔ He should plan to test his blood glucose very frequently during the competition, as often as every 30 minutes. He may want to wear a continuous glucose monitor (see Chapter 7) so that you both can see how his glucose trends during play.

✔ Test his glucose several times in the hours after he competes. The exercise will make him very sensitive to the insulin and prone to hypoglycemia.

✔ Follow the nutrition guidelines for any competitive sport: Have him load up with carbohydrates for a few days before the competition so that there's plenty of stored energy in his muscles and liver. He also should be prepared to consume more carbohydrates throughout the competition at regular intervals.

✔ Should he become hypoglycemic, he shouldn't hesitate to stop and treat it. Not finishing is not the worst thing that can happen. Allowing his body to be damaged because he can't think clearly is. There will be many more competitions.

A good pick for everyone: Walking 10,000 steps a day

The great thing about walking is that just about anyone without a physical limitation can do it — and enjoy it, particularly if you're lucky enough to have a beautiful park or path nearby. If you throw in a little uphill walking, you benefit even more.

You and your child need a way to count your steps. Enter the *pedometer,* a little device worn on your belt that adds a step every time you do (see Figure 9-1). Some fancy pedometers are able to convert your steps into miles after you enter into the pedometer the distance you go with each step, but you really don't need more than a step counter.

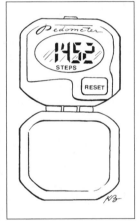

Figure 9-1: A pedometer tracks the number of steps you take.

If your pedometer doesn't keep track of mileage, you can do the math to figure it out yourself. Just multiply your stride length (the distance you go each time you take a step) in feet by the number of steps you took to get your total distance in feet. Divide that by 5,280 to get your miles. If you walk about a foot each time you step, you go about 2 miles every 10,000 steps. This is a good goal for children older than 12 and adults. Younger children between ages 8 and 12 may set 5,000 steps; children younger than 8 should be encouraged to just keep beating their previous daily average.

Accusplit pedometers work very well. The model I like is the Accusplit Eagle, which does nothing but record your steps. You can find it at www. accusplit.com/product.html. You also can find pedometers at sporting goods stores.

Here's how you and your child can use your pedometers to get up to 10,000 steps a day:

- ✔ Record your daily step count for a week. Remember to reset the steps after you have your daily total. Divide your seven-day step total by seven to get your average number of daily steps. Then try to add 500 steps to your daily total, and don't go to a higher level until you have seven days of 500 more. Once your average is 500 higher, move up another 500.

- ✔ Walk, don't ride, whenever you possibly can.

- ✔ Choose some favorite walks, and count the steps to complete each one. When you need a certain number of steps, select the walk that will give you that number.

- ✔ Use stairs instead of the elevator, whether you're going up or down.

Although affordable and accurate, a pedometer isn't essential to keep track of your steps. If you prefer not to use one, use these average conversions to get up to 10K (10,000) steps a day:

- ✔ 1 mile = 2,100 average steps

- ✔ 1 block = 100 average steps

- ✔ 10 minutes walking = 1,200 steps on average

- ✔ Biking or swimming = 150 steps per minute

- ✔ Weight lifting = 100 steps per minute

- ✔ Roller skating = 200 steps per minute

Training with weights

In addition to exercises for cardiovascular fitness, encourage your child to lift weights. Have him select lighter weights that he can lift repetitively. This is called *weight training*. (He should avoid very heavy weight lifting, which is anaerobic; refer to the earlier section "Developing (And Sticking to) an Exercise Plan" for an explanation of aerobic versus anaerobic exercise.)

Weight training improves muscle strength. The exercises I recommend in this section work his upper body muscles, which are neglected with most aerobic exercises that involve only his legs.

Your child's choices of exercises are numerous. I like seven specific upper body exercises because they get most of the different arm muscles. These exercises are the bicep curl, shoulder press, lateral raise, bent-over rowing, good mornings, flys, and pullovers. (I like these exercises for adults with T1DM, too.)

Anyone attempting these exercises, which I describe in the following sections, should choose weights that allow them to do three sets of ten exercises with a rest in between each set.

To try some other weight-training exercises, see the book *Weight Training For Dummies,* 3rd Edition, by Liz Neporent, Suzanne Schlossberg, and Shirley Archer (Wiley). You also can consult an exercise trainer in a fitness club to find out how to do these exercises and others safely.

Bicep curl

To do the bicep curl, follow these instructions and refer to Figure 9-2:

1. **Hold the dumbbells along the sides of your body, palms facing forward.**

2. **Raise the dumbbells until your elbows are fully bent.**

3. **Slowly lower the dumbbells to the original position.**

Shoulder press

To do the shoulder press, follow these instructions and see Figure 9-3:

1. **Hold the dumbbells with your palms facing each other and your elbows bent.**

2. **Raise the dumbbells over your head, turning your palms to face forward.**

3. **Lower the dumbbells to the original position.**

Lateral raise

To do the lateral raise, follow these instructions, illustrated in Figure 9-4:

1. **Hold the dumbbells along the sides of your body, palms facing each other.**

2. **Lift the dumbbells to the sides, palms facing the floor, until they are above your head.**

3. **Lower the dumbbells to your sides.**

Bent-over rowing

To do bent-over rowing, follow these instructions and see Figure 9-5:

1. **Hold a dumbbell in each hand, arms hanging down, with your legs straight and back parallel to the floor.**

2. **Raise the dumbbells to your chest.**

3. **Lower the dumbbells back toward the floor.**

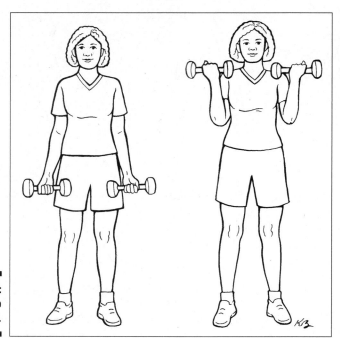

Figure 9-2:
The bicep
curl.

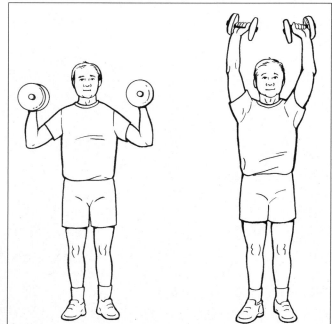

Figure 9-3:
The
shoulder
press.

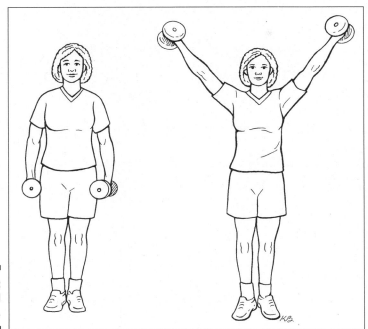

Figure 9-4:
The lateral
raise.

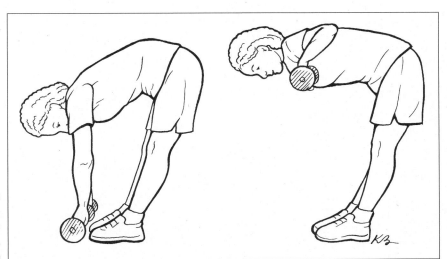

Figure 9-5:
Bent-over
rowing.

Good mornings

To do good mornings, follow these instructions and refer to Figure 9-6:

1. Hold the ends of one dumbbell above your head, arms straight.

2. **Lower the dumbbell forward as you bend forward so that your back is parallel to the floor.**

3. **Stand upright and raise the dumbbell to the original position.**

Flys

To do flys, follow these instructions, illustrated in Figure 9-7:

1. **Lie on your back, and hold the dumbbells out to each side at the shoulder level.**

2. **Lift the dumbbells together until they're above your head.**

3. **Lower them to the sides again.**

Pullovers

To do pullovers, follow these instructions and refer to Figure 9-8:

1. **Lie on your back holding one dumbbell with both hands straight up above your head.**

2. **Lower the dumbbell with your arms straight to the floor behind your head.**

3. **Raise the dumbbell back above your head.**

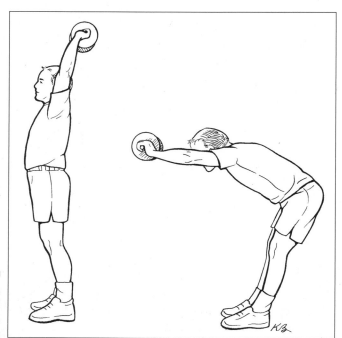

Figure 9-6:
The good
morning.

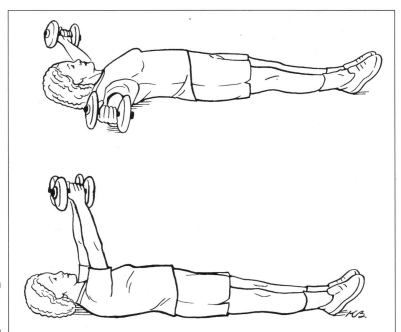

Figure 9-7:
The fly.

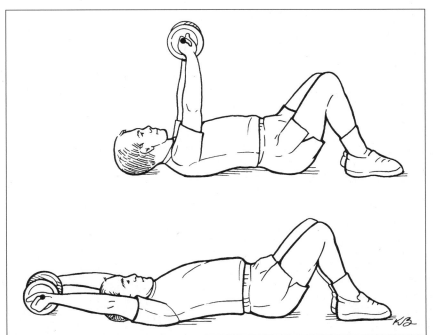

Figure 9-8:
The pullover.

Chapter 10

Understanding the Basics of Using Insulin

In This Chapter

▶ Looking at the purpose and types of insulin

▶ Doing the math on insulin doses

▶ Administering insulin with injection methods

▶ Breathing in inhaled insulin

*I*nsulin is the key substance that every patient with type 1 diabetes (T1DM) must take in order to live. The day it was successfully extracted by Dr. Frederick Banting and his assistant Charles Best in 1921 marks the great divide between the days of certain death for every person with T1DM and greatly extended life. In a matter of days after receiving the first insulin shots, weak, emaciated children were able to stand, eat normally, and look forward to many more years of life. But it turned out that there was still one small problem.

Beginning around ten or more years after developing T1DM and starting on insulin, many patients were found to have one or more of several long-term complications of diabetes as described in Chapter 5. Controversy grew as to why this was happening until the Diabetes Control and Complications Trial was published in 1993. That study confirmed that the complications were caused by levels of blood glucose that were too high over many years. The study also indicated that the long-term complications could be prevented by keeping the blood glucose as close to the normal range as possible.

The story of insulin since 1993 has been about finding ways to keep the blood glucose normal by balancing food intake and exercise with consistent insulin administration. In this chapter, you find out how you can administer it either to your child or yourself to successfully prevent both short-term (see Chapter 4) and long-term complications of diabetes. (Head to Chapter 11 for details on an exciting new method of delivering insulin: the pump.)

The Purpose and Types of Insulin

So you know that your child needs insulin (or you need it yourself), but do you know anything about what it does in the body and the types of external insulin available for patients with diabetes? Fear not; I explain what you need to know in the following sections.

What does insulin do?

Insulin is a *hormone,* a chemical that's made in one organ of the body — in this case, the pancreas — and travels throughout the body via the bloodstream performing its task. Insulin's task is to permit the entrance of *glucose* (the sugar in the blood that provides energy) into the cells of the body, especially muscle and liver cells.

Think of your insulin as an insurance agent who lives in San Francisco (which is your pancreas) but travels from there to do business in Seattle (your muscles), Denver (your fat tissue), Los Angeles (your liver), and other places. This insulin insurance agent is insuring your good health.

Wherever insulin travels in your body, it opens up the cells so that glucose can enter them. After glucose enters them, the cells immediately use it for energy, store it in a storage form of glucose (called *glycogen*) for rapid use later on, or convert it to fat for use even later as energy.

After glucose leaves your blood and enters your cells, your blood glucose level falls. Your pancreas can tell when your glucose is falling, and it turns off the release of insulin to prevent unhealthy low levels of blood glucose called *hypoglycemia* (see Chapter 4). At the same time, your liver begins to release glucose from storage and makes new glucose from amino acids in your blood to raise the level again.

If your insurance agent (insulin, remember? — stick with me here!) doesn't show up when you need him (meaning that you have an absence of insulin, as in type 1 diabetes), your insurance coverage may be very poor (in which case your blood glucose starts to climb). In other words, a lack of insulin means that glucose in the blood isn't allowed to enter cells in the body, and the amount of glucose in the blood rises to an unhealthy level. High blood glucose is the beginning of all your problems. (Flip to Chapter 2 for more information about the overall role of insulin in type 1 diabetes.)

If all insulin did was permit glucose to enter cells, that would be enough. But insulin has a number of other actions. These include the following:

✔ Uptake of amino acids by cells. Amino acids are the building blocks of proteins, and proteins make up muscle.

✔ Conversion of glucose into glycogen, its storage form in muscle and the liver.

✔ Synthesis of fat in fat cells, the liver, and muscle for further storage of energy.

✔ Regulation of the growth of beta cells, in which insulin is made, as well as protection of the beta cells from death.

✔ Regulation of the release of insulin from the beta cells. It does this by allowing glucose to enter the beta cell, where it stimulates the release of more insulin.

✔ Synthesis of DNA, the building blocks of chromosomes, which carry genetic material.

Is insulin important? This list of essential actions leaves little doubt about that.

What are the different types of external insulin?

The person with T1DM is entirely dependent upon an external source of insulin. Since it was originally extracted from the pancreas of fetal calves in 1921, scientists have attempted to alter external insulin's activity so that it can duplicate the activity of *native insulin,* the insulin in the bodies of people who don't have T1DM. And researchers have come pretty close to that goal.

External insulin comes in several forms, and each one has a different purpose:

✔ **Rapid-acting insulin:** Taken before a meal to control the carbohydrate in that meal

✔ **Regular insulin:** An earlier form of pre-meal insulin that's active longer

✔ **Intermediate insulin:** Has activity for 12 hours and therefore is given twice a day to act as a basal insulin

✔ **Long-acting insulin:** Has activity for 24 hours and therefore is ideal as a basal insulin

✔ **Insulin mixture:** Combines the actions of the two insulins that are mixed

Table 10-1 shows all the different kinds of insulin that are currently available along with the amount of time that passes between taking them and their onset of action as well as the peak and duration of activity.

Table 10-1	Types of Insulin and Their Actions		
Type and Generic Names	**Onset of Action**	**Peak Activity**	**Duration**
Rapid-acting (Aspart, Glulisine, Lispro)	15 min	1–2 hrs	3–4 hrs
Regular	30 min	2–3 hrs	3–6 hrs
Intermediate (NPH [protamine])	2–4 hrs	4–10 hrs	10–16 hrs
Long-acting (Detemir, Glargine)	2–4 hrs	No peak	20–24 hrs
Mixtures (50% lispro protamine/50% lispro; 70% NPH/30% regular; 75% lispro protamine/ 25% lispro; 70% aspart protamine/30% aspart)	Same as components	Same as components	Same as components

Make sure you get exactly the same brand and type of insulin each time (for yourself or for your child). There are small differences even in the insulins that are grouped together as the same type. To make sure you're getting the right insulin, Table 10-2 lists the brand names for the types listed in Table 10-1.

Table 10-2	Generic and Brand Names of Insulin
Generic Name	**Brand Name**
Aspart	NovoLog
Glulisine	Apidra
Lispro	Humalog
Regular	Humulin R or Novolin R
NPH	Humulin N or Novolin N
Detemir	Levemir
Glargine	Lantus
50% lispro protamine/50% lispro	Humalog Mix 50/50
70% NPH/30% regular	Humulin 70/30 or Novolin 70/30
75% lispro protamine/25% lispro	Humalog Mix 75/25
70% aspart protamine/30% aspart	NovoLog Mix 70/30

The Details of Insulin Doses

When your child takes insulin (or you do), the objective is to duplicate the secretion of insulin by the normal pancreas. This secretion has two parts:

- ✔ Under normal circumstances, there's usually a small amount of insulin called the *basal secretion* circulating in the blood at all times. This amount can be duplicated in a patient with T1DM by taking either long-acting glargine or detemir insulin. (The other way of getting a small amount of insulin constantly is with an insulin pump, a relatively new technique that I describe in Chapter 11.)

- ✔ The pancreas secretes a larger amount of insulin at the time of the meals called the *bolus secretion*. This amount is duplicated by taking rapid-acting insulin (like aspart, glulisine, or lispro) just before the meal or regular insulin 30 minutes before meals. These days, the convenience of taking insulin just at the time your child is eating results in more frequent use of rapid-acting insulin.

Insulin is manufactured in strengths of 100 units per milliliter. The first time a patient takes insulin, the dosage is based upon a calculated total daily dose consisting of a basal dose and a bolus dose. Your child's doctor will make this determination, but he'll usually follow these steps:

1. **Multiply the weight of the patient in kilograms by 0.3.**

   For example, a 35-kg patient requires 10.5 units of insulin per day, or approximately 10 units.

2. **Divide the total daily dose into the basal dose and the bolus doses by simply dividing it in half.**

   So 5 units is used as the basal dose and 5 units as the bolus dose.

Your child takes the basal dose and the bolus dose at different times of day.

- ✔ The basal dose is taken once or is sometimes split into two times a day, usually in the morning and/or at bedtime. I like to divide the basal dose into a large number of units in the morning and a few units at bedtime. In this case, I would use 4 units in the morning and 1 unit at night.

- ✔ The bolus dose is taken before meals. It's divided up so that 40 percent is taken before breakfast, 20 percent before lunch, and 40 percent before supper. In this case, that would be 2 units, 1 unit, and 2 units.

The final determination of the insulin dose your child (or you) takes at any given time is usually based upon trial and error. Your child takes a specific dose of insulin and you check his blood glucose for the result (see Chapter 7 for full details on measuring blood glucose). If the glucose is high, he takes an extra unit next time. If the glucose is low, you reduce the insulin dose by a unit next time. A calculation like the one in the preceding list is approximate but a good starting point. After the initial dose is determined, it can be adjusted in order to achieve the levels of blood glucose shown in Table 10-3. These levels are for children and adults.

Table 10-3	Goals of Insulin Therapy	
Time	*Ideal Glucose Level (mg/dl)*	*Acceptable Glucose Level (mg/dl)*
Before meals	70–110	70–130
1 hour after meals	80–120	80–180
2 hours after meals	80–120	100–140
2–3 a.m.	80–120	100–140

In the following sections, I explain the considerations you should make when calculating the bolus and basal doses for yourself or your child.

The dosing information that I present in this chapter is approximate; no matter what type of insulin you or your child takes, be sure to get a dosing plan from your doctor and ask questions.

Calculating the bolus dose

Three major factors must be taken into account in determining the final bolus dose of insulin necessary to reach the goals in Table 10-3, based on the initial bolus dose that I show you how to calculate earlier in this chapter:

- ✔ The level of the blood glucose before a meal
- ✔ The amount of carbohydrate about to be consumed
- ✔ Whether exercise has been or is about to be done

The level of the blood glucose before a meal

The blood glucose level before a meal must be measured with a glucose meter (see Chapter 7). Because the goal is a blood glucose of about 100 to 120 mg/dl after the meal, the question is how much extra insulin to take to get there based upon the before-meal blood glucose. You add units of insulin if the pre-meal blood glucose is higher than the ideal, and you decrease units of insulin if the pre-meal blood glucose is lower than the ideal.

One way to do this is with the rule of 1500. Divide 1500 by the total daily dose, in this case 10 units, and the result is 150. That's approximately how many milligrams per deciliter (mg/dl) 1 unit of insulin will lower the blood glucose. If the glucose before the meal is 250 mg/dl and the goal is 100 mg/dl, the excess is 150 mg/dl. Dividing 150 by 150 gives 1, which is the number of units you must add to the current bolus dose to achieve a level of 100 mg/dl after the meal. On the other hand, if glucose before the meal is 70 mg/dl, you want to subtract 1 unit from the bolus dose to get to 100 mg/dl after the meal.

Some patients, especially thin ones, find that 1 unit of insulin can bring the blood glucose down by more than 150 mg/dl. Others find that 1 unit only brings the glucose down 75 mg/dl. This fine-tuning permits you and your child to achieve your goal of excellent glucose control.

The amount of carbohydrate about to be consumed

In order to adjust the insulin dose before the meal to take into account the amount of carbohydrate to be consumed, you must know how much carbohydrate your child is about to eat. Chapter 8 contains an extensive discussion of carbohydrate counting. You can only adjust your child's bolus insulin for the carbohydrates in the meal if you know how many there are.

The amount of adjustment varies for different people at different ages. One person may find that he can handle 15 grams of carbohydrate with 1 unit of insulin, whereas another may need 1 unit for every 20 grams of carbohydrate. Again, this is a matter of trial and error. If your child starts with a blood glucose around 100 mg/dl before a meal and consumes 45 grams of carbohydrate, you can figure out how to adjust for the carbohydrate at the next meal based on the glucose level an hour after the meal.

You may find that the amount of insulin that covers your child's carbohydrate intake differs at different meals. At breakfast, because of all the hormones from overnight that tend to raise glucose, he may need 1 unit for 10 grams, but at lunch, 1 unit may control 15 grams. Suppose he takes an extra 3 units of the bolus dose at dinner for the 45 grams of carbohydrate based on 1 unit per 15 grams. If his blood glucose after the meal is 140, he may try taking four extra units based on a ratio of 1 unit to 10 grams of carbohydrate at breakfast the next day.

The effect of exercise

Exercise generally lowers the blood glucose (but not always). If your child exercises but doesn't have enough insulin in his blood, the glucose can rise, sometimes to high levels.

Chapter 9 offers a number of suggestions for including exercise in your child's life (and yours too!). Here are a few other recommendations in regard to bolus insulin:

- ✔ Check blood glucose just before your child exercises. If exercise is prolonged for several hours, check every hour.

- ✔ Try to maintain a blood glucose of about 150 mg/dl during exercise.

- ✔ Take glucose in the form of three to four glucose tablets if the blood glucose falls below 100 mg/dl.

- ✔ Take rapid-acting insulin and wait to exercise if the blood glucose is over 300 mg/dl.

- ✔ Take half the usual dose before a meal before exercise if the blood glucose is satisfactory.

- ✔ Try to exercise around the same time each day.

As your child trains more, his blood glucose will tend to remain more stable during exercise.

Adjusting the basal dose

At what point do you adjust your child's basal insulin? The following adjustments are best done in consultation with your child's doctor. However, if you're unable to see the doctor, you can put your knowledge to use and make the adjustments on your own.

- ✔ **Bedtime basal insulin:** If you find that several mornings in a row your child's fasting blood glucose is too high (above the levels in Table 10-3), you may add a unit or two to his bedtime basal insulin. If it's too low, you may reduce his bedtime basal insulin by a unit or two or get him to eat a small bedtime snack.

- ✔ **Morning basal insulin:** A high blood glucose level throughout the day is an indication to raise the morning basal insulin by 1 or 2 units. Getting hypoglycemia at different times of day is a reason to lower the morning basal by 1 or 2 units.

Several weeks after starting insulin, you may find that you can lower your child's dose (of both bolus and basal insulin) more and more and even go off it for as long as six months. This is the *honeymoon phase*. It's a period of remission when the insulin in his pancreas is controlling the glucose. He may need little or no insulin for this period, but there usually comes a time when he has to start insulin again. It's extremely important to measure your child's glucose frequently so you know when to reestablish the insulin.

Injecting Insulin

Many companies have extended an enormous amount of effort to make taking insulin as painless and convenient as possible. The following sections present a large number of tools available to you, but the information here is by no means exhaustive. New devices are coming on the market almost daily.

Before you begin: Selecting an injection site

Figure 10-1 shows the various sites that you can use to inject insulin into your child, including the abdomen, the legs, and the hips/buttocks. For all injection methods, you can wipe the area with alcohol, but it's not necessary (and some may be pulled in with the needle, causing pain). If necessary, your child can even take an injection through his clothes.

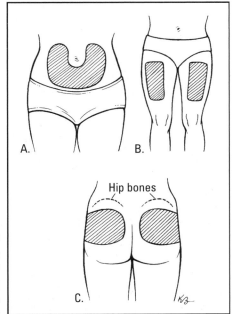

Figure 10-1: Sites for injecting insulin.

Need help in picking an injection site? Some variables that determine the speed of uptake of the insulin are the following:

✔ **Where the insulin is injected:** Uptake from the abdomen is fastest, followed by the arms and legs, and then the buttocks. If your child's blood glucose is high, inject in the abdomen so that the insulin is taken up rapidly.

✔ **Whether your child exercises:** Injecting into his leg when he's about to move speeds uptake.

✔ **Use of the same site:** Uptake slows when the same site is used repeatedly. Rotate sites.

✔ **The depth of the shot:** The deeper the shot at the site, the faster the insulin is taken up. You can use this knowledge to slow down the onset of the insulin when your child isn't eating immediately or is eating low-glycemic foods (see Chapter 8 for more about these types of foods).

Syringes and needles

More and more, people are using insulin pens to administer their insulin (I discuss these devices later in this chapter). Compared to a syringe and needle, the pen is just more convenient and easier to determine the correct dose. However, you and your child still need to know how to measure and deliver insulin with a syringe and needle (the oldest and still most common method for delivering insulin) in case you run out of pens or pen refills.

Numerous different brands of syringes and needles are available. Here are some of their common features:

✔ Syringes come in sizes of 1 ml (100 units), 0.5 ml (50 units), and 0.3 ml (30 units). Disposable syringes may be reused as long as the needle remains sharp.

   If you're using less than 30 units of insulin for all shots, the 0.3 ml syringe is easiest to use. If you use more than 30 but less than 50 units, the 0.5 ml syringe is best.

✔ Needle size is either ½ inch or ⁵⁄₁₆ inch. Children usually use the shorter needle.

✔ Needle gauge is 28, 29, 30, or 31. The higher the number, the thinner the needle. The thinner needles are less painful and are preferred for children and adults alike.

✔ Packages contain 100 needles and syringes already connected.

The syringe shown in Figure 10-2 is a 1-ml syringe that can hold a maximum of 100 units of any insulin. There are ten longer lines along the barrel that mark the syringe each time ten more units of insulin are added and that read 10, 20, 30, and so forth. Between the longer ten lines are ten shorter lines representing 1 unit each. At the fifth unit, the line is longer than the 1-unit line but shorter than the 10-unit line.

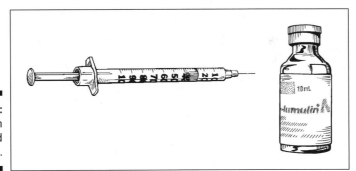

Figure 10-2:
An insulin
syringe and
bottle.

The bottle in Figure 10-2 is a typical bottle of insulin. When it's new, the top is covered by an aluminum cap that you break off and discard when using the insulin. Under the cap is a rubber stopper through which you push the needle to obtain the insulin. The stopper neatly seals itself when the needle is removed.

Every bottle of insulin has an expiration date on it. You can keep it in the refrigerator until that expiration date, and then discard it. You can have it at room temperature for four weeks before the expiration date, but then you must obtain new insulin. Insulin that has been stored at temperatures above 86 degrees F loses its potency; you can still use it, but discard it as soon as you can get new insulin. Insulin that has been frozen should be discarded.

Taking (or giving) a shot

If the insulin is rapid-acting or regular, it should be clear, and you don't have to roll the bottle. Intermediate-acting insulin (NPH) is cloudy, and you need to roll the bottle a few times to suspend the tiny particles in the liquid. A new bottle has a cap on the top, which you break off and discard. When you're ready to give insulin to your child (or take it yourself), wipe the rubber stopper in the top of the bottle with an alcohol wipe.

Make sure that you've selected the correct type of insulin before you draw it up into the syringe. Suppose that you need to give (or take) 25 units. Follow these steps to load the syringe with insulin:

1. **Pull the plunger of the syringe out, pulling in air, until the end of the plunger is at the 25-unit mark, the line exactly between 20 and 30 units.**

2. **Turn the insulin bottle upside down, and insert the needle into the soft rubber stopper until it's in the liquid insulin.**

3. **Push the plunger so that the air in the syringe goes into the insulin bottle, and then pull the plunger out to the 25-unit mark. Leave the needle inside the bottle.**

4. **Make sure there's no air in the syringe; you can tell by looking for air bubbles. If there is air, push the plunger back in to discard the insulin.**

5. **Pull the plunger out again to the 25-unit mark, and repeat Step 4 if necessary.**

6. **Pull the syringe and needle out of the insulin bottle.**

After you select an injection site (refer to the earlier section "Before you begin: Selecting an injection site"), push the needle into the skin until it goes no further. Push the plunger down to zero. You've successfully given insulin.

If you're giving your child an insulin shot, he's probably had many shots in the hospital. He should know that they're just about painless, and he shouldn't put up much of a fuss about receiving them.

Mixing two types of insulin

You can mix two different kinds of insulin in one syringe with the exception of long-acting insulin glargine and detemir insulin. You may need to mix insulins if you're giving NPH insulin combined with a rapid-acting insulin, for example. Here are the steps to follow to mix insulin:

1. **Wipe both bottles with alcohol wipes.**

2. **Pull out the plunger on the syringe to draw up the total units of air corresponding to the total insulin you need, both rapid- and long-acting.**

3. **Turn the long-acting insulin bottle upside down, and insert the needle into the soft rubber stopper until it's in the liquid insulin.**

4. **Push the units of air into the long-acting insulin bottle that correspond to the number of units of long-acting insulin you need, and withdraw the needle.**

5. **Turn the rapid-acting insulin bottle upside down, and insert the needle into the soft rubber stopper until it's in the liquid insulin.**

6. **Push the rest of the units of air into the rapid-acting insulin bottle, and then pull the plunger out to withdraw the correct number of units of rapid-acting insulin.**

7. **Insert the needle into the upside-down long-acting insulin bottle, and pull out the plunger to withdraw the correct number of units of long-acting insulin.**

It's important to follow these steps to mix rapid- and long-acting insulin so that you don't contaminate the rapid-acting insulin with the additive in the long-acting insulin.

Aiding the use of syringes and needles

Many people are a bit squeamish and have difficulty looking at the syringe and needle they're about to use. The following injection aids either hide the tools or turn inserting the needle into pushing a spring-loaded button that pushes in the needle and then pushes in the plunger to give the insulin. Some of the injection aids on the market are

- Autoject and Autoject 2: A spring-loaded plastic syringe holder
- BD Inject-Ease Automatic Injector: A spring-loaded plastic syringe holder
- Inject-Ease: A spring-loaded plastic syringe holder
- Instaject: A syringe injector and blood lancet device
- NeedleAid: A device that hides the needle of the syringe or insulin pen (which I discuss later in this chapter)
- NovoPen 3 PenMate: A device that conceals the needle of an insulin pen

Some devices magnify the syringe so that a visually impaired patient can easily see the dose he's taking while holding the syringe and needle firmly. Some of them include:

- BD Magni-Guide: A magnifying device
- Count-a-Dose: A device that converts pulling up the plunger of the syringe into audible clicks so that you can hear the dose
- Syringe Magnifier: A magnifying device
- Tru-Hand: A magnifying device

Some devices hold a syringe and needle firmly so that a physically handicapped patient can easily pull up the correct amount of insulin. The best of these include:

- Holdease: A device that holds the needle and syringe together
- Inject Assist: A device that holds the needle and syringe together
- Inject Safety Guard: A device to protect the hand
- NeedleAid: A device that stabilizes an insulin syringe or pen at the time of the injection

Many of these injection aids are available at pharmacies, and you can also find most of them on the Internet at diabetes supply Web sites. Two such sites are

- www.diabeticexpress.com
- www.diabeticsupplies.com

Disposing of syringes and needles

It's essential that you dispose of needles, syringes, and disposable pens (see the next section) in proper containers so that others don't reuse the syringes or stick themselves on the needles. Several companies make containers or other items to accomplish this important safety precaution (you can find them at the Web sites mentioned in the preceding section).

- BD Home Sharps Container holds 70 to 100 syringes or 300 pen needles.

- BD Safe-Clip clips and stores up to 1,500 needles.

- BD Sharps Disposal by Mail allows you to mail in 70 to 100 syringes or 300 pen needles.

- UltiGuard Syringes and Disposable Container Unit is a combination of syringes in various sizes and needle gauges with a disposal unit.

Firmly close any disposal unit you use. When the unit is full, dispose of it according to your local waste disposal rules.

Insulin pens

An insulin pen consists of a device filled with insulin that allows you to dial the dose shown in a window (with audible clicks) and make the injection by pushing in a plunger. Pens come in two different styles:

- The pen contains the insulin already and is discarded when you use up the insulin.

- You put a cartridge of 1.5 or 3 ml of insulin in the pen as needed and reuse the pen.

Also, some pens allow you to dial back down if you dial too much insulin. Check out an insulin pen in Figure 10-3.

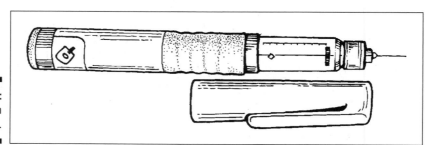

Figure 10-3:
An insulin
pen.

Many patients find that dialing a dose in an insulin pen is much simpler than taking insulin from a syringe and needle. Of course, with the exception of the mixtures that are already on the market in pen form, you can't mix two types of insulin when you use pens. Pens are probably the best option for children with T1DM because they're so easy to use and so accurate.

A number of different companies make pens for their own insulin. Available pens include the following:

- ✔ Autopen, which is available in four different models. Two contain a 1.5-ml cartridge, and two contain a 3-ml cartridge. Within each size, one pen delivers insulin in 1-unit increments, and the other pen delivers insulin in 2-unit increments.

- ✔ Humalog Mix 75/25, Humalog Mix 50/50, Humalog Pen, Humulin Mix 70/30, and Humulin N, all of which are prefilled, disposable pens containing 3 ml of the particular kind of insulin you use.

- ✔ HumaPen Luxura HD, used for Humalog insulin when half-unit doses are needed, particularly in children.

- ✔ HumaPen Memoir, a new pen that remembers the 16 most recent doses, their times, and dates; and is used with 3-ml lispro cartridges.

- ✔ Levemir FlexPen, a prefilled disposable pen containing 3 ml of Levemir insulin.

- ✔ NovoLog FlexPen and NovoLog 70/30 FlexPen, which are prefilled disposable insulin syringes containing 3 ml of insulin.

- ✔ NovoPen Junior, which takes NovoLog cartridges containing 3 ml of insulin and can be measured in half-unit doses.

- ✔ NovoPen 3, which holds NovoLog 3-ml cartridges.

- ✔ SoloStar, a disposable pen that contains 3 ml of Lantus insulin.

- ✔ Opticlix, which uses 3 ml glargine or glulisine cartridges.

Insulin pens require needles, and you must match the pen with the proper needle in order for the pen to work properly. If the needles don't come with the pen, the instructions with the pen tell you which needle to use.

The technique for injecting insulin with a pen is the same as injecting with a syringe and needle. The age of your child when you turn injections over to him depends on your assessment of his capability.

Insulin infusers

Insulin infusers are needles or catheters placed in the tissue under the skin and taped there for two to three days. When insulin needs to be given, the syringe is attached to the infusion set and injected into it by you or your child.

An infuser is useful when your child just hates the idea of three or four needle sticks a day and prefers to have something already under the skin into which you inject the insulin. The downside is that the infusion site sometimes gets infected, in which case you have to remove it and select another site.

An example of this device is the Button Infuser, which has a needle that penetrates the skin once. The insulin is delivered into the button each time it's needed. Another product called Insuflon has a catheter that remains under the skin; syringes and needles pierce a membrane instead of the skin, and insulin is injected through it.

Jet injectors

Jet injectors use a puff of air under pressure to release a jet stream of insulin that's forced through the skin by the pressure of the air. There's no needle involved. You simply draw up the amount of insulin needed, and you can use the device again and again. Figure 10-4 shows a typical jet injection device.

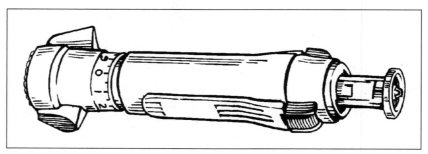

Figure 10-4: A jet injector.

Although jet injection devices avoid the use of a needle, they still cause some bruising. For many patients, they're a satisfactory substitute for a syringe and needle. Jet injectors may be used on children, and parents must decide when the child is mature enough to take on the responsibility of administering his own insulin using the device.

There are several jet injectors to choose from, including:

✔ Advanta Jet, which delivers ½ to 50 units of all types and mixes of insulin

✔ Advanta Jet ES, which is useful when the skin is particularly tough

✔ Gentle Jet, which is a low-power version of the two Advanta Jet devices above for children

✔ Medi-Jector Vision, which delivers all types of insulin from 2 to 50 units in 1-unit increments

Avoiding side effects, no matter the method

There are a few side effects that can be minimized or avoided when injecting insulin. Following are the common side effects and suggested ways of avoiding them, if possible:

- **Blocked needles** usually result from injecting insulin too slowly. Inject faster.

- **Bruises** are due to puncturing a small blood vessel. The blood is reabsorbed rapidly and causes no lasting discoloration.

- **Insulin leakage** is frequent. A drop or two found on the skin when the needle is withdrawn represents less than a unit of insulin. One trick is to pull out the needle halfway, wait, and then pull it out the rest of the way.

- **Lipohypertrophies or fatty lumps** occur when you inject in the same site each time. Rotate the sites to avoid this, and remember that the insulin is absorbed more slowly through these lumps.

- **Lipoatrophy** is an indentation under the skin that's probably the result of an immunological reaction to the insulin. Inject insulin along the edge of the cavity to cause fat to be laid down.

- **Pain** is caused by hitting a nerve. You may want to withdraw the needle completely and insert it elsewhere.

A Major Advance: Inhaled Insulin

For years various companies have looked for a way to get insulin into the body that doesn't require injections. An obvious site is the lung, which has an absorbing surface the size of a tennis court (singles, not doubles). The major difficulties have been the concern over possible damage to the lungs caused by the insulin and finding a way to change the dose by small amounts when necessary.

In 2006, the FDA gave approval to Pfizer to market inhaled insulin, which the company calls Exubera. The following sections discuss this major advance in insulin administration and how you can use it to control your diabetes.

As this book was going to press, Pfizer announced that it would no longer sell Exubera because sales were less than satisfactory. There have been no adverse effects of inhaled insulin. Pfizer is returning the product to the designer of the inhaler, Nektar Therapeutics, which is seeking another company to market it. Several other companies are about to come to market with inhaled insulin, and the information in the following sections, with the exception of the information about the particular device used for the insulin, applies to their insulin as well.

The limits on potential patients

The studies done on inhaled insulin prior to bringing it to market didn't show any permanent damage to patients' lungs. However, the studies were short term. The FDA requires that all potential users have their lungs checked before use, at six months after use begins, and every 12 months, or more often if lung symptoms develop. The lung test, called *spirometry,* involves the patient blowing all the air out of his lungs as rapidly as possible. If the patient can successfully blow out 70 percent or more of the air in his lungs in one second, he passes the test.

A number of patients aren't permitted to use inhaled insulin for one reason or another. These include:

- **Children:** The long-term effects of inhaled insulin aren't known yet, and if children were to use it, they'd have many decades of exposure. Until doctors and researchers have years of experience in prescribing inhaled insulin and seeing its effect on patients, it will remain off-limits to children with diabetes.

- **Pregnant women:** The risk to the fetus is unknown, so for now pregnant women aren't permitted to use inhaled insulin.

- **Patients with chronic lung disease:** Uptake of the inhaled insulin is too variable in these patients, so it can't be used.

- **Patients exposed to secondary smoke regularly:** These diabetes patients also have irregular uptake.

Determining the dose

Inhaled insulin takes the place of rapid-acting insulin. Its onset is a little slower than that of rapid-acting insulin, but it's faster than the onset of regular insulin. It lasts longer than rapid-acting insulin and almost as long as regular. You take inhaled insulin just before the meal begins or after the meal.

Inhaled insulin isn't basal insulin. A person with T1DM who takes inhaled insulin continues to need a shot of long-acting insulin such as glargine in order to provide the basal insulin.

The device used to inhale the insulin, manufactured by Nektar Therapeutics, is in Figure 10-5. The insulin comes in two different doses called *blisters* and is measured in milligrams rather than units. The 1-mg blister is equal to 3 units of rapid-acting insulin, whereas the 3-mg blister is equal to 8 units of rapid-acting insulin.

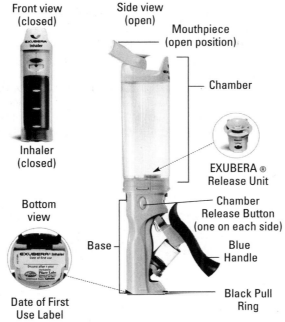

Figure 10-5:
The device
used to
administer
inhaled
insulin.

The initial dose taken before each meal is based on your weight. If you need
more than one blister, you take it immediately after the first blister. Table 10-4
shows the starting dosage for inhaled insulin based on weight in pounds. For
example, if you weigh 90 pounds, you start with two 1-mg blisters before each
meal and adjust this dose based upon your blood glucose reading before the
next meal or at bedtime in the case of supper.

Table 10-4	Doses of Inhaled Insulin According to Body Weight
Body Weight (pounds)	*Exubera Dose before Each Meal*
66–87	1 mg
88–132	1 mg, 1 mg
133–176	3 mg
177–220	1 mg, 3 mg
221–264	1 mg, 1 mg, 3 mg
265–308	3 mg, 3 mg

When it comes to inhaled insulin, 1 plus 1 plus 1 does not equal 3. If you run out of blisters with 3 mg, don't substitute with three 1-mg blisters. Use two 1-mg blisters instead.

After you establish a starting dose, you need to continually measure your blood glucose so that you can change the dose as needed. The desired blood glucose levels are the same for inhaled insulin as they are for rapid-acting insulin; see Table 10-3. For example, if you're getting readings that are too high before lunch, add a 1-mg blister to the dose before breakfast. Stay at that dose for a few days and adjust it again if your readings still aren't satisfactory.

Curiously, despite the inability to give less than 3 units as the lowest dose, getting to the right dosage of Exubera has not been a problem with my patients. Nor have they experienced excessive amounts of hypoglycemia.

Inhaling the insulin

The steps for actually taking inhaled insulin are as follows:

1. **Pull the base out of the chamber by pulling the black pull ring at the bottom of the chamber down until you hear a click.**

2. **Load the proper-sized blister into the slot above the blue handle, with the pocket containing the insulin facing down, and push it in as far as it will go.**

3. **Make sure the mouthpiece is closed. To pressurize the system, pull out the blue handle from the bottom as far as it will go and squeeze it until it snaps shut.**

4. **Hold the inhaler upright with the blue button facing you. Press the blue button until it clicks. A cloud of insulin fills the chamber.**

5. **Without delay, stand or sit up straight, and breathe out normally.**

6. **Turn the mouthpiece around to face you, place it in your mouth, and form a seal around it. In one breath, slowly and deeply breathe the insulin cloud in through your mouth.**

7. **Remove the mouthpiece, close your mouth, and hold your breath for five seconds. Then breathe out normally.**

A little insulin may escape when the mouthpiece is turned around, and there may be a little left in the chamber after you breathe in. Neither fact affects your dose. The insulin isn't pushed into your lungs by pressure but rather is breathed in by your inhalation.

My experience with inhaled insulin

I have patients with both type 1 and type 2 diabetes taking inhaled insulin. Some of my discoveries about using it include:

✔ Patients with T1DM using inhaled insulin are generally happier than they were on insulin shots.

✔ There has been no loss of diabetic control; in fact, those who were well controlled before using inhaled insulin remain that way, and those who weren't as well controlled have improved.

✔ The patients haven't had more hypoglycemia since starting on inhaled insulin.

✔ The patients feel that their quality of life has improved as a result of the inhaled insulin.

✔ None of them is embarrassed to use their inhaler in public, although some say that it's a large device.

I'm generally very satisfied with the results of using inhaled insulin and plan to expand my use of it to more patients.

A few notes on inhaler maintenance and usage

Instructions for maintaining an inhaled insulin inhaler come with it. Because the insulin is in the form of a dry powder, it's extremely important that the inhaler is dry when you take your insulin. Otherwise, the powder will stick to the moisture and you won't get the proper dose.

Inside the inhaler is the Release Unit, which is what punctures the blister. You must change the unit every two weeks. The refill kits come with a month's supply of blisters and two release units. The month's supply is divided among 1- and 3-mg blisters in two ways, depending upon how much of each type you use: You get either a package with 90 blisters of each type or a package with 180 1-mg blisters and 90 3-mg blisters.

Here are the answers to a few frequently asked questions about inhaled insulin:

✔ If you don't eat a meal, you don't have to take the insulin.

✔ If you forget to take the insulin before the meal, take it immediately after the meal but don't wait any later.

✔ Don't put any part of the inhaler in a dishwasher.

✔ You can use the insulin if you have a cold.

✔ You need to replace the entire inhaler once a year.

✔ Keep the insulin blisters at room temperature. If they find their way into the refrigerator, discard them.

✔ Keep used blisters away from children and pets because they still contain some insulin.

Chapter 11

Delivering Insulin with a Pump

*Y*our child doesn't like sticking himself with a needle, pen, or injector several times a day. Does he have an alternative? He sure does. It's called the insulin pump. About the size of a deck of cards, it uses a slowly turning screw to push the plunger of a small syringe full of rapid-acting insulin. The insulin goes through a tube and exits under the skin of your child's abdomen from a needle or plastic cannula — the infusion set — that you replace every three days or so.

This chapter covers the pros and cons of insulin pumps. You find out how to determine the insulin doses for a pump, and I also run through the different insulin pump devices on the market. See Chapter 10 for the basics of insulin, including the types of insulin available, information on dosages, and traditional methods of delivering insulin several times a day.

Keeping a Few Considerations in Mind before Using an Insulin Pump

Most people who have type 1 diabetes (T1DM) prefer using a pump over other methods of delivering insulin. If you ask the experts, about 60 percent of members of the American Association of Diabetes Educators who have T1DM use a pump instead of needles; about 50 percent of the members of the American Diabetes Association who have T1DM use an insulin pump rather than needles. There are more than 300,000 people with both types of diabetes using pumps.

Studies comparing the control that patients achieve with multiple injections versus the pump show little difference, which means that your child can use a pump to get the right amount of insulin without having to worry about using needles. Here are five additional reasons that people who like the pump cite for using one:

- ✔ The pump delivers insulin to the body much like the pancreas does.

- ✔ Your child can adjust the amount of insulin by fractions of a unit and have many different amounts at different times of day. The insulin pump easily adapts to a patient's lifestyle.

- ✔ Taking a larger dose before meals is as easy as pushing a button on the pump.

- ✔ Your child can be more flexible with meals because he's constantly getting a small dose of insulin. That's great news for today's active youngsters.

- ✔ There's less risk of hypoglycemia because your child is getting small amounts of insulin at a time (see Chapter 4 for details about this complication).

On the other hand, here are five equally significant reasons that people don't like to use an insulin pump:

- ✔ It's much more expensive than conventional syringes and needles.

- ✔ The pump is visible, especially when your child wears less clothing on hot days. Also, if there's a blockage, an alarm goes off. Essentially, it makes diabetes more obvious to others.

- ✔ If the pump fails for any reason that doesn't set off an alarm, such as a leak, your child has so little insulin in his body that he may rapidly go into ketoacidosis (see Chapter 4). (I explain how to handle problems with a pump later in this chapter.)

- ✔ Your child must monitor his blood glucose more frequently, sometimes more than four times daily, to properly use the pump. And right now, monitoring still means finger sticks. (Chapter 7 has the scoop on monitoring blood glucose.)

- ✔ The pump is attached to the body 24 hours a day, making sleeping and physical activities like sports less convenient. (I explain ways to live comfortably with the pump later in this chapter.)

- ✔ Pump wearers who engage in sex may find the pump inconvenient because it's attached to the body.

Not everyone is a good candidate for an insulin pump. The best candidates have the following characteristics:

- ✔ They're highly motivated.

- ✔ They're willing to stick themselves multiple times a day to check their blood glucose.

✔ They can afford the costs involved because many insurances pay only a part of the pump expenses.

✔ They understand how the pre-meal glucose and the carbohydrates about to be consumed are used to determine the insulin dose (see Chapter 10).

✔ They have a good understanding of the complications of diabetes, especially signs of ketoacidosis.

Kids of all ages can use the insulin pump. Parents usually manage the pump until they feel the child can do it.

Using an Insulin Pump Properly

Because your child's body requires different amounts of insulin at different times of day and night, you can set the pump to deliver many different amounts of insulin depending on your child's particular pattern. The syringe within the pump contains rapid-acting insulin — Humalog, Novolog, or Apidra. The pump delivers insulin constantly over 24 hours at what's called the *basal rate*. Just before each meal, your child pushes a button to deliver a larger dose depending upon the current blood glucose and the amount of carbohydrates he's about to eat. This larger dose is called the *bolus*.

There are a number of different insulin pump manufacturers, each claiming that their pump has the features that make it the best, but they all work in the same basic way, as you find out in the following sections. (I discuss the different types of pumps on the market later in this chapter.)

Going from a syringe and needles to a pump can take some adjustment. When in doubt, call your child's doctor with any questions or concerns about dosages, wearing a pump, and other related issues.

Taking the right doses

Some people recently diagnosed with T1DM can use a pump immediately, but most people who decide to start using a pump are switching from the following routine:

✔ Long-acting insulin once or twice a day, which corresponds with the basal insulin of the pump

✔ Multiple daily injections with rapid-acting insulin before meals, which corresponds to the boluses given by the pump

The total insulin dose from a pump is about 20 percent less than the amount of rapid-acting plus long-acting insulin from needles or other types of injection methods. This reduction is due to the fact that a constant infusion of insulin is more effective than multiple shots.

A pump can be started with a few or many durations of different basal rates, but in the beginning, the basal rate for most patients is broken down into these time frames: midnight to 3 a.m., 3 a.m. to 7 a.m., 7 a.m. to noon, noon to 6 p.m., and 6 p.m. to midnight. The rate of flow of the insulin, whether 1 unit per hour, 0.5 unit per hour, or whatever a particular patient needs, is determined by the measurement of the response with finger-stick blood glucose tests. For example, the patient may be started on 0.5 unit per hour throughout each time frame. If the morning blood glucose is above the desired fasting level listed in Chapter 10, the infusion of insulin in the time frame prior to that time may be increased to 0.6 unit per hour.

If you're the type 1 diabetes patient and your schedule is different than that of most people, you can adapt the schedule to your life. For example, if you work the night shift, you may reverse the preceding schedule.

Suppose that your child takes 5 units of rapid-acting Lispro insulin before meals and 5 units of long-acting glargine insulin at bedtime. The total is 10 units. With an insulin pump, he should start with 20 percent less, so his total dose starts at 8 units.

- ✔ He may take 0.2 unit per hour from midnight to 3 a.m. for a total of 0.6 unit.

- ✔ He needs more insulin just before awakening to deal with the *dawn phenomenon,* the tendency to have higher blood glucose tests first thing in the morning (see Chapter 4), so he takes 0.3 unit from 3 a.m. to 7 a.m. for a total of 1.2 units.

- ✔ At 7 a.m., he takes a bolus to cover his breakfast carbohydrates, assuming he's eating within ten minutes. Suppose that he takes 1 unit before breakfast.

- ✔ From 7 a.m. to noon, he takes a little less, say 0.2 units per hour for a total of 1 unit.

- ✔ At noon, he again takes a bolus to cover his lunch — 1 unit again.

- ✔ Your child continues the basal insulin at the same time. He may drop his basal rate to 0.15 unit between noon and 6 p.m. for a total of 0.75 unit and keep it to 0.15 unit again from 6 p.m. to midnight for 0.75 unit. The total units from noon to midnight is 1.5.

- ✔ He shouldn't forget to take that pre-supper bolus, perhaps 2 units.

Adding up your child's basal and bolus insulin, he's taking 8.3 units initially. Then it becomes important to check his blood glucose before meals and occasionally one hour after eating and in the middle of the night (see Chapter 7 for details on monitoring blood glucose). With the readings and knowing the amount of carbohydrates he's about to eat, you and your child can adjust the size of his boluses to achieve the levels in Chapter 10.

How often should you and your child make changes in the basal rate? If all is well, you can fine-tune it once or twice a month. If his body is changing rapidly due to sickness, increased daily physical activity, and so forth (or due to pregnancy if you're the patient), changes may need to be made much more often than that, perhaps even daily.

One way to easily determine if your child's basal rate is correct is to check his blood glucose before he would normally eat a meal, don't take a bolus and don't eat the meal, and then check his glucose an hour later. If his glucose remains about the same, his basal rate is good. Do the same thing with each meal over a day, if possible, to get the complete picture.

Changes made in the basal rate affect your child's blood glucose two hours later. For example, a change made at 2 p.m. is felt at 4 p.m. To counteract the delay, a bolus dose equal to two hours' worth of the basal rate will result in a more immediate response of blood glucose. In contrast, stopping the pump for two hours rapidly reduces the effect of the basal rate on blood glucose. If you want to rapidly affect the blood glucose, do it by giving a bolus dose, not by changing the basal rate.

Setting temporary doses

Most of the latest pumps offer the ability to set temporary doses. Here are a few instances when a temporary change in a dose may be useful:

- ✔ Your child's sick and his blood glucose begins to rise. You may want to set his basal rate temporarily higher until he's better (see Chapter 15 for details on handling sick days on a pump).

- ✔ Your child's going to bed and his glucose is higher than you'd like. A temporary addition of a few tenths of a unit of insulin may be all he needs for the night, and his glucose can return to its usual rate the next night.

- ✔ Your child is going to do a very strenuous exercise on a once- or twice-a-week basis, so a temporary reduction in the bolus rate by as much as half may be necessary on the day of exercise to compensate.

- ✔ If you're an adult patient who works nights a few days a week, you may want to have a temporary program to manage the nights you're up late. You can switch back to your usual program when you're sleeping at night again.

Changing the needle and insulin

Most of the time, you put the pump's needle or cannula in your child's abdomen, taking care not to put it where it will be under pressure, such as at his belt line. In particular, you shouldn't place the needle or cannula within a 2-inch circle around the belly button.

It's important to rotate the site to avoid fatty lumps and infections. You can do that by creating an imaginary "W" to one side of the belly button. Start at the upper left of the "W" the first time. Move to the lower left the second time, then up to the top middle of the "W" the third time, and so forth. When you finish with that "W," move to the other side of the belly button and start another "W." When you finish with the second "W," return to the upper right of the first "W" and proceed accordingly.

You change the needle or cannula every three days at first and less often with time and experience. Here are the general steps to follow when you insert a new needle or cannula (*always* read the instructions for your particular pump for specific instructions):

1. **Wash your hands with soap and water.**

2. **Remove the needle or cannula from its packaging.**

3. **Don't touch the end of the needle or cannula, the tip of the pump syringe, or the top of the insulin bottle; you want everything to remain sterile.**

4. **For a child, prepare the site with a topical anesthetic, especially early on.**

   You don't want pain to discourage the child from using the pump. Applying ice to the injection site just before inserting the cannula or needle also works for children less sensitive to the pain.

5. **Clean the site with antiseptic, such as an alcohol swab.**

6. **Before inserting the tubing or needle, give a priming dose of insulin to rid the tubing of air. Make sure that you see a bit of insulin coming out at the end of the tubing or needle.**

   For signs of a malfunctioning pump, see the later section "Dealing with problems."

7. **Insert the needle or cannula by pushing it through the skin.**

8. **Apply a sterile dressing, such as a sterile gauze and tape.**

Change the needle or cannula early in the day so that you have a few hours to verify that it's working properly. You don't want your child to go to bed and miss a night of insulin.

Check the site for infection several times a day and change it if infection is present or if the blood glucose is more than 250 mg/dl twice in a row. Signs that suggest an infected cannula include:

- ✔ Elevated blood glucose
- ✔ Redness at the site
- ✔ Tenderness at the site
- ✔ Heat at the site
- ✔ A lump under the skin
- ✔ Pus at the site
- ✔ Fever

If you suspect a severe infection, contact your child's doctor for advice. "If in doubt, take it out" is a good way of avoiding serious infections associated with your child's insulin pump. Put the infusion set in another site, and start pumping again.

With all this information on changing the needle, you may forget to switch the insulin, too. The reservoir of insulin in the pump needs to be changed every three days or so to keep the insulin fresh. If your child's in a hot climate, he may need to change it even more often. Every pump requires a different method for changing the insulin, so be sure to read the manufacturer's instructions carefully. Keep the insulin he's not using in the refrigerator.

Living comfortably with the pump

Living with an insulin pump requires some changes, but after a while, it will be second nature. Here are some tips to guide your child (or you, if you're the patient):

- ✔ Your child can wear the pump in a number of different places, and numerous items are available to make it easier. Your child may find that belts with pump pockets, socks or stockings that can hold a pump, and even a bra with a pump pocket are great aids.

- ✔ During sleep, the pump can be placed next to your child on the bed assuming that he doesn't move a lot during sleep. Another possibility is to turn off the pump and disconnect it during sleep, although it's a time when the pump can be especially useful to reduce the dawn phenomenon.

- ✔ Some pumps may be worn in the shower, but others require that you cover them or even disconnect them before coming into contact with water. Check the manufacturer's instructions!

✔ Your child can disconnect the pump for up to two hours while playing contact sports. The exercise helps to bring down the glucose, so he doesn't have to make up the insulin he didn't get from the pump. And your child should still be checking his blood glucose before and after heavy exercise and making adjustments as needed. For example, if he eats and plans to exercise while wearing the pump two to three hours later, he should reduce the pre-meal bolus by 50 percent and see what blood glucose results he gets. Check out Chapter 9 for more about the relationship between exercise and type 1 diabetes. If he wears the pump during exercise, he must protect it with some sort of covering.

If your child's feeling well in terms of overall health yet his blood glucose is rising on the pump, consider the following possibilities:

✔ **His pump is malfunctioning:** Visually check that insulin is coming out as the pump is working.

✔ **His insulin reservoir isn't providing insulin:** Look at the reservoir.

✔ **The infusion set is leaking, blocked, or has come out:** Check the placement of the infusion set and look for leaks along its length.

✔ **The needle or cannula has been inserted into a fat pad:** Visually inspect the site of the set.

✔ **There's something wrong with the insulin, such as it's expired or was exposed to very hot temperatures:** Use new insulin.

Whenever your child can't hold down food or fluids, head for the nearest emergency room. He may need a tune-up.

Switching from the pump in special cases

There will be times when your child needs to use a syringe and needles (or another injection method) instead of the pump. For example, if the pump breaks down, if it's lost or stolen, or if he runs out of supplies for it. How do you figure out how much insulin he should take to replace the insulin in the pump?

Assuming your child's using rapid-acting insulin in the pump, the doses before meals remain the same with injections as they were in his boluses. The basal insulin is replaced by glargine or detemir insulin. Just calculate how much basal insulin he was taking, and replace it with a dose of glargine or detemir of the same amount. You'll probably find that you have to increase the dose over the next few days by about 20 percent because these insulins don't lower the glucose as efficiently as continuous insulin. Adjusting the insulin is always done by measuring the blood glucose.

Checking Out Various Insulin Pumps

A number of companies make insulin pumps, and each one promotes its product's own good points. In clinical practice, all the pumps on the market are useful and can help your child to control his diabetes. Figure 11-1 shows a typical pump.

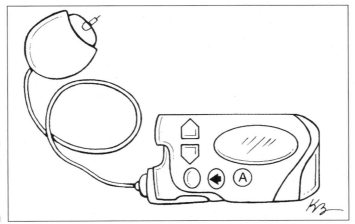

Figure 11-1:
A typical insulin pump.

In the following sections, I describe some of the most popular pumps on the market and give you some guidelines for selecting the right one for your child's needs (or your own).

MiniMed Paradigm pumps

Medtronic, the maker of the MiniMed pump, claims to manufacture the number-one prescribed pump for diabetes patients. I don't doubt it. The company has been around the longest and has the most experience in this field. Medtronic is very reliable and is set up to offer maximum help to the patient who uses its product.

As of this writing, Medtronic sells four different pumps: the MiniMed Paradigm 522 and 722, and the MiniMed Paradigm 515 and 715. The difference between the first set of pumps (the 522 and 722) is that the 522 reservoir holds 176 units of insulin and the 722 holds 176 or 300 units (and has to be slightly larger, therefore). That's also the difference between the 515 and 715 — the 515 holds 176 units and the 715 holds 176 or 300 units. The difference between the two sets is that the 522 and 722 work with the Guardian REAL-Time Continuous Glucose Monitoring System (see Chapter 7), whereas the 515 and 715 do not.

The future of insulin pumps

In the beginning, insulin pumps were just pumps. Now they're systems because insulin pump manufacturers are trying to combine glucose monitoring with insulin pumping. Ideally, this system would detect the level of the blood glucose and change the rate of insulin infusion based on that. This would be a *closed system,* just like the normal pancreas with no intervention by the patient. There are a few obstacles to this pump capability at the present time.

✔ The pump can't know the amount of carbohydrate that the person is about to eat and adjust for that.

✔ The pump can't know the exercise the person is about to do and adjust for that.

✔ The continuous glucose monitors that are currently available (see Chapter 7) aren't accurate enough to direct action on the basis of their readings. A finger-stick blood glucose check is necessary before changing insulin dosages. For example, when the blood glucose is falling rapidly, the continuous glucose monitor may lag behind the finger-stick blood glucose reading by as much as 30 to 45 minutes.

✔ The insulin infused by a pump has an effect on the blood glucose two hours later — too far behind the need for it. In contrast, insulin from the pancreas acts immediately.

Nevertheless, I have to give credit to the pump manufacturers for trying. One future solution is an implanted pump that would deliver insulin right into the bloodstream rather than under the skin, but that would only solve the insulin lag problem, not the measurement lag problem.

Some of the important features that all four MiniMed pumps share include:

✔ Changes can be as small as 0.05 units of insulin.

✔ The pumps store up to 90 days worth of information about insulin dosages, which can be downloaded to a computer.

✔ The accuracy of the delivery of insulin is plus or minus 5 percent.

✔ An occlusion alarm rings when the line of insulin is blocked.

✔ An over-delivery alarm prevents delivery of too much insulin.

✔ Remote controls are available to remotely give the bolus dose without exposing the pump.

✔ A Bolus Wizard Calculator combines blood glucose readings that you enter (515/715) or that are transmitted from the continuous glucose monitor (522/722) with food information that you enter to calculate the proper bolus.

✔ The bolus can be delivered immediately, either as a square wave (it's delivered slowly over 30 minutes to eight hours) or as a dual wave (part is delivered immediately and the rest by square wave).

✔ The smallest bolus is 0.1 unit.

- The basal rate range is between 0.05 to 35 units per hour.

- You can set up to 48 different basal rates (the day can be broken up into 48 different time periods) in three patterns.

- Temporary basal rates can be programmed to manage special circumstances like sickness or prolonged exercise.

- You can set up to eight blood glucose testing alarms per day as a reminder.

- The keypad can be locked to prevent accidental changes or children changing the dosages.

- An alert can be set to notify you when the reservoir of insulin is low or when a certain amount of time remains before it runs out.

- They're water-resistant (but can't be worn in a shower or when swimming).

- They require one AAA alkaline battery.

Accu-Chek Spirit Insulin Pump System

The Accu-Check Spirit insulin pump is made by Diesetronic, which is owned by Roche Diagnostics. Here's a rundown of this pump's the specific features and requirements:

- The reservoir holds 315 units of insulin.

- You can set up to 24 basal hourly rates in five different patterns. You also can set temporary rates.

- The basal rates range from 0.1 to 25 units per hour.

- The smallest bolus dose is 0.1 units.

- It can recall the last 30 boluses, daily insulin totals, and temporary rate increases and decreases.

- Multiple alarms indicate malfunctions of the pump.

- You can download information about daily insulin totals, boluses, and alarms to a computer.

- It requires one AA battery.

Animas pumps

The Animas IR 1250 and the Animas 2020 have many of the same features as the Medtronic pumps. The newer 2020 model is the first insulin pump to have a flat panel, high-contrast color screen. The Animas 2020 also can store the last 500 blood glucose values and carbohydrate counts. Here are some key points about the Animas pumps:

- It holds 200 units of insulin.
- The basal range of doses is 0.025 to 25 units per hour.
- You can set up to 12 basal rates in four personalized programs in 24 hours as well as a temporary basal rate.
- The smallest bolus is 0.05 units.
- They have a program called CarbSmart that stores up to 500 food items and allows calculation of insulin for the blood glucose and carbohydrates to be eaten.
- The battery is an AA lithium or an AA alkaline.
- They're waterproof up to 12 feet.

CozMore Insulin Technology System

This system consists of the Deltec Cozmo insulin pump and the CoZmonitor Blood Glucose Monitor, which attaches to the pump in the back and communicates with the pump via infrared technology to display the result on the pump screen. Some of this pump's features include:

- The smallest bolus is 0.05 units.
- It alerts you of a missed bolus before a meal.
- It holds 300 units of insulin.
- It alert you to test blood glucose.
- It has a site change alert to notify you to change the infusion set.
- It comes with *CoZmanager PC Communications Software,* which allows you to connect the pump with your computer and either print or e-mail the pump program as well as view the history of pump programs.
- It uses a proprietary 3.6 V battery.
- It's waterproof.

Dana Diabecare II pump

Made by Sooil Development, this pump is the lightest weight of the ones I cover in this section — it weighs a mere 1.8 ounces. Some unique features of this pump include:

✔ It holds 300 units of insulin.

✔ It allows you to set preset meal boluses (standard boluses for standard meals).

✔ It's about 20 percent less expensive than the other pumps.

✔ It has a proprietary luer lock connection between the infusion set and the pump, so you must use the specific infusion set.

✔ You can set up to 24 basal rates in 24 hours in a single pattern. You also can set a temporary basal rate.

✔ It uses a 3.6 V battery.

✔ It has multiple alarms to warn of malfunctions.

✔ It keeps track of daily insulin totals, boluses, and alarms that you can download.

✔ It is watertight.

OmniPod Insulin Management System

A product of the Insulet Corporation, the OmniPod is unique in that it consists of a wireless two-part design: the OmniPod and the Personal Diabetes Manager. The OmniPod has a disposable insulin reservoir, an angled infusion set, an automated inserter, a pumping mechanism, and power supply. It lasts for three days and is then discarded. The Personal Diabetes Manager is the device that programs the delivery of the insulin, and it has a Freestyle glucose monitor (see Chapter 7) built into it.

Here are some of the features of the OmniPod pump:

✔ The reservoir holds up to 200 units of insulin

✔ It can be set for 24 rates in 24 hours with seven possible basal patterns. There are also temporary basal rates.

✔ The basal range is between 0.05 and 30 units per hour.

✔ The smallest bolus is 0.05 units.

✔ The Personal Diabetes Manager has a built-in food database with over 1,000 common food items.

✔ It can store 90 days of downloadable data.

✔ The OmniPod has an integrated battery, and the Personal Diabetes Manager uses two AAA batteries (making it the heaviest of the pumps covered in this section).

Choosing the right pump

Given this wealth of choices, how do you choose the pump that's best for your child? You're about to purchase a device that costs more than $6,000 and will require more than $1,500 worth of supplies per year, so take your time and don't select the first pump you look at. Take these factors into consideration:

- ✔ Your child's doctor may be very familiar with one or two pumps and feels most comfortable using them. That may be a very important part of your choice unless you want to choose a new doctor with your child's pump.

- ✔ Your insurance company may prefer that you select one particular pump. However, if your child prefers another, don't give up easily on the pump of his choice. Many insurance companies will permit the purchase of an insulin pump that isn't on their preferred list if you provide convincing evidence that your child needs the special features of that particular pump.

- ✔ The need for a waterproof pump influences which pump you can use.

- ✔ If you or your child have problems with your hands, some pumps are easier to program than others.

- ✔ Your child may prefer a pump that's silent rather than a pump that clicks as insulin is delivered.

- ✔ A pump that can be set to deliver the smaller basal rates is better for small children.

- ✔ Representatives of the pump company will work with you to help you understand how to program the pump, so you should be comfortable with them.

- ✔ You should know ahead of time if the pump uses any infusion set or requires a special one that you have to order.

- ✔ Whether or not you receive a backup pump immediately if there's a problem is an important detail.

Your child can wear the different pumps (without insulin) to get the feel of them for a few days. You can get them from the pump manufacturers.

I find that my insulin pump patients use very few of the special features that their pumps provide. They average about five different basal rates in 24 hours and don't change patterns very often. They don't use temporary settings very often either. The tendency is to use lots of features when the pump is new and then back off after you've been using it for months.

Chapter 12

Getting a Grip on Other Drugs and Treatments

Although insulin, which I describe in Chapter 10, is the lifesaving drug for type 1 diabetes (T1DM), there's a world of other drugs out there, some of which can profoundly affect your child's (or your) diabetes. Some may be helpful, whereas others are damaging to blood glucose control. In this chapter I tell you about all the important drugs that may affect your child's diabetes, both positively and negatively. In addition, I discuss a few treatments that have proved useful for diabetic complications.

Boosting Insulin's Effect: Pramlintide

Since the end of the 19th century, doctors have known about a red-staining, waxy material called *amyloid* in the insulin-secreting beta cells of the pancreas (see Chapter 2 for the basics of beta cells). In 1987, this material was extracted and dubbed *amylin*. Researchers found that the beta cells secreted amylin at the same time that they secreted insulin, but the amylin was secreted in a much smaller amount. Amylin has some valuable properties that help the person with diabetes; among them:

✔ It blocks the secretion of glucagon, a major hormone that tends to raise blood glucose (see Chapter 2 for details).

✔ It slows the emptying of the stomach so that glucose is absorbed more slowly.

✔ It causes loss of appetite and weight loss.

Amylin, therefore, has an important effect on the rate at which glucose appears in the blood after eating. These effects occur when amylin reaches certain centers in the brain.

Because amylin comes from the same cells that make insulin, it's absent in T1DM just as insulin is absent in T1DM. It was thought that providing amylin to a patient with T1DM may improve the blood glucose. However, naturally occurring amylin has chemical properties that make it unusable as a pill or an injection. Mainly, it couldn't be made to dissolve in any liquid. A small change in the chemical structure made it possible to dissolve the new chemical while retaining all the properties of amylin. The new chemical is called *pramlintide.*

Pramlintide is available for use in diabetes under the brand name Symlin. It's given before meals as an injection but can't be mixed with insulin in the same syringe. It works with regular and rapid-acting insulin. Pramlintide prolongs the emptying of the stomach for up to an hour after an injection, although it has no effect on the next meal. Less glucose enters the blood from the intestine because the stomach empties more slowly and from the liver because glucagon is reduced by pramlintide's blocking action.

When pramlintide was given for over a year, it improved blood glucose control with a significant reduction in the hemoglobin A1c (see Chapter 7 for more about hemoglobin A1c). There was also a decrease in the amount of insulin that patients needed and a reduction in weight in many patients.

Like all drugs, pramlintide has its problems, although they don't seem to be too severe.

- ✔ Nausea is the most common side effect and is worse with higher doses. It's usually mild, starts when pramlintide is started, and usually stops after a month of therapy. It can be minimized by gradually increasing the dose of pramlintide once a week.

  The insulin dose should be reduced by 50 percent before meals when pramlintide is started. The usual starting dose of pramlintide is 15 micrograms before each meal, and it's raised by 15 micrograms every three days as long as the nausea is tolerable. The maximum dose is 120 micrograms.

- ✔ Hypoglycemia (see Chapter 4) is also a problem at the beginning of treatment; it usually ends after a month of therapy, when the insulin dose has been properly adjusted. It may be that the nausea prevents eating, leading to hypoglycemia at first (within three hours of the pramlintide injection).

- ✔ Other more rare side effects include dizziness, indigestion, stomach pain, tiredness, and vomiting.

- ✔ Pramlintide has not been studied in pregnancy and breast feeding, and it should probably not be used under these conditions. (I discuss the treatment of T1DM during pregnancy in Chapter 16.)

> ✔ It slows down the uptake of other medications as well as glucose being used to treat hypoglycemia.

Pramlintide may be used in adults and children with T1DM when the control of the blood glucose isn't satisfactory. Your or your child's doctor must prescribe this medication.

You should probably not use pramlintide if you have hypoglycemia unawareness (see Chapter 4) or a form of diabetic neuropathy called gastroparesis (see Chapter 5), which makes the stomach empty slowly.

Surveying Different Treatments

In the last few years, several treatments have been found to help to make the blood glucose more normal or control symptoms of type 1 diabetes. These treatments may be used for children as well as adults. Other treatments, while common, haven't been found to be useful, and I want to make sure that you know about them (and steer clear of them).

Acupuncture

In the past few decades, diabetes has become more common and complications have appeared more frequently. Acupuncture is often promoted as a treatment for these complications, especially painful neuropathy and gastroparesis (see Chapter 5). Not surprisingly, most of the information about the usefulness of acupuncture comes from China. The literature on acupuncture and diabetes goes back hundreds of years, but here are some of the latest findings on the role of acupuncture in diabetes (both type 1 and type 2).

> ✔ **For neuropathy:** An article in *The Journal of Traditional Chinese Medicine* in March 2006 compared acupuncture with Western treatments in groups of 30 diabetes patients. It showed that the patients receiving acupuncture not only improved in terms of pain from the neuropathy but their blood glucose and blood fats improved as well. Unfortunately, it's next to impossible to repeat these studies in the West because few practitioners perform acupuncture here.
>
> ✔ **For gastroparesis:** Gastroparesis, which is delayed emptying of the stomach due to diabetic neuropathy, can cause hypoglycemia and difficulty with glucose control because the insulin doesn't have its peak activity when the blood glucose is highest. In a study published in *The Journal of Traditional Chinese Medicine* in September 2004, groups of diabetes patients with gastroparesis were treated with acupuncture or medication. The patients receiving acupuncture fared much better, with significant improvement in gastroparesis.

If you or your child suffer from these painful conditions and can't find relief from traditional medical treatment, it's definitely worth trying acupuncture for whatever relief it may give.

Be sure that your acupuncturist is qualified by the state. You can find qualified acupuncturists in your area at www.medicalacupuncture.org/findadoc/index.html. Also, the treatment is rarely associated with infection, but you should be sure to check the needle sites afterward in case there's a problem.

Biofeedback

Biofeedback is a technique in which a machine detects an internal body function like your heart rate or your body temperature that's supposed to be involuntary. When you're aware of the function, you can attempt to alter it. Experiments with biofeedback techniques show that people have more control over so-called involuntary bodily functions than they realize.

Biofeedback has been shown to relieve stress in patients with type 1 and type 2 diabetes with a significant fall in hemoglobin A1c, muscle tension, and average blood glucose. A study in *Diabetes Care* in May 1991 found that type 1 patients who did biofeedback had significantly more normal blood glucose levels than a comparable group that didn't undergo biofeedback.

You can find a practitioner at the Web site of the Association of Applied Psychophysiology and Biofeedback, www.aapb.org.

Chromium

Many studies from China and Taiwan suggest that chromium can improve the blood glucose in patients with type 2 diabetes. For example, a study in *Metabolism* in July 2006 found that the average blood glucose and hemoglobin A1c were lowered in the group that got chromium compared to the group that did not. However, an article in *Diabetes Care* in May 2007 indicated that chromium had no effect on blood glucose in a Western group of patients with type 2 diabetes after six months of treatment compared with a group that received no chromium. Due to concern about the toxicity of chromium, the article recommended against supplementing the Western diet with chromium.

I haven't found any studies that suggested that chromium has a role in the treatment of type 1 diabetes.

Cinnamon

Cinnamon was first described as a possible treatment for diabetes in *Diabetes Care* in December 2003. Sixty patients with type 2 diabetes were given 1, 3, or 6 grams of cinnamon daily or a placebo. They received cinnamon or a placebo for 40 days, and the levels of fasting glucose, LDL cholesterol, total cholesterol, and triglycerides were measured. All three amounts of cinnamon reduced all these measurements in patients with type 2 diabetes.

In 2006, an article in the *European Journal of Clinical Investigation* confirmed these findings. Seventy-six patients with type 2 diabetes were given 3 grams of cinnamon daily or a placebo. Cinnamon reduced the plasma glucose significantly more than the placebo. The higher the initial glucose, the more the cinnamon reduced it.

This result called for a study of patients with type 1 diabetes, which was published in *Diabetes Care* in April 2007. Patients took 1 gram of cinnamon daily. Unfortunately, the study didn't show an improvement in hemoglobin A1c, total daily insulin usage, or the number of hypoglycemic reactions.

The bottom line as of this writing is that cinnamon isn't useful for blood glucose control in patients with T1DM.

Ginseng

Ginseng is a traditional Chinese herb that has been shown to have some glucose-lowering properties. For example, an article in *Phytomedicine* in October 2003 showed that ginseng lowered blood glucose and hemoglobin A1c in patients with type 2 diabetes. However, no controlled trials have shown that ginseng lowers the blood glucose in people with type 1 diabetes, and it's not recommended as a treatment for this condition.

Vanadium

Vanadium is a chemical found in tiny amounts in plants and animals. Studies have shown that animals with both type 1 and type 2 diabetes respond to vanadium with a lowering of the blood glucose. However, no study has compared a group taking vanadium with a group that isn't.

The verdict on vanadium's benefits to people with diabetes is still out, but if you want to get a bit more of it into your diet, have a glass of red wine a few times a week. Perhaps this practice is the explanation for the decreased occurrence of heart disease in the French compared to Americans, and as I explain in Chapter 5, heart disease is a major complication of T1DM. Anything you can do to lower your chances of heart disease is a step in the right direction. But remember, a person with T1DM needs to watch his alcohol intake like a hawk; I discuss alcohol in the next section.

Drinking Alcohol Safely

Alcohol is a drug that may be okay in small amounts but can ruin you when it's abused, especially if you have T1DM. Your child hopefully won't drink alcohol until he has reached the permissible age in your state. However, as an adult, he may drink, and you and he have to understand the role of alcohol in diabetes. Of course, if you're an adult patient, you need to be wise about alcohol intake, too. In the following sections, I advise you on safe amounts to drink, the dangers of drinking too much, and resources for getting help kicking the habit.

Your child's drinking habits will be a direct reflection of your drinking habits. The less you encourage excessive drinking and back it up by not drinking yourself, the more likely it is that your child won't drink either.

The maximum amount of alcohol allowed

The best way to start a discussion of the maximum amount of alcohol permissible for someone with T1DM is to define *acceptable amounts*. Here's the scoop:

- For a man, an acceptable amount of alcohol means a maximum of two glasses (5 ounces each) of wine or its equivalent (24 ounces of beer or 3 ounces of hard liquor) every 24 hours. The maximum amount permissible is ten glasses a week.

- For a woman, an acceptable amount means one glass (5 ounces) of wine or its equivalent (12 ounces of beer or 1.5 ounces of hard liquor) every 24 hours. The maximum amount permissible is five glasses a week.

The difference results from the fact that women metabolize alcohol much more slowly than men.

You don't have to adjust your insulin before drinking these amounts of alcohol, but eat something when you drink. And don't only drink alcohol, especially last thing before going to bed.

Wear a bracelet or necklace identifying you as a person with diabetes. If something goes terribly wrong and someone finds you unconscious after drinking, he'll smell the alcohol on your breath and assume you're drunk even if the real problem is that your blood glucose is dangerously low.

The dangers of excess alcohol

If you have type 1 diabetes, here's what alcohol does to complicate your condition (and your life):

- It provides *empty calories,* which are calories with no nutritional value that have to be counted in your diet. The approximate numbers of kilocalories that various forms of alcohol contribute to your diet are

  - Beer (12 ounces): 90 calories for light and 160 calories for regular

  - Hard liquor (1.5 ounces): 100 calories

  - Wine (5 ounces): 110 calories

- It doesn't have an immediate effect on the blood glucose when you drink it because it isn't a carbohydrate. As the carbohydrates in the food you have eaten decline, alcohol has its effect, especially if you drank too much.

- It prevents the liver from forming new glucose. If taken without food by a person who has taken a shot of insulin, the glucose can fall to severely hypoglycemic levels. This usually happens overnight when the patient is asleep. The result can be coma and brain damage.

- It reduces the secretion of growth hormone and cortisol, substances that typically raise the blood glucose.

- The more you drink, the longer it takes the liver to break down the alcohol, so the effects of a bottle of wine, for example, may be felt for the next 10 to 12 hours.

- It interferes with your understanding of how to take the proper amount of insulin in the proper way.

- It interferes with your better judgment about the fact that you must eat. If you have T1DM and don't eat as you drink alcohol, you're at great risk for a severe hypoglycemic reaction.

- It impairs your ability to recognize hypoglycemia, especially when you're drunk.

Finding help

Alcohol abuse has numerous physical and mental consequences, including cirrhosis of the liver (when the liver loses its ability to function properly and you die of hemorrhage or liver failure) and degeneration of the brain (when you lose coordination and develop severe emotional instability). Alcohol also is a home wrecker.

For the person with T1DM, alcohol abuse makes it impossible to control the blood glucose to prevent complications. The abuser takes in enormous quantities of empty (non-nutritious) calories and usually fails to eat good food. He fails to take his insulin either because he's drunk or because he forgets to take it when sober. All this is a prescription for diabetes disaster.

How do you know if you have a serious problem with alcohol? Here are the key tip-offs that suggest you need help with a drinking problem:

✔ You crave alcohol.

✔ You have tolerance to alcohol, so you require more alcohol than a non-alcoholic to reach the same state of inebriation.

✔ You have a physical dependence on alcohol and go through withdrawal symptoms like nervousness, shakiness, and headaches if you don't drink.

✔ You can't stop drinking after you start.

You can stop your heavy drinking, but you need help to do it. Only a small percentage of alcoholics stop on their own, but 90 percent of alcoholics who go through a combination of the following are typically sober after one year:

✔ **Treatment,** which is an intervention during which the patient totally gives up alcohol

✔ **Participation in Alcoholics Anonymous,** a program in which alcoholics meet regularly and declare their inability to control their alcohol intake

✔ **Aftercare,** which consists of attending regular weekly meetings in which the patient's alcohol abuse continues to be addressed

There are a number of drugs that the alcohol abuser with T1DM can use to avoid drinking, particularly disulfiram and varenicline. If you're a heavy drinker and a smoker, which is a common combination, varenicline may allow you to kill two birds with one stone. (See the later section "Kicking the habit" for more about this drug.)

The resources for the alcohol abuser are enormous. Here are the best (in addition to talking to your doctor):

✔ **Alcoholics Anonymous** offers publications and instructions for finding meetings that take place everywhere. Call 212-870-3400 or visit `www. alcoholics-anonymous.org` for more information.

✔ **The Internet Alcohol Recovery Center** has resources on everything you need to know about alcohol abuse and treatment. Call 215-243-9959 or visit `www.uphs.upenn.edu/recovery`.

Avoiding Dangerous Drugs

If you have type 1 diabetes, you should avoid a number of drugs. They can make your blood glucose worse or set you up for horrendous complications of diabetes like amputation. The following sections tell you about these dangerous drugs and offer some suggestions for getting off them if you're already hooked.

Prescription medications

For someone with T1DM, prescription medications are divided into two categories:

✔ Those medicines that affect T1DM by interfering with insulin

✔ Those medicines that affect T1DM by raising blood glucose on their own

Whatever drugs you take, check to see whether the drug has a side effect or interacts with a drug you're already taking that may cause your blood glucose to increase or decrease. Your doctor has the information to help you to do this, but if you want to do some sleuthing on your own, try these Web sites:

✔ `www.drugs.com`: Here you'll find numerous ways to look up a drug, but the simplest is to type the name of the drug in the box at the top of the page and click on Drug Search. If you want information on that drug from other Web sites, click on Internet Search. But beware, a lot of the information on the Internet isn't based on science but rather is an attempt to sell you something. Evaluate your findings closely.

✔ `www.drrubin.com`: On my Web site, you can find enough authoritative Web sites about diabetes to find the answer to just about any question you have. Select Diabetes under Related Websites on the left side of the home page, and you're off!

No matter what, if you start a new drug and notice that your blood glucose is suffering, be sure to talk to your doctor.

See Chapter 15 for information on taking care with over-the-counter medications when you (or your child) are ill.

Tobacco

Whether it's smoked, snorted, chewed, or inhaled as secondhand smoke, tobacco kills. If it were a quick killer like rat poison, it wouldn't last on the market for a day. But tobacco kills slowly, and by the time you realize that there's a problem, the damage has been done, whether it's lung cancer, stomach cancer, chronic lung disease, amputation, or a combination of these. Unfortunately, too many people wait until they have an irreversible disease to put away their cigarettes or other forms of tobacco for good. And at that point, it hardly matters anymore.

In the following sections, I explain the dangers of smoking for folks with T1DM and give you guidelines for quitting.

If you're a young person (or a not-so-young person) with or without diabetes, don't make the biggest mistake of your life and start using tobacco in any form. If you've started already, stop today!

The dangers of tobacco

Some of the ways that tobacco hurts the person with diabetes include:

- ✔ It increases *arteriosclerosis,* the condition of changes in arteries that lead to heart attacks, strokes, and loss of blood supply to the legs that results in amputations. (See Chapter 5 for details on T1DM complications that affect the heart.)

- ✔ It increases blood pressure, which also leads to worsening of arteriosclerosis and the tendency to have a stroke.

- ✔ It increases the clustering of *platelets,* the tiny disks in the blood that normally prevent a small cut from becoming a hemorrhage. Increased platelet clustering causes clumping within the arteries, blockage of blood flow, and death of tissues, especially the heart, brain, and arteries.

- ✔ It increases pain in the legs and heart in people with diminished blood flow.

- ✔ It reduces blood flow in arteries immediately in addition to contributing to the long-term worsening of arteriosclerosis.

Kicking the habit

Can you stop smoking? Forty-six million Americans have done it, so why not you? There are numerous ways you can go about it. You may be able to do it the first time you try, but don't give up if that doesn't happen. Many people manage to quit for good on their second, third, or fourth attempts. The important thing is to keep trying!

Some people can stop "cold turkey," making up their minds to quit immediately and never touching another cigarette. Others require a scare like chest pain or shortness of breath. Still others find success in nicotine replacement therapy because the nicotine in cigarettes is what's so addictive. Some of the forms of nicotine replacement therapy include:

- ✓ **Nicotine gum:** Available without a prescription, you chew the gum for a while until the need for a cigarette is gone. Then you park the gum in your cheek until you again feel the urge and chew some more. Each day, you decrease the number of pieces of gum you chew, and finally you reach a day when you don't need it at all.

- ✓ **Nicotine inhaler:** You need a prescription to get a nicotine inhaler. It delivers a vapor into the mouth, and the tissues in the mouth absorb the nicotine. Sometimes it causes irritation in the mouth.

- ✓ **Nicotine nasal spray:** Available by prescription, you use the nicotine nasal spray whenever you feel the urge for a cigarette. Over time, the urge diminishes. People with sinus problems have trouble using this form of replacement therapy.

- ✓ **Nicotine patches:** You can buy patches over the counter or with a prescription if you need a higher dose. The nicotine is absorbed through the skin, and you decrease the strength of the nicotine in the patch as your need for nicotine diminishes.

There are also certain drugs that block the addictive power of nicotine in your brain. Among the drugs that are safe for folks with T1DM are

- ✓ **Bupropion SR (brand name Zyban):** Takes away the craving for nicotine, but researchers don't know exactly how it does it. You take this prescription-only drug twice daily. The dose should be no greater than 300 mg daily, and no single dose should be greater than 150 mg to avoid the risk of seizures.

- ✓ **Varenicline (brand name Chantix):** Seems to be more effective than bupropion in helping people stop smoking. This new drug blocks the places in the brain to which nicotine attaches, so there's less craving and a reduction of the pleasurable effects of nicotine. Here's how you use varenicline:

  - You set a date to quit smoking and then start taking this drug a week earlier.

- You take it after a meal with 8 ounces of water.

- The dose is 1 mg twice daily for 12 weeks. If you haven't stopped smoking after the first 12 weeks, you'll benefit from another 12 weeks on the drug.

Varenicline can cause drowsiness, so you shouldn't drive or use heavy machinery until you know how you react to the drug. Elderly people may be particularly sensitive to its effects, and it shouldn't be used in children under 18 or breastfeeding mothers. Pregnant women need to discuss use with their doctors before they start the drug.

The combination of bupropion and nicotine replacement therapy may be even more effective than either alone. However, the safety and effectiveness of combining varenicline and nicotine replacement hasn't been studied.

If you want more help to accomplish the critical task of giving up tobacco in any form, talk to your doctor and consult these great resources:

- **The American Cancer Society** has all kinds of pamphlets and other materials as well as books and tapes on quitting smoking; call 1-800-227-2345 or visit www.cancer.org.

- **The American Lung Association** has information and clinics to help you to stop smoking; call 1-800-586-4872 or visit www.lungusa.org.

Illegal drugs

Use of illegal drugs makes it difficult to impossible to take care of your type 1 diabetes properly. You don't eat properly, take your insulin, or exercise when you're high. Just the expense of keeping up with your illegal drug habit may interfere with buying your medications. In addition, each illegal drug has its own negative side effects that can make you sick or complicate your diabetes. Here are the specific negative consequences of various illegal drugs:

- **Marijuana** (grass, weed, bud, cannabis) increases appetite, so you take in too many calories.

- **Amphetamine** (speed, Dex, crank, whizz, sulph) and **Ecstasy** (E, eckies, MDMA, X, adam, bean, roll, doves) speed up the metabolism, leading to hypoglycemia because you usually aren't eating properly while you're on the drug.

- **Cocaine** (coke, snow, nose candy, dust, toot) and **freebase cocaine** (crack, rock) cause diminished food intake and failure to take medications.

- **Heroin** (dope, junk, smack) has the same effects as cocaine but also involves an injection through which hepatitis and HIV/AIDS can be passed.

The best way to avoid the consequences of illegal drugs is never to start them. They're powerful enough that just one experience can get you hooked.

For much more information about illegal drug use, try either of these valuable Web sites:

✔ www.drug-rehabs.org/illegal-drugs.htm: At this site, you can find rehabilitation centers for every type of drug abuse, including alcohol. It also contains information about the various illegal and legal drugs that are abused.

✔ www.drugabuse.gov/OtherResources.html: This Web site from the National Institute on Drug Abuse tells you where to find information on every aspect of drug abuse and its consequences.

Chapter 13

Surveying Kidney, Pancreas, and Pancreatic Islet Transplants

● ●

In This Chapter

▶ Getting a new kidney and pancreas

▶ Receiving new beta cells

▶ Recovering from all types of transplants

● ●

*I*f there's such a thing as a "cure" for type 1 diabetes (or T1DM), it will be found in the information in this chapter. Three types of transplants are available to adults who have severe long-term complications from T1DM or who suffer from severe hypoglycemia and hypoglycemic unawareness. These surgeries generally are off-limits to children under the age of 18, who typically don't have such complications. The surgeries are as follows:

✔ **Pancreas transplant:** Some folks, if their complications are severe enough, require a whole new pancreas. No matter how hard doctors and researchers try, they can't precisely mirror the function of the pancreas — either through insulin shots or continuous insulin infusion with an insulin pump. Only the pancreas works so well. What an organ!

✔ **Kidney transplant:** If you bought this book too late to use the information to prevent kidney damage, this chapter tells you what you need to know about having a kidney transplantation or, even better, combining it with transplantation of the pancreas.

✔ **Pancreatic islet transplant:** A new way of "curing" type 1 diabetes is transplanting just the cells that make insulin, the beta cells found in the islets of the pancreas (see Chapters 2 and 10 for more about these cells). This technique was first reported in 1974 but had little success until a report in 1990 from Edmonton, Alberta, Canada, which described a new way of preventing rejection of the islets without using steroids.

Receiving a New Kidney

When your kidneys are failing, a kidney transplant can be a lifesaving move that lets you avoid the difficulties of dialysis. See Chapter 5 for more about long-term kidney complications.

Recognizing when you need a new kidney

The time to do a kidney transplant is when your kidneys are beginning to fail. Don't wait until they no longer function. As soon as you have to start dialysis, your life span is reduced compared to the person who has a kidney transplant early on, before the need for dialysis.

The signs that your kidneys have reached the stage where transplantation is essential are

- ✔ Chronic fatigue
- ✔ High blood pressure
- ✔ Swelling of your legs
- ✔ Elevation of the serum creatinine (this blood test reflects the current level of kidney function; as kidneys fail, blood creatinine rises)

Your doctor evaluates you and determines when the signs and symptoms have reached the point that you need to see a kidney specialist about a transplant.

Knowing when you can't have a kidney transplant

Even if you fulfill the criteria in the previous section, you may not be a candidate for a kidney transplant if any of the following are true for you:

- ✔ Severe heart disease
- ✔ Failure of other organs such as the lungs and liver
- ✔ Active cancer
- ✔ Abuse of drugs or alcohol
- ✔ Psychological instability
- ✔ Body mass index (BMI) greater than 40
- ✔ Age greater than 75

These risk factors make the transplant much more dangerous; you're more likely to die from the surgery or quickly reject the kidney.

The pros and cons of a kidney transplant

The biggest advantage of having a kidney transplant is that your quality of life is much improved compared to dialysis. For one thing, you no longer need dialysis if it has been started. For another, you're likely to be able to resume your regular life activities, even becoming pregnant if you're female. (I explain the precautions for women with T1DM to take when they're trying to conceive in Chapter 16.)

The success rate of a kidney transplant is quite high, too. Ninety percent of transplanted kidneys are working well after one year, 80 percent after four years, and 50 percent after ten years. Some transplants have lasted as long as 40 years. Now that's something to cheer about!

When you have a transplant, however, you have to take drugs to prevent rejection. This is the biggest disadvantage because drugs to prevent rejection may

- Make you more susceptible to infection
- Slowly damage the transplanted kidney
- Cause osteoporosis or soft bones

It's important to continue to monitor your kidney function after the transplant to make sure that your body isn't rejecting the kidney. The best test for this is the creatinine. If it starts to rise, you have to temporarily increase the dosage of your immunosuppressive drugs. (See the later section "Following up and treating your diabetes" for more information.) Post-transplant, your doctor also continues to monitor your bones for osteoporosis and your skin for skin cancers that are more common after a kidney transplant. He or she does this with blood tests and observation of your skin.

Occasionally, the transplanted kidney fails and another transplant is necessary. The same evaluation and precautions apply to this new kidney.

Understanding the costs

The average cost for a kidney transplant is less than $40,000. Compared to continuous need for dialysis, a kidney transplant becomes cost-effective after less than three years. Put simply, a lot of money could be saved if more kidney transplants were done, not to mention the improvement of more patients' quality of life.

Most kidney transplant patients are eligible for Medicare, which pays 80 percent of the cost of the transplant. Medicare also pays up to 80 percent of the cost of ongoing care, such as the antirejection drugs, but this only continues for 36 months. If you're eligible for Medicare because of your age or disability, it continues to cover ongoing care costs as long as you remain eligible. Speak to your doctor and insurance company about your eligibility for payment of these costs.

Undergoing an evaluation

So you've weighed the pros and cons, figured out how to pay for a kidney transplant, and decided to go ahead with the procedure; that's great news! Before you go under the knife, you need to complete a number of steps in the evaluation process:

- ✔ You see a cardiologist to make sure that your heart is healthy enough to handle major surgery.

- ✔ You meet the surgeon, who informs you of the risks and complications.

- ✔ You see a psychologist or social worker to evaluate your emotional state.

- ✔ You check with your insurance company to confirm your coverage.

After you accomplish these tasks, you do the actual work of finding a proper donor with the following steps:

- ✔ Your blood type is checked to match you with a donor. A donor with type O blood can donate to anyone. A recipient with type O blood can only receive a kidney from another type O. (See the next section for more about donors.)

- ✔ Your blood is checked for *human leukocyte antigens* (HLA), substances on white blood cells that show how close the match is between donor and recipient.

- ✔ Your blood is checked for human leukocyte antibodies to the donor HLA. If these are present, you're said to have a positive crossmatch and the transplant isn't done due to a much higher risk of rejection of the kidney. If they're not present, you're ready to go.

Finding a donor, living or deceased

A kidney transplant is better done with a living donor, someone who's willing to give up a kidney to save your life. Generally, a living donor is someone you know who's willing to give up a kidney — your spouse, brother, sister, and so forth. Using a living donor has advantages and disadvantages. Kidneys from living donors tend to last longer than kidneys from deceased donors, and you're likely to get your transplant before kidney failure damages your body. But you have to find a related donor willing to give up a kidney, and the donor is giving up one of two kidneys in a major operation that requires recovery time.

Many more kidneys have become available from living donors since the development of the *expanded criteria donor* (ECD) policy. ECD kidneys come from an older population (older than 60) and from younger donors who may have a history that previously would have ruled them out as donors, such as high blood pressure or elevated serum creatinine.

If you have to go on a list to receive a kidney from a deceased donor, the wait may be long, and you don't get to choose the source.

The process of surgery and recovery

During a kidney transplant, the native kidneys are left in place. The new kidney is attached by its blood vessels in the pelvic area, and its ureter goes into the bladder. Surgery takes about three hours.

During recovery, you're tested for your kidney function. You're in the hospital for two to three days after the transplant, but the recovery doesn't end there. See the later section "Dealing with Continuing Issues after Any Transplant" for more information.

Getting a New Pancreas (Alone or with a New Kidney)

The failure of the pancreas to produce insulin is the major problem in type 1 diabetes. The simple solution is to transplant a new pancreas into the patient with T1DM. A person can receive a new pancreas in one of three ways:

✔ A pancreas transplant can be done simultaneously with a kidney transplant, which is the most common procedure in 80 percent of cases.

The survival of the simultaneous kidney and pancreas transplant is greater than the other types in this list and similar to the survival of a kidney transplant alone (see the earlier section "The pros and cons of a kidney transplant" for details). A person with T1DM having a kidney transplant should be considered for a pancreas transplant at the same time.

✔ Sometimes the pancreas is transplanted after the kidney, such as when a kidney is immediately available for transplant and a pancreas isn't. This occurs 15 percent of the time.

✔ In 5 percent of pancreas transplant cases, the pancreas alone is transplanted. This is done when the patient has severe and frequent hypoglycemia or hyperglycemia (see Chapter 4 for more about these complications).

I outline the process of receiving a new pancreas in the following sections. Keep in mind that the evaluation process for a pancreas transplant is similar to that for a kidney transplant, which I cover earlier in this chapter.

Recognizing when you need a new pancreas

If you suffer from severe hypoglycemia or hyperglycemia that doesn't respond to treatment, or if you have severe hypoglycemic unawareness, you're a candidate for a pancreas transplant. Often, the pancreas transplant is done in conjunction with a kidney transplant.

Knowing when you can't have a pancreas transplant

The same criteria that prohibit you from having a kidney transplant are true for a pancreas transplant or a pancreas-kidney transplant (refer to the earlier section "Knowing when you can't have a kidney transplant"). If you have other severe diseases or abuse drugs or alcohol, you're not a candidate for a pancreas transplant.

The pros and cons of a pancreas transplant

Are you nervous at the thought of undergoing a pancreas transplant? Fret not; here are several advantages of receiving a new pancreas:

✔ The benefit of needing no insulin injection and no dialysis after a combined kidney and pancreas transplant is enormous. Your quality of life improves tremendously.

✔ With a combination kidney and pancreas transplant, your new kidney doesn't suffer the same deterioration as the original, damaged kidney. Without the healthy pancreas, the new kidney would deteriorate.

> ✔ If you suffer from hypoglycemic unawareness (see Chapter 4) with severe resultant low blood glucose, you resume hypoglycemic awareness after a transplant of the pancreas.
>
> ✔ Glucose levels that are very brittle smooth out after pancreas transplantation.
>
> ✔ Early complications like eye disease, nerve disease, and heart disease reverse after pancreas transplantation.

Keep in mind, though, that a pancreas transplant isn't without risks. The newer drugs used to suppress rejection of a pancreas don't cause osteoporosis, as corticosteroids (the traditional antirejection drugs) do, but they have their own problems. In addition, the surgery on the pancreas is technically more difficult than kidney surgery, which leads to other possible complications. Some of the specific risks of pancreas transplant include:

> ✔ Surgical complications that require removal of the graft in 10 percent of transplants
>
> ✔ Bleeding and infection in as many as 25 percent of transplants
>
> ✔ Damage to the kidney from the antirejection drugs (if you're receiving a combined kidney and pancreas transplant)
>
> ✔ High blood pressure due to the drugs
>
> ✔ High blood glucose due to the drugs
>
> ✔ Diarrhea and gastrointestinal bleeding due to the drugs

Looking at the costs

The cost for a kidney transplant alone varies widely; I've seen figures from $25,000 to $150,000 for this procedure. A pancreas transplant costs from $51,000 to $135,000. Concrete information on the cost of the combined organ transplant isn't available, so you need to talk to your doctors and insurance company for specific estimates.

If you're eligible for Medicare, it provides coverage for a combined pancreas-kidney transplant. Be sure to check with your insurance company to find out what will be covered beyond Medicare.

Finding a pancreas donor

The pancreas donor is always deceased, and you don't get to choose. If you're eligible for a pancreas transplant, you're placed on a list and get the transplant when you reach the top of the list.

The process of surgery and recovery

Figure 13-1 shows the appearance of the abdomen after simultaneous kidney and pancreas transplant.

✔ As in a regular kidney transplant, the native kidneys are left in place. The new kidney is attached by its blood vessels in the pelvic area, and its ureter goes into your bladder.

✔ The pancreas is attached to your intestine so that the digestive enzymes can go into the intestine where they belong. Its blood vessels are attached to nearby arteries and veins. Your own pancreas is left in your body to continue to provide digestive enzymes to your intestine. (A pancreas-only transplant also looks like this.)

Surgery takes about four to six hours for a simultaneous kidney and pancreas transplant; a pancreas-only transplant takes two to four hours. The drugs that prevent rejection of the kidney and pancreas are introduced after surgery, and their concentrations are measured by blood tests. You must stay in the hospital for 7 to 12 days after the combined transplant; if you're in the hospital for just a pancreas-only transplant, you'll stay a similar number of days. I discuss additional follow-up later in this chapter.

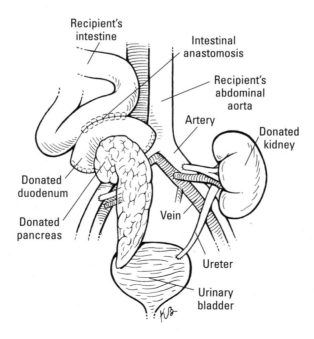

Figure 13-1:
A combined kidney and pancreas transplant.

On the Cutting Edge: Pancreatic Islet Transplantation

When you think about it, kidney and pancreas transplants (which I discuss earlier in this chapter) are pretty straightforward; simply speaking, a donor's organs are sewn into your body so that all the organs, old and new, work together. But as you find out in the following sections, you also have a new and exciting method of "curing" T1DM at your disposal: transplanting only the pancreatic tissue that contains the insulin-secreting beta cells. That's what's done in *islet transplantation*.

As I explain in Chapters 2 and 10, insulin is made in beta cells in the pancreas, which are found in areas of the pancreas called *islets*. The islets make up only 2 percent of the pancreas, but there are a million of them. Pancreatic islet transplantation involves the extraction of the islets from the donor pancreas and the injection of the islets into the liver of the recipient with T1DM. Islet transplantation is much simpler than whole pancreas transplantation because the more-major surgery is limited to the donor, who's deceased. (For details on the actual transplant, see the later section "The process of surgery and recovery.") The objective is to eliminate the need for insulin injections.

As of this writing, islet transplantation in the United States is being done only in the form of clinical trials. If you're interested in joining a clinical trial on islet transplantation, go to www.clinicaltrials.gov. Enter "islet transplantation" in the search box, and you'll be taken to a listing of studies, one of which may be near you.

Recognizing when you need islet transplantation

The indications for islet transplantation are the same as those for whole pancreas transplantation: The patient suffers from debilitating hypoglycemia or hyperglycemia or has significant complications of diabetes. If you want to join a clinical trial, you'll be fully evaluated by a doctor before undergoing the procedure.

Islet transplantation is most successful when the patient is taking a low dose of insulin. Any patient whose insulin use is 40 units daily or less is an excellent candidate for this procedure.

Knowing when you can't have an islet transplant

The same contraindications for having one of the other transplants are true for this type of transplant. If you have a debilitating disease like severe heart disease or cancer, or if you abuse alcohol or drugs, you can't have this treatment.

The pros and cons of an islet transplant

The advantages of the islet transplantation include

- ✔ Freedom from the need for insulin injections
- ✔ Reversal of long-term diabetic complications
- ✔ An end to hypoglycemia and hyperglycemia
- ✔ A return of hypoglycemic awareness

Several risks are associated with islet transplantation. They include the following:

- ✔ Danger of bleeding because heparin is given to prevent clotting of the portal vein for the injection
- ✔ All the risks of the antirejection drugs used for intact pancreas transplantation (which I cover earlier in this chapter), including increased blood pressure, increased blood fats, and decreased kidney function
- ✔ Potential worsening of diabetes-related eye disease, requiring laser surgery

The outcome for islet transplantation isn't nearly as good as intact pancreas transplantation. At one year after surgery, 70 percent of patients don't need insulin injections, but at four years, the number drops to 20 percent. For intact pancreas transplantation, the continued success at four years is 70 percent.

Even partial success in an islet transplant makes a big difference in the quality of life of the patient with diabetes who has severe up-and-down blood glucose or hypoglycemic unawareness.

A few variations on islet transplantation

Three new developments in the transplantation of islets are experimental, just like the original procedure.

✔ Microencapsulated islet cells have been used for transplantation. The cells are coated with gum-like materials so that other cells that promote rejection as well as the antibodies that attempt to do the same are prevented from getting to the islets. If this were successful, there would be no need for antirejection drugs.

✔ *Stem cells,* the cells in the body that haven't yet changed for a specific function, have

been made to evolve into beta cells. However, scientists are having difficulty generating sufficient numbers of stem cells to eliminate the need for insulin.

✔ Animal islets, particularly from pigs, are being evaluated for transplantation into humans. However, the body would try to reject these islets even harder than it tries to reject human islets.

The problems associated with the last two possibilities mean it will be years before doctors and researchers see the benefits of stem cell or animal islet transplantation.

Considering the costs

Patients currently don't pay for the islet transplantation procedure because it's in clinical evaluation.

The donation of islets

Islets are obtained from a deceased donor who had previously agreed to donate his pancreas. It takes six to eight hours to extract the islets from a pancreas. The recipient needs 10,000 islets per kilogram of body weight to be free of the need to take insulin shots. For a 150-pound male, for example, that would be 700,000 islets.

Even though each pancreas has a million islets, the extraction process isn't perfect, and it takes two to four pancreases to get the required number. However, even the islets from a single pancreas will greatly improve diabetic control, converting a person with very unstable blood glucose levels into a much more stable patient.

The process of surgery and recovery

If you're receiving an islet transplant, an area of your abdomen is numbed with anesthesia. Under radiologic observation, the radiologist injects the donated cells into your portal vein, which drains into the liver. (Figure 13-2 shows the process of extracting and transplanting islets.) The transplanted islets stick to the liver. They take days to weeks to make enough insulin to supplant the external source of insulin, which is gradually tapered down to nothing.

An uncomplicated islet transplant takes one hour and should keep you in the hospital no more than a few days.

The use of antirejection drugs followed in the clinical trials is based upon the Edmonton Protocol. However, several of the drugs in this formulation make the blood glucose higher.

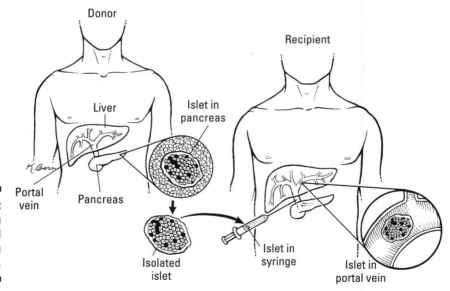

Figure 13-2: Extracting and injecting islets.

Dealing with Continuing Issues after Any Transplant

It would be wonderful if you could forget about your diabetes after you've had any type of transplantation. Unfortunately, you need to remain alert to several issues, as I explain in the following sections.

Following up and treating your diabetes

The follow-up is similar for all types of transplantation:

- ✔ You go back to the clinic for tests of function and any need for insulin injections.

- ✔ You measure your blood glucose frequently, looking for signs of a sudden need for more. An increase indicates that the transplant is failing, probably due to rejection.

- ✔ At first, the levels of the antirejection drugs in your blood are measured. After blood levels have stabilized, they're checked once a month.

The need for insulin diminishes immediately or within days of a transplant. It's important to measure your blood glucose frequently to know when you may reduce your insulin shots. Hypoglycemic episodes and brittleness of the diabetes (frequent and unexpected ups and downs in the blood glucose) improve within one month of the transplant.

Checking for long-term complications

Obviously, depending on how long you've had T1DM, you may have some evidence of diabetic complications after a transplant. The following is still necessary to watch for potential problems:

- ✔ Eye exams must continue once a year even though your blood glucose is now normal because the progression of eye disease doesn't stop abruptly after transplantation.

- ✔ Foot exams must continue, especially if you've had neuropathy (see Chapter 5). You must have your feet checked for sensation and examine them regularly for cuts and infections that you may not be able to feel.

Check out Chapter 7 for general information on eye and foot examinations.

Avoiding infections

After transplantation, you're on potent drugs that block immunity, so you're at risk for severe infection. Make sure that you get immunized for pneumonia with pneumococcal vaccine and that you get an annual influenza vaccination. Washing your hands regularly and practicing good dental care are also ways of preventing the occurrence of infections.

Being careful with conception

Antirejection drugs have been associated with reduced fertility in women. If they do get pregnant, they have more complications of pregnancy than women who don't take these drugs. They may have more infections, high blood pressure, swelling, and even loss of the transplanted organ. For these reasons, it's suggested that women who want to become pregnant after transplantation of the kidney and/or pancreas wait at least one year until their condition stabilizes. There aren't sufficient studies of pregnancy in women who have undergone islet transplantation, but common sense suggests that waiting a year for stabilization of the transplant is a good idea.

As far as breastfeeding is concerned, the effect of the drugs on the infant has not been clarified. The drugs do enter the breast milk, so monitoring the levels of antirejection drugs in the baby is recommended.

Flip to Chapter 16 for general information on handling pregnancy smoothly when you're a T1DM patient.

Watching out for cancer

The overall incidence of cancer after transplantation is low (less than 1 to 2 percent). However, the risk still exists, so it's wise to know the possibilities:

- The antirejection drugs increase your risk for cancer, especially a form called *posttransplant lymphoproliferative disease* (PTLD). PTLD has the following characteristics:

    - It's more common in patients under age 18.

    - Caucasian males have a higher incidence than others.

    - It can occur in a single site or multiple sites in the body.

    - Treatment may require stopping the antirejection drugs.

- Cervical cancer occurs more frequently after transplants and should be prevented by regular pelvic exams.

Finding More Information Online

Before you have a transplant, you may want to find out where they're having the best results and a lot more. The place to go is the U.S. Registry of Transplant Recipients at www.ustransplant.org. Here you can find national transplant statistics as well as annual reports that address waiting lists, immunosuppressive drugs, survival of the organs, survival of the patients, and a lot more.

Another valuable site for more information on kidney and pancreas transplantation is the National Diabetes Information Clearinghouse at `diabetes.niddk.nih.gov`. You should be able to find answers to all your questions at this site. But if not, I recommend heading to one more Web site: the National Kidney Foundation at `www.kidney.org`.

The National Kidney Foundation's site has a search box to help you locate information quickly and easily. (When I entered "kidney transplantation," it came back with 2,800 articles on the topic!)

These three sites will keep you busy until you're notified that your kidney and/or pancreas is ready and waiting for you so that you can begin your new life free from injections and free from dialysis.

Part IV
Living with Type 1 Diabetes

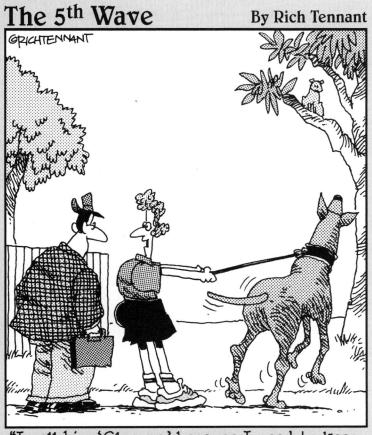

The 5th Wave — By Rich Tennant

"I call him 'Glucose,' because I need to keep him under control every day."

In this part . . .

People don't live in isolation. They have jobs and families, parents and children. They go through many stages in their lives: childhood and school, adulthood and work, fertility and menopause, and finally the "golden" years. Type 1 diabetes affects every one of those stages in different ways. Part IV provides you with a roadmap of your child's life as someone with type 1 diabetes and what direction to go at every turn. (This also applies to you if you're the patient.)

Chapter 14

Adjusting to School, Work, and Other Activities

....

In This Chapter

▶ Accommodating diabetes in school

▶ Making diabetes work in the workplace

▶ Hitting the road safely: Driving with diabetes

▶ Getting insurance coverage

....

*Y*our child with diabetes not only has to deal with the medical consequences of type 1 diabetes (T1DM) but the social and economic
consequences as well. You want him to get the best education possible —
the same as a child without diabetes. And when he gets older, you want your
child not to face discrimination in getting a job. Then there's the issue of
health insurance for your child with diabetes; you want a rate that doesn't
bankrupt you, and you want him to have the same reasonable rate when the
time comes that he's dealing with his own insurance.

Relax! Those who have come before you have faced all these problems, and
with the help of a beneficent government prodded by many organizations
like the American Diabetes Association and the Juvenile Diabetes Research
Foundation, most of the issues have been managed in a very satisfactory
manner. (I provide contact information for these organizations and others
in Appendix B.)

There's plenty of help out there for you, the parent of a child with diabetes,
but you have to be assertive and make sure your child gets all that is coming
to him. I think you'll be satisfied with the result. This chapter tells you what
you need to know to be the best possible advocate for your child (or yourself).

Dealing with Diabetes in School

If you're the parent of a child with T1DM about to enter school, you're probably concerned about whether your child will get the same education as a child who doesn't have diabetes. The answer is a definite yes if your child goes to a school (public or private) that gets federal funding assistance. In return for these funds, schools have agreed to abide by federal laws concerning the treatment of students with any type of handicap. Three key laws apply to your child entering school:

- ✔ **The Americans with Disabilities Act** says that schools and day care centers can't discriminate against handicapped children.

- ✔ **Section 504 of the Rehabilitation Act of 1973** prohibits discrimination against anyone in an activity that receives federal funding. Children with T1DM qualify for protection under this act. It states that the parents of a qualifying child have the right to develop a Section 504 Plan with the school for their child.

- ✔ **The Individuals with Disabilities Education Act** mandates that the federal government help state and local agencies provide a "free, appropriate education" to any child who qualifies. Under this act, the parents of a qualifying child have the right to develop an Individualized Education Program, which is similar to a Section 504 Plan but more detailed.

In the following sections, you come to understand what a Section 504 Plan is, how to set one up for your child, and how to follow through to make sure that your child gets the excellent education he deserves.

Developing a Section 504 Plan

Essentially, a Section 504 Plan stipulates how your child's diabetes will be handled at school; it gets into specifics about certain allowances that will be made for your child as well as adults at the school who will be expected to monitor your child's condition and help him if needed. You create a Section 504 Plan together with the school officials and any expert you bring to the meeting. For example, you may want to bring a Diabetes Educator or even an attorney if you sense some resistance on the part of school officials.

The following sections tell you what to do to get a Section 504 Plan in place for your child and also what types of clauses the plan should include.

Working with teachers and school staff

A Section 504 Plan doesn't create itself. So how do you get the ball rolling on the road to a safe and accommodating school experience for your child with type 1 diabetes? Follow these steps:

1. **As a parent, you bring the fact that your child qualifies for a Section 504 Plan to the attention of the school's administrators.**

2. **You give consent for the school to evaluate your child and determine if he qualifies for a plan.**

3. **Assuming he qualifies, a team of regular and special education teachers, nurses, and others such as dietitians and diabetes educators meet to develop a plan with you and your child if he's mature enough to participate.**

4. **The plan is carried out and reviewed at a minimum of three-year intervals.**

A typical Section 504 Plan requires at least two adults at a child's school to be educated and trained to deal with the child's diabetes; the school is responsible for assigning these adults and making sure they're properly trained. You can find a valuable resource to help from the Juvenile Diabetes Research Foundation at www.jdrf.org. Select "Life with Diabetes," and then click on "Type 1 Diabetes in School." You'll find a School Information Packet containing everything your school needs to know about the child with diabetes. You can order the packet from the Web site and take it to the school as part of setting up the Section 504 Plan.

Getting down to plan specifics

If you aren't happy with the complete Section 504 Plan, you can sign only those parts that you agree with while you continue to negotiate other parts. As your child's needs change, you need to change the plan together with the school officials.

The Section 504 Plan should be as detailed as possible, leaving little room for interpretation. Here are some of the clauses that need to be in your plan:

- ✔ The child may use the bathroom without restriction.

- ✔ The child may have immediate access to water, including a water bottle at his desk.

- ✔ The child may have snacks at his desk or at any school location, including on the school bus.

- ✔ The child may see the school nurse at any time, and hypoglycemia should be treated immediately.

- ✔ The child may test his blood glucose and use insulin (if appropriate to the child's age) during school hours. He also has permission to carry these items at all times.

- ✔ Blood glucose tests may be done anywhere in school.

- ✔ The child may participate in all field trips and extracurricular activities.

- ✔ If the child takes a break for his diabetes during a classroom assignment or test, he will be given an opportunity to make up the missed work.

✔ If the child's blood glucose is greater than 240 mg/dl before heavy exercise, he may be excused, checked for ketones, and given water and insulin as necessary.

✔ The child won't be penalized for being absent or late due to medical appointments or activities involved in controlling his blood glucose.

✔ The child's blood glucose meter and insulin must accompany him during a fire drill.

✔ Two adults (a primary caregiver and a back-up) must be trained to recognize hypoglycemia and to administer glucose, glucagon, or insulin as needed.

✔ The school nurse will have a copy of the plan.

This is a typical plan for a small child who takes insulin shots. If your child switches to an insulin pump (see Chapter 11 for pump particulars), you and school officials must add the various requirements for that form of treatment, including pump training for an adult.

To see a typical 504 Plan for a child at every age from 4 to 17, visit www. childrenwithdiabetes.com/504. Just click on the age of the child and the type of treatment. Remember that these plans are simply illustrations and the plan for your child will depend upon his special needs.

Considering an individualized education program

If T1DM makes your child unable to learn with the rest of his class (because he suffers from frequent hypoglycemia or frequent hyperglycemia, for example), he may need an individualized education program. This is a detailed program for his education based on the requirements of his diabetes as well as his special education needs. It's more of an education program than a health program, which is why I don't get into it extensively in this book. The need for this type of program is determined by parents and school officials working together. For a complete guide to the individualized education program and a program document template, visit www.ed.gov/parents/needs/speced/iepguide/index.html#form.

Handling diabetes in college

After your child has gotten through high school, it's assumed that he's old enough and responsible enough to take care of his diabetes. If he's heading off to college, encourage him to notify the health team at the college of his diabetes. Health officials need to know about his medications, the history of his diabetes, and his treatment plan. He also should take his college roommate into his confidence so that someone very close to him is aware of his condition and in a position to help if needed. A student living in a dorm should notify the dorm staff and make sure that someone there knows about high and low blood glucose problems. He doesn't have to tell his professors as long as the student health program knows about him and his condition.

Living with Diabetes as a Working Adult

Type 1 diabetes affects all aspects of life if you're the patient. In this section, you discover the professional limitations that T1DM causes you as a working adult. You also find out how to use the legal protections that exist for you.

Understanding limits and protections

Today, diabetes isn't the obstacle that it once was, but there are still a few jobs that you (or your grown child) can't have if you have T1DM. These jobs have a blanket ban against people with diabetes, so if you have the disease, you can't have the job no matter what your condition. Among these jobs are:

- ✔ Armed forces
- ✔ Commercial airline pilot
- ✔ Fire services
- ✔ Jobs requiring a large goods- or passenger-carrying vehicle license
- ✔ Police services
- ✔ Train driving
- ✔ Working at heights

Advancements in diabetes management and glucose control are slowly but surely wiping out the blanket ban. For example, there used to be a blanket ban on people with diabetes working as any type of airline pilot. Then it was recognized that with proper precautions, a person with T1DM can safely fly a private plane. It's expected that soon the door will be opened to working as a commercial pilot as well.

As a person with T1DM, you're protected in the workplace by the Americans with Disabilities Act. The U.S. Court of Appeals ruled in 1998 that the act, which applies to employers with 15 or more employees, protects people with diabetes. It's illegal for your employer to ask if you have diabetes, but he can request that you undergo a physical examination to determine if you're well enough to do the job. Years earlier, the Federal Rehabilitation Act of 1973 accomplished the same thing for anyone applying for a federal job or a job with a company that receives federal aid.

These laws put the burden on the employer to show that the employee isn't qualified to do the job. If the employee is qualified for the job (just like anyone else) and his diabetes requires some reasonable accommodation, like allowing him to eat on the job as necessary or go to the bathroom, the employer must comply.

 With all the different kinds of insulin and delivery systems that are available now (see Chapters 10 and 11), it should be possible for you to accommodate any work schedule. It's true, however, that you'll have difficult time keeping your blood glucose normal if you have to constantly change work shifts, so a job with a changing schedule may not be the best choice for you if you have T1DM.

The real risk of hypoglycemia in the workplace

A study in *Diabetes Care* in June 2005 represents an important accomplishment for people who take insulin. In this study, researchers looked at 243 employees (ranging in age from 20 to 69) who were taking insulin for diabetes. Over a 12-month period, researchers recorded the frequency, severity, and consequences of hypoglycemia occurring at work or elsewhere. (They focused on hypoglycemia because it's the most common complication that employers point to as the reason they don't want to hire people with diabetes.)

During the period of study, there were 1,995 episodes of hypoglycemia that were mild and could be treated by the patients. There were an additional 238 severe episodes that required help from someone else. Of the severe episodes, 62 percent happened at home, 15 percent occurred at work, and 23 percent occurred elsewhere. (Fifty-two percent of the severe episodes occurred during sleep.)

As for the consequences of severe hypoglycemia, 14 percent of the patients being studied lost consciousness, 9 percent had seizures, 2 percent had head injuries, 2 percent had other injuries, 1 percent injured someone else, and 1 percent damaged property. Severe hypoglycemia in the workplace was associated with six episodes of minor soft-tissue injury.

The authors concluded the following about severe hypoglycemia in the workplace:

- ✔ It's uncommon.
- ✔ It seldom causes disruption.
- ✔ It rarely causes serious health effects to the patient or others.
- ✔ Its infrequency and mild effects in the workplace don't justify restriction of employment for people with diabetes who take insulin.

Taking action if you suspect discrimination related to diabetes

If you feel that you're suffering from discrimination in the workplace because of your diabetes, you have several options for handling it. Begin by talking to your supervisor. If that doesn't work, you can

- ✔ Hire an attorney and sue the company.
- ✔ Ask your union to file a grievance.
- ✔ Contact the U.S. Equal Employment Opportunity Commission (EEOC) at www.eeoc.gov or call 800-669-4000.

Unfortunately the Bush administration has reduced the staff of the EEOC by 20 percent and a reduced budget in the EEOC has resulted in a huge backlog of cases at present. You may want to turn to one of the other options listed here to get your complaint handled in a timely fashion.

Most employee complaints related to diabetes are surprisingly modest. For example, perhaps the employer won't allow the employee to snack when his glucose is low, give him a place to do a blood glucose test, or provide predictable hours.

Employers win more cases than employees. The employee has to prove that he's disabled for the law to be on his side, and that can be difficult. In past cases, judges have decided that a store manager who couldn't walk because of poor circulation and a security guard who had lost vision in one eye and was losing vision in the other were not disabled.

Working together: Helping employers integrate employees with diabetes

If you have T1DM, you can help your employer meet the standards for helping you and others like you to be as productive as everyone else. I recommend that you bring the information in this section to the attention of your employer.

There's an enormous amount that a company can do to integrate its employees with diabetes. After all, they're some of the most skillful employees and their loss would be felt in the company's bottom line.

The government has set up a Web site to help employers hire and accommodate people with diabetes successfully. At www.diabetesatwork.org/ diabetesatwork, you can find many case studies of companies that have successfully integrated people with diabetes into their staff. Some of the other valuable information you'll find on the site includes:

✔ Guidance on making a case for and developing a diabetes prevention and management program.

✔ Recommendations for healthier eating in the workplace.

✔ Suggestions for controlling obesity in the workplace.

✔ A way to estimate the number of people with diabetes in your company. This information gives the employer an idea of the magnitude of the problem, and he'll be much more accommodating when he realizes how common it is.

✔ A formula for determining the cost of health care for the people with diabetes in your company. (At the time of the writing of this book, this formula was being revised to reflect the fact that diabetes is generally better controlled than in the past, thus avoiding the higher costs for complications of diabetes.) This information helps your employer to plan appropriate health insurance for his employees.

The case studies show how a company can save a lot of money on medical expenses while greatly increasing the health and morale of employees with diabetes. For example, the clothing and outdoor equipment retailer Lands' End, which has more than 7,000 employees, adopted a Diabetes Prevention and Management Program that included:

✔ Support groups and talks on general health as well as diabetes-specific topics

✔ A disease management module

✔ Regular A1c testing (see Chapter 7) and screening for diabetes

As a result, the company was able to slow the increase in medical costs to 3 percent compared to a national average of 12 percent in 2002. The next year, Lands' End's medical costs increased only 2 percent compared to a national average of 13 percent. The company's diabetes program continues to have great success.

Driving Safely with Type 1 Diabetes

When your child has diabetes and is of driving age, he can't just hop in the car and hit the open road like someone without the disease. T1DM shouldn't hold him back; it just requires that he take a few extra steps and monitor himself along the way. (If you're the patient, the same goes for you!) Share these keys to driving safely with diabetes with your child:

- Know your blood glucose before you start to drive. If it's below 90 mg/dl, eat something before you drive.

- Keep a source of glucose that won't spoil where you can reach it as you drive.

- Check your blood glucose at least hourly by pulling over and using your meter.

- If there's any question in your mind that you may be hypoglycemic, pull off and test your blood glucose. If it's low, take glucose and make sure that the level is above 90 mg/dl before you resume driving.

Check the stats on diabetes and car crashes

In 2003, seven diabetes clinics in the United States and four in Europe pooled the results of an anonymous questionnaire about diabetes and driving given to both type 1 and type 2 diabetes patients. The study was published in *Diabetes Care* in August 2003. Here are the highlights of the findings:

- Drivers with T1DM reported more crashes, moving violations, severe hypoglycemia, and need for assistance while driving compared to drivers with T2DM and their non-diabetic spouses.

- Drivers with T2DM (including those who took insulin) had no more frequent crashes than their non-diabetic spouses.

- The drivers with T1DM who crashed tested their blood glucose less often than drivers with T1DM who didn't crash.

- Drivers with T1DM who used insulin pumps crashed less often than those who used injections.

- Nearly half of the drivers with T1DM had never spoken with their doctors about diabetes and driving.

- Despite the higher frequency of crashes in patients with T1DM than with T2DM, it's less than half the frequency of crashes in patients with other medical conditions that have no driving restrictions, including sleep apnea and attention deficit/hyperactivity disorder.

- Crashes involving a driver with T1DM are far less frequent than crashes involving a person under the age of 20 as a percentage of the numbers in each group.

Individual states issue drivers' licenses, and the applications don't consistently ask about diabetes. They usually ask about any general condition that would impair safe driving. In California, where I live and practice, the Department of Motor Vehicles requires a doctor to certify that the person with T1DM follows a good medical plan with frequent blood glucose testing, is free of frequent hypoglycemia, and can safely operate a motor vehicle.

You can find out the regulations concerning driving with T1DM at the Bureau of Motor Vehicles in your area. Having T1DM doesn't usually have any adverse effect on your auto insurance.

Tackling Insurance Issues

Health insurance and life insurance are tough issues for anyone with a chronic disease. Insurers don't like risks and resist insuring people who may actually use their insurance. Nevertheless, although it may take longer to find a policy and it may cost more, you *can* get insurance for yourself or your child with T1DM.

Health insurance

A child with T1DM is insured under your policy as his parent, and the health insurance usually comes through your job. When your child becomes an adult and enters the workforce, his company is likely to have a group insurance policy that he enrolls in, generally without penalty for being a person with diabetes. No law mandates that health insurance must be provided to employees; in many cases, employer health insurance coverage arose as an incentive to attract employees and keep them with the company.

You can turn to *Insurance For Dummies* by Jack Hungelmann (Wiley) for more coverage of health insurance than I have room to provide here. This section looks at health insurance specifically as it applies to coverage for someone with T1DM.

When it comes to getting insurance as a person with type 1 diabetes, there are plenty of protections in place if you understand them and know how to use them. One such protection is the Employee Retirement Income Security Act (ERISA), which regulates employee group health plans. If your child has T1DM (or you do), the ERISA rule that you can appreciate the most is that an employer health plan can't discriminate against your child (or you) by refusing to let him join or charging you more if he has an illness.

The Health Insurance Portability and Accountability Act (HIPPA) limits the time that you can be excluded from a company health plan because of a prior illness. That means that if you have T1DM when you join the company, the company must offer you health insurance within a reasonable time if all other employees have it.

There are basically two types of health insurance:

- **Fee-for-service plans** pay the provider (a doctor or hospital) based on the number of services provided. It's to the provider's advantage to perform more services.

- **Health Maintenance Organizations (HMOs)** charge the same for all members, dividing the risk among more expensive and less expensive patients. The fewer services that the provider actually performs, the more the provider takes home, so HMOs try to enroll the healthiest population possible to avoid the higher costs of sickness.

It's common for companies to give employees the choice between a fee-for-service plan and an HMO. As someone looking to insure either your child or yourself with T1DM, you need to anticipate using your insurance coverage more than someone without diabetes. Under those circumstances, you need to keep in mind that generally the HMO costs you less but the fee-for-service plan allows you a much wider choice of doctors and hospitals. The following are some particularly important considerations to make and questions to ask about insurance coverage when choosing a plan:

- What's the total annual cost of the plan? How much does your employer pay, and how much do you pay?

- Do you have to pay a certain amount (called the *deductible*) before the insurance kicks in and begins to pay?

- Do you have a *co-payment* (an amount you pay every time you use a provider), and how much is it?

- Will your plan pay for durable medical equipment like an insulin pump, which is expensive?

- Will your plan pay for diabetes medication and supplies?

- Is your physician restricted to prescribing certain medications?

- Can you get a 90-day supply of drugs, or do you have to go back to the pharmacy (and pay another co-payment) every 30 days?

- Are you covered for specialists like eye doctors, neurologists, and kidney doctors?

- Are you limited to using certain doctors or hospitals that may not be convenient?

- Is home health care included?

Each state also has its laws about how medical insurance can be offered. The best place to find the information for your state is the Web site of the Georgetown University Health Policy Institute at ihcrp.georgetown.edu. Go to healthinsuranceinfo.net to access the consumer guide for health insurance for your state. The Health Policy Institute site also has a lot of information about social and health issues that may apply to you, like the Center on an Aging Society and the Long-Term Care Financing Project. It's amazing how much valuable information is at your fingertips!

Life insurance

As you would expect with T1DM, it's a little harder and more expensive to obtain life insurance than if you (or your child) had no medical condition, but it is out there. One bright spot is that premiums are coming down as insurance companies realize that people with diabetes can live a lot longer than they used to.

Because you (or your child) have T1DM, you're said to have an *impaired risk*. Some insurance agents specialize in obtaining insurance for people who have an impaired risk. The best way to find these agents is to just pick up the phone and start calling. Briefly explain your condition, and ask if they can get insurance for you.

One of the best things you can do to make yourself more attractive to life insurance providers is maximize the control of your blood glucose, blood pressure, and blood fats. Insurance companies look favorably on someone who has these elements of T1DM under control and therefore is in better health than someone who doesn't. Turn to Chapter 7 for information and advice on managing blood glucose and other key elements.

Chapter 15

Managing Illness and Travel

In This Chapter

▶ Taking care on sick days

▶ Hitting the road with type 1 diabetes

*T*wo situations are particularly challenging for both the parent of a child with type 1 diabetes (T1DM) and adults with T1DM: days in which the patient is sick with some other illness and days in which the patient travels. In this chapter, I tell you everything you need to know to manage these two difficult situations.

Although the emphasis in this book is on controlling the blood glucose as tightly as possible, it's better to err of the side of looser control when the patient is sick with another illness or is traveling because the scenario doesn't usually last long. A person with T1DM who's sick or is traveling through time zones and is very tired is much better off with a blood glucose of 225 mg/dl than a blood glucose of 25 mg/dl. A few days of above-normal glucose levels don't cause any lasting damage.

Dealing with Sick Days

Three of the basic tools of good diabetes care become even more important when your child with T1DM is sick or traveling: frequent monitoring of the blood glucose, careful food choices, and timely medication. During sickness, blood glucose levels tend to be higher than expected and you can't know that unless you measure it. Food may be limited to a few items that your child can tolerate, and he may need surprisingly more insulin than you expect, especially because he's eating little.

Discuss how to handle illness with your child's doctor before it happens. Make a sick-day plan and find out the doctor's rules for contacting him in case of illness.

Children whose diabetes is under good control (that is, hemoglobin A1c is less than 8 percent; see Chapter 7 for details) don't develop illnesses any more frequently than children without diabetes. In any case, preventing illness is much better than treating it. One major preventive measure is making sure that your child gets a flu shot every year. This section covers other ways to prevent and deal with illness in your child with T1DM.

Monitoring the blood glucose

You may think that a sick child should have lower blood glucose, especially if he has nausea and vomiting. This isn't the case, however. Don't assume that your child's blood glucose falls because he can't eat. Illness provokes the body to secrete hormones such as cortisol and glucagon that tend to raise the blood glucose. Illness also increases insulin resistance, so a given amount of insulin doesn't lower the blood glucose as much as usual.

When your child is sick, allowing looser control of his diabetes is perfectly okay; a slightly higher blood glucose reading is safer than a reading that's too low. That said, it's also true that the more the blood glucose is kept within the normal range, the more rapidly a child (or an adult, for that matter) can recover from any illness. White blood cells, which fight bacteria and viruses, function much better when the blood glucose is normal.

Measure the blood glucose every two hours when your child is sick, and give extra rapid-acting insulin if necessary. (Readings above 250 mg/dl require more insulin, but don't give it any more often than every four hours because a shot lasts the same amount of time.) How much extra insulin you give depends upon your child's size, his usual insulin dose, and his response to insulin when he's sick. The smaller the usual dose, the smaller the increase needed to keep the glucose under control. A fever that's over 100 degrees F requires an even greater increase in insulin, sometimes as much as 25 to 50 percent more than usual.

A child who's getting his basal insulin from long-acting insulin such as glargine or detemir (see Chapter 10) may need a temporary increase in the dose of that medication. If the blood glucose is higher throughout the day, more long-acting insulin is indicated. The increase is proportional to the amount he's taking already. For example, a child taking 10 units of glargine may need 12 units during the illness, and a child taking 20 units may need 25 units during the illness. Remember, these are approximations. Your child's needs may be different.

Is your child on an insulin pump (or are you, if you're the patient)? Elevated blood glucose levels above 200 mg/dl throughout the day suggest the need for an increase in the basal rate. If his usual basal rate is 1 unit per hour, he may go up to 3 units per hour during a period of illness. The blood glucose should respond within one to two hours. If it doesn't, he may not be getting the insulin, and a switch to insulin shots temporarily may be in order. (Refer to Chapter 11 for full details on using an insulin pump.) Talk to your child's doctor before making this switch.

One illness that may call for *less* insulin is gastroenteritis. The usual symptoms are vomiting and diarrhea, both of which decrease the amount of food that stays in the body. And that means that the blood glucose may fall significantly. If your child has gastroenteritis, measure his glucose every two hours, and don't give rapid-acting insulin if the glucose is below 100 mg/dl. You may need to reduce the dose of long-acting insulin as well; the reduction is proportional to how much he takes already. If your child can hold down small sips of drinks containing glucose, such as apple juice or ginger ale, and can maintain a glucose level over 100 mg/dl, he doesn't need to go to the hospital. If he can't do these things, call the doctor.

When the glucose goes up to 250 mg/dl or higher, you should measure the urine ketones as I explain in Chapter 7, especially if your child's vomiting. A high ketone reading is highly suggestive of diabetic ketoacidosis (see Chapter 5). This is one reason to call your child's doctor or take him to the hospital emergency room. Other reasons include:

- Vomiting more than one time
- Diarrhea more than four times or persisting longer than 24 hours
- Stomach pain
- Rapid, hard breathing with a fruity odor to the breath
- Increasing weakness and drowsiness

As your child begins to eat normally and has a more normal temperature, and as his blood glucose stays down under 150 mg/dl, cut back on extra doses of rapid-acting insulin, long-acting insulin, or the increased basal rate on a pump. He should be back to baseline medication levels in two or three days.

Measuring blood ketones

Blood ketone testing may prove even more useful than urine ketone testing during illness. It's done with a finger stick drop of blood applied to a blood ketone test strip. At present, only two home meters provide blood ketone readings: the Precision Xtra Blood Glucose Meter (refer to Chapter 7) and the CardioChek Blood Testing Device (which can test blood glucose, blood ketones, cholesterol, HDL cholesterol, and triglycerides when the proper test strip is used).

The advantage of blood ketone testing is similar to the advantage of blood glucose testing: Ketones rise in the blood earlier than in the urine, so the earlier the ketones are noted to be abnormal, the earlier treatment can proceed. A study published in *Diabetic Medicine* in March 2006 showed a large reduction in patient time spent in the hospital when blood ketone testing was done compared to urine ketone testing. Another advantage is the ease of obtaining a drop of blood compared with urine from a small child.

The disadvantages at present are the cost (about $3 to $4 per test compared to less than 20 cents for urine testing) and the fact that only two meters can do the test.

If you test for ketones with the blood test, the interpretation for adults and children is as follows:

- Above 1.5 mmol/L with high (greater than 250 mg/dl) blood glucose means that your child is at high risk to develop diabetic ketoacidosis. Call your doctor immediately.

- 0.6 to 1.5 mmol/L with high blood glucose means less risk. Treat with fluids and insulin, and let your doctor know that your child is showing this level.

- Less than 0.6 mmol/L is normal.

Modifying the diet

Most illnesses in children don't last more than a few days. During that time, the emphasis should be on keeping the blood glucose from going too high (above 250 mg/dl) or too low (below 80 mg/dl) — not on whether the child is getting enough protein, fat, vitamins, or minerals. (See the previous section for details on carefully monitoring the blood glucose during illness.)

If your child's illness allows him to eat normally, by all means encourage that. If he experiences nausea, vomiting, or both, focus on getting him carbohydrate that's rapidly absorbed into the bloodstream (see the following list). It's also important to keep him well hydrated, but he probably can't tolerate a lot of fluid at one time. Give him small sips of tea with sugar, fruit juice, or soft drinks with real sugar, not diet drinks, encouraging him to drink four times an hour.

The following contain 15 grams of carbohydrate that's rapidly absorbed:

- 1 tablespoon honey
- 4 teaspoons granulated white sugar
- ½ cup fruit juice
- ⅓ cup plain pudding

> ✔ ½ cup ice cream
>
> ✔ One small frozen juice bar

Give your child the honey or table sugar in particular if his glucose is low (under 80 mg/dl). You can use the other items in the list to encourage some nutrition when the child refuses to eat regular food.

If your child becomes dehydrated, give him a drink that consists of 4 cups water, ½ teaspoon salt, and 2 tablespoons granulated white sugar. (If the child has a blood glucose level over 250 mg/dl, reduce the amount of sugar in the concoction to 1 tablespoon.) Give him 1 ounce of this drink per year of age per hour. For example, an 8-year-old should drink 8 ounces of this drink per hour or 2 ounces every 15 minutes. Adults can drink apple juice or ginger ale to maintain their hydration.

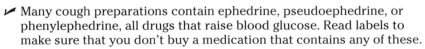

Taking medications

If your child has a cough, you may want to give some over-the-counter medicine to suppress it, but keep the following points in mind:

> ✔ A cough helps to get rid of secretions in the lungs that make breathing more difficult, so you shouldn't suppress it completely.
>
> ✔ Most over-the-counter cough preparations contain a lot of sugar and alcohol. These ingredients may provide some of the calories the child is missing, but they also may raise an already high blood glucose even higher.

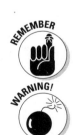

> Many preparations of cough medicine don't contain sugar, so *read the label!* Also, if you see "DM" in the name of the medicine, it usually means that it doesn't contain sugar.
>
> ✔ Many cough preparations contain ephedrine, pseudoephedrine, or phenylephedrine, all drugs that raise blood glucose. Read labels to make sure that you don't buy a medication that contains any of these.

If your child has a fever, you can use acetaminophen (Tylenol) to bring it down. If you or your child needs antibiotics, ones that lower the blood glucose and are safe for folks with T1DM include chloramphenicol (brand name Chloromycetin) and the sulfa drugs with brand names like Gantrisin, Septra, and Bactrim.

Ibuprofen is sometimes used for inflammation, but it can cause kidney failure in people with diabetes who already have kidney damage. Check with your doctor before giving this to your child.

You can give your child medication for his illness at any time it's needed because it doesn't interfere with his diabetes medications.

Traveling with Type 1 Diabetes

Traveling with a child is hard enough, but when the child also has T1DM, the challenges are that much greater. Be sure to think about the considerations in the following sections before you travel.

Carrying the necessities

Whether you travel by car, train, plane, or boat, make sure that the essentials of diabetes care are easy to access. If you're flying, all diabetes medications and equipment must be in carry-on baggage. You definitely don't want your child's insulin to end up in Chicago when you and he are in New York. In addition, checked luggage may be in an exceedingly cold part of the airplane, and freezing destroys insulin.

You have to follow the rules of the Transportation Security Administration (TSA) if you fly within the United States. (Airlines operating outside the U.S. may have different rules; check with your airline before you travel overseas.) The TSA instructs that you should "make sure injectable medications are properly labeled (professionally printed label identifying the medication or a manufacturer's name or pharmaceutical label). Notify the screener if you are carrying a hazardous waste container, refuse container, or a sharps disposable container in your carry-on baggage used to transport used syringes, lancets, etc." Updated information is available at the TSA Web site, www.tsa.gov/public/display?theme=1.

Although it's not essential, a letter from your doctor stating that your child has diabetes and needs to carry the following list of medication supplies and testing equipment may be helpful and especially useful should he get sick while traveling. Carry twice as much of each item as you think you'll need; supplies can get lost, or you may be delayed or decide to stay longer.

- ✔ Insulin (long-acting and rapid-acting for syringe injection if necessary)
- ✔ Syringes or insulin pens
- ✔ Insulin pump supplies

    If your child uses an insulin pump, take an alternative form of insulin administration (such as an insulin pen or a bottle of insulin and a syringe) in case the pump breaks.

- ✔ Rapidly acting sugar source (glucose tablets are most convenient)
- ✔ Glucagon emergency kit with emergency shot (see Chapter 4)
- ✔ Medications for nausea (prochlorperazine) and diarrhea (loperamide)

✔ Medication for fever (acetaminophen)

✔ Glucose meter and spare batteries

✔ Test strips for glucose and ketones

✔ Lancets

✔ A container that allows you to keep insulin at the proper temperature, whether it's very cold or very hot

In addition, I recommend that you do the following:

✔ Carry the telephone numbers for your child's health care providers at home, and compile a list of English-speaking doctors at your destination if possible. At the least, have the name and address of the local American consulate and the local American Express office; either usually can arrange for you to see English-speaking doctors.

Consider taking advantage of free membership in the International Association for Medical Assistance to Travelers; on the association's Web site, www.iamat.org, you can sign up for membership and get the names of English-speaking doctors in most countries. You don't have to be a member to read about the latest medical alerts and problems in various countries.

✔ Make sure that your child is always wearing a bracelet or necklace identifying him as someone with T1DM.

✔ Take snacks to eat while traveling, and carry some bars or other packaged food to eat after arriving, too.

✔ Check your insurance policy to make sure that it covers your child at your destination. If it doesn't, get coverage that does. (I discuss the basics of insurance in Chapter 14.) Carry your insurance card, and leave photocopies of your card at your hotel.

Adjusting insulin intake in a different time zone

The old saying, "Go West, young man" could be altered to "Go West, young person with type 1 diabetes." When T1DM is involved, it's a lot easier to travel west than east over several time zones. Here are the differences in insulin intake depending on your child's time zone changes:

✔ You add hours to your day when you head west, so all your child has to do is check his blood glucose an extra time or two and add short-acting insulin to cover those hours. He doesn't change the long-acting insulin but resumes his usual schedule when he gets to the new time zone.

✔ When you head east, you lose hours. Given that, your child may have too much insulin when the long-acting combines with the rapid-acting to lower his blood glucose. He has to be proactive and reduce the long-acting insulin he takes just before the trip. The rule is to reduce it by 4 percent for every hour lost. For example, if his usual dose is 10 units of Lantus and he's traveling east through six time zones, he should take 6 × 4 percent, or 24 percent less insulin. That comes to 7½ units if the insulin can be measured in ½ units, or just 7 units if it can't be. Err on the side of conservatism. Give less rather than more insulin.

Folks using insulin pumps have the easiest time going through time zones. If your child (or you) uses a pump, he should continue the basal insulin as usual, taking boluses only when he eats meals. At the new time zone, he should change the time on his pump so that his basal schedule corresponds to the old time zone. (See Chapter 11 for details on using a pump.)

At your new time zone, no matter whether you've traveled east or west, your child will undoubtedly feel sleepy if the difference is more than four hours. Obviously, that's jet lag. Get your child back on his usual regimen of long-acting insulin but hold the rapid-acting insulin if he's going to sleep through a meal.

I find that I can acclimate myself to the new time zone, especially the more difficult eastern direction, if I exercise as early as possible in the new "morning." Thirty minutes on a treadmill or elliptical trainer allows me to stay awake in early morning meetings. Try this with your child to see if you both can overcome some jet lag. Early morning exercise also provides all the benefits of general exercise described in Chapter 9.

Eating sensibly

It's very difficult to know how much carbohydrate your child is eating when all the meals are in restaurants. You can start the trip carrying prepared nutrition bars that tell you how much carbohydrate is in each one, but you have to deal with unknown foods sooner or later.

If you're traveling in the United States, get online and search the Web sites of popular restaurant chains to see which ones exist at your destination. The sites should contain a list of the nutritional values for all the chain's menu items. Record what looks okay for your child and note the carbohydrates so that you can calculate his bolus dose for each meal.

Traveling outside the U.S. or eating in non-chain restaurants is a different matter. You can simplify the problem by sticking to the following menu items (and avoiding the fried foods and rich desserts!):

> ✔ **Breakfast:** Fresh fruit, yogurt, eggs, oatmeal, and whole-wheat toast with-out butter are all good choices. Avoid pancakes or waffles with syrup.
>
> ✔ **Lunch:** Grilled chicken, tuna, fresh green salad, fresh steamed vegetables, and egg salad without mayonnaise are all good choices. Avoid creamy dressings high in fat.
>
> ✔ **Dinner:** Turkey, tuna, salmon, whitefish, grilled chicken, fresh green salad, and fresh vegetables are all good choices.

Be careful about portions in restaurants. They're usually too large, even the children's sizes. Educate yourself on proper portion sizes of meat, chicken, pasta, and so forth before you leave home.

Of the various kinds of restaurants, probably the easiest place to find good choices for your child is a seafood restaurant. Just focus on fish dishes and stay away from fried anything (including French fries), tartar sauce, butter, and creamy dressings.

Keep some meal replacement bars handy for the times when you can't get to a restaurant. You also can give them to your child as snacks between meals to smooth out the blood glucose.

Alternately, you can try to stay in places where you have your own kitchen to make meals in, such as an extended-stay hotel or a rental house. Of course, making meals is hardly a vacation for you, but it won't be the first (or last) sacrifice you'll make for your precious offspring.

Ensuring a smooth journey

Here are some additional pointers for having a safe and enjoyable trip with a child with T1DM:

> ✔ Visit www.cdc.gov/vaccines to find out if your child (and you) needs vaccines for any of the countries you'll be visiting.
>
> ✔ If your child uses an insulin pump, consider switching him to insulin pens that don't require all the extras associated with the pump (like infusion sets). Talk to his doctor about it, and make the switch at least a week before you leave so that your child can transition smoothly in a setting where everything is more or less under your control.
>
> ✔ Have supplies sent to your various destinations or brought along by people you'll be meeting there so that they're fresh and you don't have to carry so much. (Bring enough supplies with you to handle any delays you encounter in foreign customs.)

✔ Learn to say "My child has diabetes" (or "I have diabetes") and "sugar or orange juice, please" in the language of your destination.

✔ Don't inject pre-meal insulin until the food comes on the plane or train.

✔ When traveling by air, have your child drink lots of fluids because airplane travel is dehydrating.

✔ Check for air bubbles that tend to form in insulin pens as a result of pressure differences in airplanes. Before using the pen, get rid of the bubbles by pushing them out of the pen as the needle points up.

✔ If you have to depend on foreign sources of insulin when you arrive, make sure that the insulin is U-100 (100 units per milliliter). U-40 and U-80 are no longer used in the United States but are still used in some foreign countries; if you can only get U-40 or U-80, you have to use U-40 or U-80 syringes to administer the proper dose.

Chapter 16

Going through Pregnancy and Menopause

*E*very pregnant woman wants a healthy baby. Before insulin, girls with diabetes rarely lived long enough to become pregnant, and if they did, their babies usually didn't survive. What a difference a hormone (insulin) makes! Today, it's possible for any woman with T1DM to become pregnant and to deliver a beautiful, healthy baby who will probably never get diabetes. There are a number of places along the pregnancy path where things can go wrong, however. The point of this chapter is to alert you to those places and get you past them with minimal difficulty.

There is one major factor that all pregnant women, diabetic or not, will agree to. They will do anything in their power to ensure the health of their growing baby. This makes excellent diabetes care during the time of pregnancy a lot easier to accomplish. Before getting to the time of pregnancy, I want you to understand what a healthy girl goes through to make her body ready for that miraculous task and what may go wrong if you have T1DM.

After the years when pregnancy is possible, the woman with T1DM has special challenges as she goes through menopause. Should she use hormone replacement therapy? What are the special considerations for the woman with T1DM as she ages so that she can enjoy a high quality of life for many years? I cover all these issues in this chapter.

Understanding Normal Female Sexual Development

A lot has to happen to prepare the body of any female to carry a successful pregnancy. It actually begins before birth and continues right up through *menarche,* the time at which female periods begin. Although T1DM occurs several years after birth, its effect on sexual development requires an understanding of how the female sex organs develop in the first place.

Starting before birth

Just six weeks after the baby is conceived, the presence or absence of a Y, or male, sex *chromosome* (the collection of genes that determine the characteristics of the body) leads to the production of testicles if present or ovaries if absent. If absent, a set of tubules present in both males and females develops into the female structures of the fallopian tubes that carry the egg to the uterus.

The lack of testosterone in the female also causes the brain to develop female sexual characteristics in a structure called the *hypothalamus,* which controls many of the body's glands, including ovaries in women and testicles in men. At puberty, the hypothalamus starts the monthly cycles that continue until menopause.

Continuing at puberty and adolescence

Puberty begins in girls around age 8 to 12. The hypothalamus causes the release of *hormones* (chemical messengers) that cause widespread body changes including the development of breasts, the rounding of the body seen in females, and the onset of menstrual periods by age 12 or 13. A girl develops underarm hair growth and more secretions from oil and sweat glands.

During adolescence, the girl begins to go through the social and emotional changes that end in adulthood. It starts around age 12 and ends around age 17. During this time, she may experience increased sexual behavior, including masturbation and sexual intercourse.

Normal menstrual function requires the coordinated release of a hormone from the hypothalamus, which causes release of hormones from the pituitary gland in the brain, resulting in the formation of a *follicle.* A follicle is a round area of cells in the ovary in which the egg rests waiting to be expelled at ovulation each month. Prior to ovulation, the follicle produces estrogen.

After ovulation takes place, the follicle transforms into a corpus luteum, which produces progesterone and estrogen, in order to prepare the uterus for implantation of a fertilized egg. If the egg doesn't get fertilized, progesterone secretion ceases and the uterus sheds its lining, producing a menstrual period.

Controlling Type 1 Diabetes before Conception

In the following sections, you find out how to manage a number of the special considerations of being a female with T1DM. I address specific topics including how to handle your glucose during the ups and downs of menstruation, how to prepare your body for a pregnancy, and how to get through the pregnancy with minimal trouble for you and your growing baby.

Handling blood glucose during your menstrual periods

Because sex organs are formed before the onset of T1DM in females, they're usually normal. However, several studies, including a paper in *The Journal of Diabetes Complications* in July 2006, have shown that the onset of menstruation is delayed in girls with T1DM to an average age of 15 (a girl without T1DM usually starts having periods around age 12 or 13). The earlier the onset of diabetes, the later the onset of menstruation.

After you start to have periods, your blood glucose levels rise and your insulin needs increase and then decrease as you go from day 1 to day 28 of your menstrual cycle. The changes in blood glucose and insulin occur because of the production of progesterone and estrogen until just before your period, when they fall dramatically. (What's the reason for this drop? If an ovulated egg isn't fertilized, progesterone secretion ceases and the uterus sheds its lining, producing a menstrual period.)

Blood glucose control tends to be worse in women with premenstrual syndrome (PMS); one possible reason for the irregularity of the control is the constellation of symptoms that accompany PMS: bloating, irritability, water retention, depression, and craving for carbohydrates.

It can be challenging to manage insulin during your menstrual cycle. As always, the best way to deal with this challenge is with more information — do more blood glucose tests! Test before meals, an hour after meals, at bedtime, and at 3 a.m., and adjust your insulin intake appropriately (see Chapter 10). You'll find that everything isn't actually random but rather that there's some sort of pattern that you can adjust to. As you adjust your insulin intake to the pattern, your overall control will improve as shown by lowering of the hemoglobin A1c. Irregularity of periods tends to be greater as your hemoglobin A1c is higher. The better you control your diabetes, the less this will be a problem. (See Chapter 7 for full details on hemoglobin A1c and testing blood glucose.)

If you suspect that PMS is to blame for tough control of your blood glucose, make some changes that may reduce the symptoms. Stick carefully to your dietary program; avoid salt, alcohol, chocolate, and caffeine; and increase the amount of exercise you do.

Dealing with sexual dysfunction

As a woman with T1DM, you may not have any problems with sexual function if you monitor and control your blood glucose tightly (especially after you figure out its pattern in relation to your monthly cycle; see the previous section). Women with poorly controlled T1DM, however, may have several problems with sexual function.

- They tend to have dryness of the vagina when the blood glucose is persistently high, making sexual intercourse uncomfortable. Creams can manage this problem; talk to your doctor.

- They may have a fungus infection of the vagina, leading to pain with intercourse. Tight glucose control eliminates this problem. Antibiotics can give only temporary relief if the poor diabetic control isn't improved.

- They tend to have orgasms less often than non-diabetic women, probably because of decreased sensation in the clitoris. No treatment has been consistently successful for this problem.

Getting a few tests if you're thinking of getting pregnant

If you're a woman with T1DM thinking of becoming pregnant, you must undergo several tests before and during your pregnancy to ensure that you don't develop or worsen diabetic complications and that your baby is healthy at birth and stays healthy afterwards (see Chapter 7 for more about these tests). They include:

- **Hemoglobin A1c testing:** Results should be less than 7 percent before conception of the baby and stay that way throughout the pregnancy. Hemoglobin A1c should be measured every one to two months because the turnover of red blood cells is more rapid in a pregnancy, and therefore, the results will change more than normal during pregnancy.

- ✔ **Kidney function testing:** The test by urine microalbumin should be performed on a normal basis before pregnancy and should be repeated once each trimester during pregnancy.

- ✔ **Eye examination:** The examination should be normal before pregnancy, and it should be done once each trimester during pregnancy.

- ✔ **Thyroid function testing:** This test is done with a thyroid-stimulating hormone (TSH). It should be normal before pregnancy and conducted once each trimester during pregnancy.

- ✔ **Blood pressure:** A blood pressure reading should be taken at each doctor's visit, and results should be normal.

- ✔ **Weight assessment:** Weight gain should be appropriate at each doctor's visit. When the weight is normal before pregnancy, the average weight gain for a woman is about 25 pounds. If you're underweight at the beginning of the pregnancy, 30 pounds is recommended. If overweight, 20 pounds is suggested.

- ✔ **Blood glucose:** Your blood glucose level should be less than 90 mg/dl before meals and less than 120 mg/dl at one hour after eating throughout the pregnancy.

If you meet these criteria, it's time to stop the contraceptive pills, hide the condoms, or take out the IUD (intrauterine device) from your uterus. You're ready to have a baby! You'll have no more trouble with your pregnancy than if you didn't have diabetes. Even if the criteria aren't completely met, the pregnancy may be normal. This is where working with a specialist who manages pregnancies in T1DM is very valuable.

The risks of conceiving before you have control of T1DM

So you've undergone some testing to see whether you're ready to conceive, but the doctor says that you need more control of your T1DM first. Thinking of disregarding this warning? Think again! The following sections explain the risks you pose to your baby and yourself if you don't have control before (and during) pregnancy. The bottom line: You can avoid all sorts of problems if you control your T1DM as I explain earlier in this chapter and throughout this book.

Risks to the baby

If a woman with T1DM conceives a child when her control is poor, the child is at higher risk than normal of having a congenital malformation, often so severe that it leads to a spontaneous abortion. Slightly less than 2 percent of normal pregnancies have an associated malformation in the baby; a pregnancy in a woman with diabetes increases the risk two or three times. Among the possible malformations are:

- Hernia of the brain
- Absence of parts of the brain, skull, and scalp
- Holes in the heart
- Small heart chambers
- Obstruction of the outlet from the heart to the blood vessels
- Severe narrowing of the major artery of the body
- Cysts on the spinal cord
- Failure of formation of the kidneys
- Cysts on the kidneys
- Abnormal closure of the duodenum or rectum

These congenital abnormalities don't occur at this higher rate if the blood glucose of the woman with T1DM is normal at the time of conception and for eight weeks after that (which is how long it takes for the baby's vital organs to form).

When the baby has gotten past the first 20 weeks of pregnancy in a woman with T1DM, the greatest risk if the blood glucose still isn't controlled is *macrosomia,* a condition that produces a very large body with deposits of fat in the shoulders, chest, abdomen, and legs. The heart, liver, and spleen are filled with fat. Macrosomia occurs because the baby is exposed to large amounts of sugar. His pancreas works and releases large amounts of insulin, the storage hormone. A baby who weighs more than 9 pounds and whose mother has T1DM is considered to have macrosomia. Figure 16-1 shows the appearance of a baby with macrosomia.

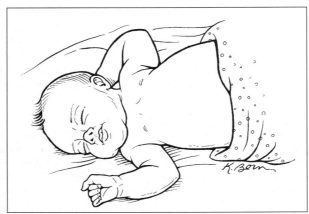

Figure 16-1:
A baby with macrosomia.

These babies are difficult to deliver because of their size; they often require cesarean sections (surgical removal of the baby through an abdominal and then a uterine incision). A baby with macrosomia may be born early and is premature even though he is so large. He may have to stay in the hospital until he's more mature. He may have breathing difficulties and will probably need immediate feeding because he has been making so much insulin and no longer has his mother's glucose. The pediatrician evaluates the newborn for specific problems and treats them.

Consistent elevation in the one-hour blood glucose after eating may be responsible for macrosomia, even though the before-meal blood glucose is normal. Taking more insulin before meals manages this problem.

The baby of a woman with T1DM may have a number of other problems related to poor control of the blood glucose. These include:

- Abnormally slow growth in the uterus, resulting in a poorly developed baby at birth.

- Decreased diameter of the large intestine and rectum.

- Increased production of red blood cells to carry the increased oxygen needed to metabolize all the extra glucose. All these extra blood cells can clog the arteries and veins and cause strokes and obstruction in veins.

- Iron deficiency because the red blood cells use up all the available iron, leaving organs like the heart and brain that need iron deficient.

- Hypoglycemia when the baby is separated from his mother. He continues to make large amounts of insulin, but large quantities of glucose are no longer available and his blood glucose falls. Several days of supplemental glucose may be needed until his pancreas stops making so much insulin.

- Low blood levels of calcium and magnesium leading to spasms of the hands and feet and abdominal cramps. At birth, the parathyroid gland normally takes over regulation of calcium and magnesium, but in babies of mothers with poorly controlled glucose, this gland is immature at birth.

- Respiratory distress syndrome, which is difficulty breathing as a result of a lack of *surfactant,* a substance made in the lungs that keeps the air tubes open for breathing. Surfactant requires cortisol from the adrenal gland, but the large amount of glucose in the baby's circulation during the pregnancy suppresses the production of cortisol. The more immature the baby, the worse the problem is, so delivering the baby as late as possible is very important.

- Jaundice due to hyperbilirubinemia. Bilirubin is the breakdown product of hemoglobin and is normally eliminated by the liver. The baby's large amount of red blood cells greatly increases the amount of bilirubin that the liver must handle. The necessary enzymes that the liver needs to handle the bilirubin aren't made in sufficient quantity in babies of women with poorly controlled T1DM. Bilirubin can cause brain damage if present in large enough amounts. Before that can happen, treatment with light rapidly lowers the bilirubin level.

✔ Neurologic problems including sleepiness, poor feeding, and decreased mental capacity as a result of the hypoglycemia, low calcium, high bilirubin, and increased red blood cells discussed in the previous bullets.

Risks to the mother

The greatest risks during pregnancy exist for women with T1DM who already have complications before becoming pregnant. Here are some examples of preexisting complications and what happens to them:

✔ Proliferative retinopathy (see Chapter 5) at conception will progress in more than half of women.

✔ Significant diabetic kidney disease (marked by more than 250 mg of albumin in the urine every 24 hours) will rapidly worsen in about half of mothers during pregnancy.

✔ Diabetic nerve disease may worsen with increased loss of sensation in the feet.

✔ High blood pressure may become worse during pregnancy. This decreases the blood supply to the fetus.

✔ About 30 percent of women with T1DM have thyroid autoantibodies and may develop hypothyroidism (decreased production of thyroid hormones) during pregnancy.

Using contraception until you're under control

Until you achieve control of your T1DM and are officially ready to conceive (meaning that your doctor has given you the go-ahead), the wisest course of action is to use contraception. For purposes of contraception, the first day of your menstrual cycle is the first day of bleeding; between the 8th and 18th days, you're most fertile and likely to become pregnant if you have unprotected sex, so contraception is absolutely crucial during this time. You're most fertile for 24 hours before ovulation and a few hours after ovulation. You can determine ovulation by taking your body temperature. When it rises 0.2 degrees F and persists at that level, ovulation has occurred. If it rises again a few days later and persists, conception has likely occurred.

As a woman with T1DM, you have the same choices of contraception as a woman without diabetes. These include:

- Condoms, which also protect against sexually transmitted diseases.

- Contraceptive implants that are removable if necessary.

- Depot injections of progesterone. These may cause an increase in blood glucose and can't be removed until they're used up, which may take months, even if you experience side effects of nausea and increased appetite.

- Diaphragm and spermicidal jelly.

- Intrauterine device, which sometimes causes infections and loss of uterine function and therefore isn't used until after a first pregnancy.

- Minipills consisting of progesterone alone, which may increase spotting.

- Morning-after pills like Plan B, which must be taken within 72 hours of unprotected sex.

- Oral contraceptives, which are a combination of small doses of estrogen and progesterone, and not recommended for smokers, people with high blood pressure, or those who suffer from migraine headaches.

Oral contraceptives are the method of choice for younger women with T1DM, and an IUD is recommended for women with T1DM who have had a child.

Ensuring a Safe Pregnancy and Delivery

Tight control in pregnancy means achieving a blood glucose level that is as close to normal as possible using insulin, diet, and exercise, just as in the person with T1DM who is not pregnant.

A study in *Diabetes Care* in August 2001 showed that a normal pregnant woman without diabetes will have a blood glucose of between 55 mg/dl and 105 mg/dl one hour after meals from the 28th to the 38th week. The study also measured the abdominal circumference of the fetus by ultrasound and found that the higher the one-hour glucose, the larger the abdominal circumference.

More recently, a study that has not yet been published was reported at the Scientific Meetings of the American Diabetes Association in June 2007. Called the Hyperglycemia and Adverse Pregnancy Outcome (HAPO) study, it showed that even pregnant women with no evidence of diabetes by glucose testing at the beginning of the study could develop complications similar to those in pregnant women with T1DM if their blood glucose rose above normal frequently during the pregnancy, even when they didn't reach the criteria for diabetes. High birth weights correlated with high blood glucose levels.

Tight control of type 1 diabetes in pregnancy means achieving a blood glucose level that's as close to normal as possible using insulin, diet, and exercise, just as in the person with T1DM who isn't pregnant. Pregnant women with no diabetes normally have blood glucose and hemoglobin A1c levels lower than non-pregnant women because the fetus takes so much of the glucose. The goal is to achieve these levels in the pregnant woman with diabetes.

Ideally, because macrosomia (see the earlier section "Risks to the baby" for more about this condition) is found when the one-hour blood glucose is consistently greater than 120 mg/dl, and normal pregnant women without diabetes have a hemoglobin A1c level up to 5 percent, the desirable levels are

- ✔ Blood glucose less than 90 mg/dl before meals
- ✔ Blood glucose less than 120 mg/dl at 1 hour
- ✔ Hemoglobin A1c no greater than 5 percent

How do you achieve these goals? Read the following sections to find out.

Using insulin during and after pregnancy

In order to keep the glucose normal, more insulin is required throughout a pregnancy, and this increase drops rapidly after giving birth. Because the goal is a blood glucose level of less than 90 mg/dl before meals and less than 120 mg/dl one hour after meals, it's necessary to test before meals, an hour after meals, and at bedtime daily. This frequency of testing gives you the opportunity to treat high blood glucose or eat for low blood glucose.

Here are a couple of exceptions to the usual increased need for insulin during pregnancy:

- ✔ **At about the 9th to 11th week of the pregnancy:** At this time, the ovaries stop making progesterone and the uterus takes over. There may be a brief period (lasting eight to ten days) during which your insulin requirement falls. This is a time to do more testing, especially before bedtime and at 3 a.m. to avoid overnight hypoglycemia if you don't reduce your insulin temporarily.

- ✔ **At 37 weeks:** Your uterus begins to contract, and you start to burn glucose that way. You should test your blood glucose at bedtime and at 3 a.m., and lower your bedtime insulin if the overnight glucose falls to less than 70 mg/dl.

You can use whatever method of insulin delivery you like, but one method that has been successful during pregnancy is the insulin pump (see Chapter 11). It allows for easy treatment if the blood glucose gets too high or too low. The trouble with the insulin pump is the rapid development of ketoacidosis if insulin isn't being given as a result of blockage, leakage, or some other problem with the pump.

Ketoacidosis in the mother is very dangerous for the fetus and often leads to fetal loss. If you feel nauseated, check your blood ketones. See Chapter 15 for coverage of this test.

Among the various kinds of insulin, the newer long-acting insulins (insulin glargine and insulin detemir) haven't been used in large numbers of pregnant women with T1DM, although the experience with insulin glargine is probably large enough, at this time, to recommend its use. Insulin NPH has been the standard longer-acting insulin up to now. As for rapid-acting insulin, there's plenty of experience with insulin lispro and insulin aspart use in pregnant women, and these are used commonly in this situation as the rapid-acting component of the insulin treatment.

Immediately after delivery, as a result of the drop in hormones, your insulin needs drop below what you needed before the pregnancy. However, as the pituitary gland produces prolactin to stimulate breast milk, your insulin needs increase. You may find that you need less long-acting insulin and more rapid-acting insulin when you breast-feed.

A number of insulin treatment schedules are available for controlling the blood glucose throughout and after the pregnancy. You should work with your diabetes doctor to develop the one that works for you. This isn't something that can or should be done on your own.

Managing your diet

The amount of carbohydrate in the diet plays a large role in a person's blood glucose level. As long as the percentage of carbohydrate in a meal is kept below 40 percent, the one-hour blood glucose will remain under 120 mg/dl. See Chapter 8 for the full scoop on eating carbohydrates.

Dividing your total daily calories over three meals and three snacks helps keep your blood sugar down. If you divide your total daily calories into 12 parts, you can eat $\frac{3}{12}$ at each meal and $\frac{1}{12}$ at each snack. Make sure that you take one of the snacks at bedtime to avoid overnight hypoglycemia.

Another important factor is the weight of the mother before pregnancy and the amount of weight gain during pregnancy. If the mother's weight is more than 1½ times her ideal body weight (100 pounds for 5 feet of height plus 5 pounds for every inch over 5 feet) before the pregnancy, she should gain no more than 15 to 20 pounds during the pregnancy to avoid a large infant birth weight. If her weight is in the ideal range (the ideal weight plus or minus 10 percent), she should gain 20 to 25 pounds; if she's underweight, she should gain 25 to 30 pounds.

Figuring out how to manage your diet and weight during pregnancy can be daunting. Make use of the knowledge of a good dietitian who's a Certified Diabetes Educator. He or she can take you through what you need to know and be there when you have questions. See Chapter 2 for help in finding a diabetes educator.

Adding exercise

Pregnant women with T1DM don't use exercise to bring down their blood glucose but rather to improve cardiovascular fitness, reduce the stress of the pregnancy, and put them in excellent physical condition for the strains of labor.

The best exercise is probably a low-impact program like walking 30 minutes daily to avoid any stress on the fetus. Get your significant other to join you so you'll be well on your way to setting a great example for your newborn, or use the time to catch up with a friend. Flip to Chapter 9 for more about exercising with T1DM.

Monitoring your baby

Your obstetrician should set up the plan for monitoring your baby during the pregnancy. You have ultrasound studies at regular intervals to follow the growth and development of the fetus.

Dealing with Type 1 Diabetes during Menopause

Menopause can be an even more difficult transition than the onset of menstrual periods for several reasons. Here are a few key changes associated with menopause:

- ✔ It's preceded by the perimenopausal years when there's a great deal of irregularity in your menstrual periods due largely to hormone fluctuations that affect your blood glucose.

- ✔ Estrogen, which makes the body more sensitive to insulin, declines during menopause, resulting in decreased insulin sensitivity.

- ✔ Other illnesses of aging begin to be develop, such as osteoporosis and heart disease.

✔ If your diabetes hasn't been controlled, complications including eye disease, kidney disease, and nerve disease (see Chapter 5) complicate control. For example, visual difficulties may make exact administration of insulin more difficult, and gastroparesis due to autonomic neuropathy, which slows emptying of the stomach, may make it harder to judge the correct insulin dose and when to take it.

✔ The symptoms of menopause, such as hot flashes, sweating, and flushing, may be confused with symptoms of hypoglycemia.

The way you manage this difficult time is no different from managing your diabetes at any other time: insulin, diet, and exercise, along with lots of self-testing of the blood glucose. You have one other consideration during menopause, however: the question of hormone replacement therapy.

One question that may occur to you as you reach this passage from menstrual function to menopause is whether your T1DM needs to be as well-controlled at age 51 as it was at age 31. The answer is a definitive yes. You may have 30 or more years of life ahead of you, so you definitely don't want to be blind in ten years or on hemodialysis for kidney failure at age 60. There are plenty of women and men with T1DM in their 70s and 80s who are free of complications of diabetes and live high-quality lives.

Sticking to good habits

Here are some key considerations for living with T1DM at this stage of your life:

✔ Test your blood glucose before meals and at bedtime to determine the right dose of insulin.

✔ Don't allow yourself to gain a lot of weight, adding insulin resistance to lack of insulin. As your metabolism declines with aging, you may have to eat less and exercise more to maintain your weight.

✔ Keep exercising to maintain your physical fitness. Don't neglect your muscle strength; weight training with moderate weights of 5 or 10 pounds increases your strength, stamina, and balance.

✔ Keep up the tests recommended in Chapter 7 to find any new problems associated with your diabetes at the earliest possible time.

✔ Stay on top of screening tests like Pap smears, mammography, and so forth so that you don't add problems like cervical cancer or breast cancer to an already full plate.

✔ Get an annual flu shot and shots to prevent pneumonia and shingles.

Considering hormone replacement therapy

In recent years, medical experts have gone from recommending hormone replacement therapy (HRT) to all postmenopausal women, to condemning it as a source of all kinds of problems like heart attacks, to a more subtle reconsideration that's currently taking place, so I don't blame you if you're confused about this subject. Because these hormones have a definite effect on your blood glucose control, you need to understand what they do and whether they're for you.

The purpose of HRT

With the onset of menopause, you're at risk for some or all of the following symptoms:

- Hot flashes
- Vaginal dryness
- Sleeplessness
- Irritability
- Short-term memory loss
- Fatigue

Some of these symptoms mimic hypoglycemia, and unless you test your blood glucose, you may eat extra calories, thinking that you're treating that condition.

Having T1DM along with menopause adds several other problems that make your blood glucose even more difficult to control; they include:

- Bacterial and yeast infections
- Urinary tract infections

Because all these symptoms seem to arise from a lack of the hormones estrogen and progesterone, it seems logical to replace them to reverse the problems. Hormone replacement therapy was the standard treatment for all these conditions up until 2002. It also was thought to protect women against osteoporosis and heart disease.

Controversies about HRT

In July 2002, a key study was published in *The Journal of the American Medical Association* under the title "Risks and Benefits of Estrogen Plus Progestin in Healthy Postmenopausal Women: Principal Results From the Women's Health Initiative Randomized Controlled Trial." The report provided the following conclusions about postmenopausal women who took HRT compared to those who did not. The users had

- A small increase in cases of breast cancer
- A small excess of heart attacks
- A small excess of strokes
- A small excess of blood clots in veins
- A small decrease in bone fractures
- A small decrease in cancer of the large intestine

The study had an immediate and enormous effect. Millions of women taking HRT stopped taking it. A typical study in *The Archives of Gynecology and Obstetrics* in August 2007 showed that the number of prescriptions for HRT dropped from 1,272 per month in July 2002 to 493 per month in July 2005 at one medical center.

Since these studies and findings, there has been some reconsideration of the rush to stop using HRT. Much of it has to do with problems in the 2002 study, especially the fact that most of the women using HRT began taking it years after they went into menopause rather than the usual custom of starting it at menopause. By age 60, women have had time to develop many of the conditions that were found in excess in that study; it's possible that HRT wasn't responsible for the increases because it was given later than it should have been.

However, there has been a significant decrease in the incidence of breast cancer since HRT usage declined in the U.S., and many experts believe that the reduction in use of HRT is the explanation. The decline was noted in 2003. It's difficult to believe that a disease that takes decades to develop like breast cancer can decline after just a year of decreased use of HRT, but the experts believe that the decline was in the cancers that depended on estrogen in HRT for growth. Given that the incidence of breast cancer increased in every year for 20 years up to 2002, it's hard to argue with the findings.

Deciding whether to use HRT

HRT can be used short term, for five years or less, without being clearly associated with the abnormalities described in the previous section. The people who can benefit from short-term use of HRT are

- Women with debilitating hot flashes, especially if they disturb sleep
- Women with vaginal dryness and hot flashes

  HRT manages both these conditions. If vaginal dryness is present but not hot flashes, local estrogen preparations can be given.

The women who shouldn't take HRT at this time are

- Women with any history of breast cancer
- Women with any history of heart attacks or strokes
- Women with a history of deep vein thrombosis

Should the woman with T1DM take HRT? My answer is if she does not fall into the second group or has debilitating hot flashes making control of her diabetes difficult, this could be a short-term consideration. If the HRT allows her to achieve good control of the diabetes with hemoglobin A1c levels under 7 percent, the benefits of short-term therapy outweigh the risks. If you're at all considering whether to use HRT, be sure to talk to your doctor.

If a woman with T1DM goes on HRT, she must continue regular mammograms and checks of her cervix. Any irregular bleeding should be reported to the doctor.

Many other treatments can be used if osteoporosis is the only reason for considering HRT. Among the safe treatments for women with T1DM are

- **Reloxifine,** a selective estrogen receptor modulator that preserves bone. Side effects include hot flashes and blood clots.
- **Alendronate and risindronate,** both belonging to a chemical group called bisphosphonates that prevent fractures and slow bone loss.
- **Calcitonin,** a naturally occurring hormone that increases bone mass and prevents bone loss. It's used for people who have definite osteoporosis at least five years after menopause.
- **Teriparatide,** a form of parathyroid hormone that may reverse bone loss.
- **Vitamin D and calcium,** necessary for bone formation.

If you're considering HRT only to protect yourself again heart disease associated with T1DM, you may want to reconsider. There are a number of things you can do instead, such as the following:

- Stop smoking or any use of tobacco.
- Control your blood pressure (less than 120/80 for diabetic patients).
- Lose weight through diet and exercise.
- Control your cholesterol (LDL cholesterol less than 100 mg/dl and a ratio of total to HDL or good cholesterol less than 4.5).

Chapter 17

Controlling Type 1 Diabetes in the Elderly

Seniors are a special breed, and there are more and more of them with each passing year. At the present time the U.S. population is 300 million, more or less. The government's projection is that by 2050 there will be 400 million Americans. Currently more than 45 million Americans are older than 65. By 2050 there will be more than 98 million, of whom over 18 million will be older than 85 and almost a million older than 100!

The prevalence of type 1 diabetes (T1DM) is currently about 1 in 300 Americans, with most of those folks under age 65. Thanks to modern medical advances, however, more and more people with T1DM are reaching senior status. (Although the definition of "senior" keeps changing as I get older, the government uses age 65 and older for statistical purposes.) The prevalence of T1DM by 2050 will be more than 325,000 in the population over age 65 (by then, there will be more than 98 million people older than 65).That's going to create a huge problem requiring enormous resources.

If you're growing older with T1DM or are the spouse or child of an elderly person with T1DM, there's a lot to know about managing the disease at this stage in life. For many reasons that I explain in this chapter, it's very different from managing T1DM when your child is 10, otherwise healthy, and has his whole life ahead of him.

A key point is that you *can* now expect to reach senior status with T1DM. In fact, so many have done so that the Joslin Diabetes Center at Harvard University along with the Eli Lilly Company (which first manufactured insulin for human use) have been giving medals to people who have been on insulin successfully for 25, 50, and now 75 years (since insulin has only been available since 1921). With so many people with T1DM now living so long, they may have to rethink their free medals. (See the nearby sidebar "The Joslin Diabetes Center: Painting a picture of seniors with type 1 diabetes" for more information.)

Making a Diagnosis

T1DM typically appears during childhood, but it's not unheard of for T1DM to make its first appearance after a person reaches age 65. In the following sections, I explain the symptoms of T1DM in a senior, certain conditions that are connected to the onset of T1DM, and the testing required to confirm a diagnosis.

The Joslin Diabetes Center: Painting a picture of seniors with type 1 diabetes

The Joslin Diabetes Center was kind enough to publish its findings with respect to the 50-year medal winners in *Diabetes Care* in August 2007. These results can help you to understand what you need to do to reach that diabetes milestone, too.

The center sent questionnaires to 500 of their medalists and got useful replies from 326. They break down as follows:

- 54.7 percent of respondents were female.

- The mean age at the time of the study was 69.5 to 78 years.

- The mean age at diagnosis was 12.6 to 19.7 years.

- The median A1c level was 7.0 percent up to 10.8 percent (see Chapter 7 for more about hemoglobin A1c).

- The average insulin dose was 0.227 units per pound of weight (so a 125-pound woman was using 28 units and a 150-pound man was using 34 units).

- The mean HDL cholesterol level (the "good" kind) was 67.7 mg/dl.

In the survey, 174 people reported microvascular complications (eye disease, kidney disease, and nerve disease; see Chapter 5 for details). They differed from those without complications in the following ways:

- Their triglyceride levels were higher.

- Their insulin doses were higher.

- They had lower HDL cholesterol levels.

However there was no difference between the people who did and did not have microvascular complications in the following parameters:

- Age

- Duration of diabetes

- Hemoglobin A1c

- Body mass index

- Total cholesterol

- LDL (bad) cholesterol

Current physical activity was highly correlated with no microvascular complications, and regular exercise was protective when the HDL cholesterol wasn't high.

In terms of the individual complications,

✔ 139 people (47.9 percent) reported retinopathy. Those without retinopathy had T1DM longer, were older, and had lower triglycerides.

✔ 22 people (6.7 percent) reported nephropathy. These people were younger at the time of their diagnosis and had higher body mass index values, lower hemoglobin A1c levels, and higher triglyceride levels. They also had heart problems more often.

✔ 164 people (50 percent) reported neuropathy. These people had lower HDL levels, used more insulin, had higher triglycerides, and had more heart disease.

Many studies in the medical literature report that the prevalence of retinopathy is more than 90 percent in patients with T1DM. Also, of course, it's an accepted fact that microvascular complications result from poor control of the blood glucose, yet among the patients in the Joslin survey, those with poor control had no greater prevalence of complications. The authors suggest that these people have something that protects them from diabetic complications. The mean HDL level may be one reason because it's considerably higher than usual for T1DM, and levels that high have been shown to protect against many causes of death.

In summary, the study is good news for people with T1DM. It shows that

✔ You can live a long time without complications.

✔ Exercise is an important component of long life with uncomplicated diabetes.

✔ A high HDL cholesterol is important as well.

Surveying symptoms

The elderly often experience many symptoms that mimic the acute and chronic complications of diabetes. However, they may be due to other illnesses, the aging process, or diabetes. Among these symptoms are the following:

✔ Anxiety

✔ Confusion

✔ Constipation

✔ Decreased sexual interest

✔ Depression

✔ Falls

✔ Loss of appetite

✔ Tiredness

✔ Tremors

✔ Urinary tract infections

✔ Weakness

If you have these symptoms, don't assume that they're due to old age. Ask your doctor to consider other possibilities such as T1DM. It's important to make the right diagnosis (see the next section for information on confirming T1DM with testing).

Many of these symptoms also may be brought on by the medications you're taking. A long list of "potentially inappropriate medications for the elderly" can be found on the Internet at `www.dcri.duke.edu/ccge/curtis/beers.html`. (It's pulled from an article that was published in the *Archives of Internal Medicine* in December 2003.) Check the list and see if your medications are there. If they are, discuss with your doctor whether you can substitute something for the "inappropriate" medication or even stop it with no ill effects.

Conditions connected to the onset of type 1 diabetes

The following diseases and conditions are associated with the onset of T1DM in the elderly:

- **Pancreatitis,** an inflammation of the pancreas, which can destroy the functional pancreas
- **Excessive alcohol use,** which can destroy the functional pancreas
- **Cancer in the pancreas,** which can significantly reduce insulin production
- **Surgical removal of the pancreas,** which brings on T1DM
- **Gallstones,** which can lead to pancreatic destruction
- **Abnormally high calcium in the blood**
- **Traumatic injury in the area of the pancreas**

In addition, aging is associated with the development of insulin resistance. Not only must the person with T1DM take insulin shots, but they're not as effective as when he was younger. This may be a time when certain drugs that would not be used in T1DM at a younger age may be helpful, as I discuss in the later section, "Medications."

Confirming the diagnosis with testing

Making a diagnosis of type 1 diabetes in the elderly is done in the same way as it's done in younger people (see Chapter 2 for details). Two or more blood glucose levels over 126 mg/dl in the fasting state or over 200 mg/dl after feeding is diagnostic.

Some have suggested using the hemoglobin A1c (see Chapter 7) to diagnose T1DM in the elderly because blood glucose levels usually don't rise so high and the threshold for spilling glucose in the urine rises with age. A hemoglobin A1c greater than 7 percent is highly suggestive of diabetes, and it can be confirmed by the fasting or fed blood glucose.

T1DM comes on a lot less rapidly in the elderly than it does in children. Seniors may be far less sick, so the onset is much less dramatic. In addition, the many confusing symptoms in the elderly may cause you to look elsewhere and not think of diabetes as a possible diagnosis. That's why it's so important to screen for diabetes annually beginning at age 35.

Recognizing the Challenges of Managing Type 1 Diabetes in the Elderly

In this section, you discover how the elderly differ from younger patients in the way they present their signs and symptoms of diabetes. Many elderly are unable to care for themselves because of their physical and mental limitations; I tell you how to measure their limitations and decide whether they're severe enough to require nursing or other care.

Realizing how the elderly differ from other patients

Managing T1DM in the elderly compares to managing T1DM in children in the same way that managing traffic in Times Square, New York, compares to managing traffic in Broken Bow, Nebraska. There's a lot more going on in the elderly.

The differences between the elderly and younger people with T1DM play a major role in complicating diabetes management. The following points apply to the elderly:

- ✓ **They may be forgetful and fail to take medications, check blood glucose levels, exercise, or eat properly.** (See the next section for information on determining whether you or your loved one can take care of his T1DM.)

- ✓ **They may take three to seven other drugs in addition to insulin.** Some of the drugs may interact with the insulin, and some may just cause confusion in timing of doses.

- ✓ **They often have decreased sensations of taste and smell, so they aren't interested in food.**

- ✔ **They often have poor teeth and a dry mouth.** The poor teeth may make diabetic control more difficult.

- ✔ **They have reduced kidney function.**

- ✔ **They often live alone and have no one to help them.**

- ✔ **They may not recognize hypoglycemia.** (If you don't recognize it either, see Chapter 4.)

- ✔ **They may be unable to afford their medications and may have to spend their limited resources on an inexpensive diet that's rich in fat rather than more low-glycemic carbohydrate and protein.** (I discuss resources for patients on fixed incomes later in this chapter.)

- ✔ **They may be physically unable to give themselves insulin shots with a syringe and needle.**

- ✔ **They're less physically fit and less physically active than younger people.**

- ✔ **They have reduced muscle mass and increased fat mass.**

- ✔ **They're more sensitive to drugs due to slower metabolism.**

- ✔ **They may have poor vision and be unable to measure their insulin properly.** Vision trouble may be due to cataracts or glaucoma, both of which are treatable.

Determining an elderly patient's ability to treat his own type 1 diabetes

T1DM can cause a reduction in intellectual function resulting from reduced blood flow to the brain, inflammation often found in diabetes, and hypoglycemia. A reduction in brain function due to diabetes can lead to behaviors that are detrimental to the health of the patient, so it's very important to have an idea of the elderly patient's ability to perform self-care for his T1DM.

To make this assessment, some form of testing of intellectual function is very valuable. It can be done at age 70 when the person is at the beginning stages of "elderly" and should be repeated at intervals, perhaps annually, to evaluate mental functioning on an ongoing basis.

An excellent test that takes just a few minutes is called the Mini-Mental State Examination. You can administer it to your loved one or even take it yourself. It was first used in 1975, and its usefulness has been validated many times since then. The Mini-Mental State Examination tests

- ✔ Whether the person knows the correct time (day and year) and where he is (address, city and state)

> ✔ Whether the person can repeat items, read, write, draw, calculate, name items, and remember items previously named

Figure 17-1 shows a typical Mini-Mental State Examination with the scoring system.

A score of less than 26 (out of 30 total points) means that the person may have trouble caring for himself. You may need a nurse in the home, or the person may have to go to an assisted living facility or a nursing home.

Effectively Treating Type 1 Diabetes in the Elderly

Treatment of T1DM in the elderly is even more challenging than it is in younger people for the many reasons described in the earlier section "Realizing how the elderly differ from other patients." Namely, it's difficult to keep them on a diet, have them get an adequate amount of exercise, and make sure they get their insulin in the correct doses. I provide some suggestions for effective treatment in the following sections.

Maximum Score	Patient Score	
		Orientation
5		What is the year, season, date, day, and month?
5		What state, country, town, hospital, and floor are we in?
		Registration
3		Examiner names three objects, and the patient must repeat them.
		Calculation
5		Start with the number 7, and add 7 five times.
		Recall
3		Ask for the three objects named in the registration section.
		Language
2		Examiner points to a pencil and watch and asks for their names.
1		Repeat the following: "No ifs, ands, or buts."
3		Follow a three-stage command: "Take a paper in your hand; fold it in half; put it on the floor."
1		Read and obey: "Close your eyes."
1		Write a sentence.
1		Examiner draws a design, and the patient must copy it.

Figure 17-1: A typical Mini-Mental State Examination.

Medications

Insulin remains the standard of care for the elderly person with T1DM (I discuss insulin use in full detail in Chapter 10). It may not be possible to achieve excellent blood glucose control, though. Attempting to force a hemoglobin A1c of 7 percent or less on the patient at this age may lead to a significant reduction in the quality of life, with multiple episodes of hypoglycemia. You and your doctor have to decide whether you're going to try for basic or intensive care with your insulin administration.

✔ **Basic care means avoiding excessive urination and thirst.** This allows you to get a good night's sleep and feel rested. An elderly person with multiple significant medical conditions who isn't expected to live very long should receive this level of care. The goal of the treatment is to keep the blood glucose under 200 mg/dl. This can be done with a single shot of insulin glargine in the morning and moderate amounts of rapid-acting insulin before meals. An even simpler regimen may be two shots of a mixture of short- and intermediate-acting insulin daily. These come in insulin pens and are easy to administer.

✔ **Intensive care means trying to lower the hemoglobin A1c below 7 percent to prevent microvascular complications.** This is done for the elderly person with T1DM who's expected to live long enough to develop microvascular complications (eye, kidney, and nerve disease) if not treated intensively. These days, that could include the 80- or 90-year old. It may be necessary to accept some hypoglycemia in order to accomplish this level of care.

An insulin pump (see Chapter 11) may be useful in intensive care because it reduces the amount that you have to remember in order to administer the right amount of insulin.

You must test your blood glucose if you use insulin. Study after study has concluded that the more a person with T1DM tests, the better their blood glucose control. In addition, your doctor should regularly test your hemoglobin A1c (every three months), your microalbumin (at least annually), your weight and blood pressure (every visit), and your blood fats (at least annually). I describe all these tests in Chapter 7.

In view of the increasing insulin resistance in the elderly, consideration should be given to using the drug metformin, which lowers the release of glucose from the liver. It's given at a dose of 500 to 1000 mg three times daily with meals.

Other drugs said to be *insulin sensitizers* (that is, they make you more sensitive to your insulin), such as the thiazoledinedione class that includes rosiglitazone and pioglitazone, are associated with a number of side effects that, I believe, make them dangerous. They cause weight gain, anemia, and osteoporosis, and rosiglitazone has been shown to cause early heart attacks. I don't recommend their use.

It's a good idea to bring your medications to the doctor's office every time you go and to keep a list of your medicines with you at all times in case you find yourself in an emergency room unexpectedly. When you see your doctor, don't hesitate to take all your medications out and ask the doctor whether you still need to take each one or if you can lower your dose. Any time you can accomplish either, you will benefit.

Nutrition

Despite the huge increase in the number of elderly people with both T1DM and T2DM, there are few studies of proper nutrition specific to that age group — most recommendations are based on younger patients. But experts do know that a major concern with respect to nutrition in the elderly is *malnutrition,* which results from inadequate amounts of calories and consuming too much of the wrong foods. The often-limited resources of the elderly cause them to have to choose between eating good foods, buying all their medications, and spending money on occasional pleasures like a book or a movie. This isn't a medical problem but rather a social and economic problem, and it's not easily fixed. (I provide some resources to help combat this problem later in this chapter.)

The following are some nutritional recommendations that are reasonable and doable for the elderly patient with T1DM:

- ✔ **Take a multivitamin and a mineral tablet daily to ensure that you're getting adequate quantities of essential nutrients.**

- ✔ **Consume a diet in which the carbohydrate content makes up 40 to 50 percent of calories.** This recommendation is reasonable based on successful control of blood glucose in other patients.

- ✔ **Keep the levels of saturated fats down and monounsaturated and polyunsaturated fats up for a healthier diet; these fats should represent about 30 percent of your daily calories.**

- ✔ **Stick to a level of protein that's 15 to 20 percent of daily calories.** This amount strikes a balance between too much protein that may hurt the kidneys and too little protein resulting in loss of muscle.

- ✔ **Get at least 20 grams of fiber in your daily diet.**

- ✔ **Avoid a low-sugar diet.** It won't improve your glucose control and may cause weight loss because of the lack of taste in the food.

- ✔ **Keep your teeth in good condition to make eating easier and to avoid infections that complicate T1DM.** Brush, floss, and visit the dentist twice a year.

Flip to Chapter 8 for general information on eating a healthy diet.

Exercise

Time and again I've been told by an elderly person with T1DM that he can't exercise because he

- ✔ Has joint problems
- ✔ Has chest pain
- ✔ Has no time
- ✔ Doesn't enjoy it
- ✔ Can't catch his breath

These are some of the reasons that an exercise program must be developed at a young age and maintained throughout life. The description of the Joslin Medal Winners in the sidebar earlier in this chapter shows that the ones who lived longest were the ones who exercised for the longest period of their lives.

At the very least, walk for 30 minutes every day if possible. If you have any problems with balance, using a stationary cycle or doing the exercise in a pool will avoid the risk of a fall. If you have joint problems but are otherwise healthy, use of an elliptical trainer is a good idea because this device gives a good workout but doesn't cause trauma to joints.

In addition to movement exercise, lifting light weights has been shown to be very beneficial to the elderly. They regain strength in their muscles, improve their balance, and increase their stamina. See Chapter 9 for illustrations of seven low-impact exercises you can do with weights to build up your upper body.

There are some risks to exercise in the elderly with T1DM, especially those just starting to get moving. (The risks usually aren't present when the person has been exercising for decades.) Risks include:

- ✔ Hemorrhage of the vitreous of the eye
- ✔ High blood glucose after strenuous exercise
- ✔ Hypoglycemia
- ✔ Increased protein in the urine
- ✔ Possible heart disease
- ✔ Retinal detachment
- ✔ Soft tissue and joint injury

You should have a thorough examination by a cardiologist if you're 50 or older and are just starting to exercise vigorously. Also, if you haven't had an eye exam within the past year, get one before you start exercise.

Checking Out Resources for the Elderly with Type 1 Diabetes

Fortunately, there are plenty of resources for the elderly with T1DM who are on a fixed income and may not be able to afford all their medications and doctor's visits. Too many people are unaware of the resources in the following sections or don't make use of them. That's a big mistake. Use all the tools at your disposal so you can continue to live a great life with T1DM, even as a senior!

Here a few more helpful resources that the elderly can use:

- Head to Chapter 2 for details on gathering a diabetes team, including a specialist, a diabetes educator, and other fine folks.

- Appendix B has Internet resources for the latest information. Every one of them has something useful for the elderly person with T1DM. If you don't have a computer or an Internet connection, get one, ask a family member or neighbor for help, or get help at the local library. You're never too old to learn to use a computer. (Plus you can e-mail your grandchildren!)

Government help

No one has to make a choice between diabetes medications and healthy food or pleasurable activities. The U.S. government operates two major programs — Medicare and Medicaid — to make sure that you have help with medical insurance coverage when you can no longer work.

Medicare

The introduction to Medicare in the government publication "Medicare and You" explains its purpose very well: "Medicare is health insurance for people age 65 or older, under age 65 with certain disabilities, and any age with End-Stage Renal Disease (permanent kidney failure requiring dialysis or a kidney transplant)." Medicare consists of four parts; the following list covers just the basics, so for more-complete information on each part, head to www.medicare.gov:

- **Part A** is hospital care. The government pays most of this, and it isn't optional. If you have Part A, medical care is not entirely free.

- **Part B** is medical office care. It's optional, and you may end up paying a lot of this bill if you don't choose doctors approved by Medicare.

> ✓ **Part C** combines Part A and Part B in "Medicare Advantage Plans" like Preferred Provider Organization plans or Health Maintenance Organization plans to help lower your costs while providing complete medical care.
>
> ✓ **Part D** is prescription drug coverage. It's optional, but if you have sizable costs for drugs every year, it may be very helpful.

The Medicare homepage (www.medicare.gov) has a "Search Tools" link that can direct you to answers to almost any question you have. You also can read through the excellent publication "Medicare and You" (www.medicare.gov/Publications/Pubs/pdf/10050.pdf), which covers all you need to know about, well, Medicare and you. The other major resource that I recommend for further information on Medicare is the AARP Web site at www.aarp.org. Consider joining the association; it's inexpensive and the benefits (in addition to a complete explanation of Medicare) are enormous and include publications and discounts.

Medicaid

Medicaid is a program of the U.S. government but is administered at the state level. As with Medicare (see the previous section), no one can explain the program better than Medicaid itself: "Medicaid is available only to certain low-income individuals and families who fit into an eligibility group that is recognized by federal and state law. Medicaid does not pay money to you; instead, it sends payments directly to your health care providers. Depending on your state's rules, you may also be asked to pay a small part of the cost (co-payment) for some medical services."

Each state establishes its own eligibility criteria for Medicaid, and if you meet your state's criteria, your health provider gets the benefits. On the Medicaid Web site, www.cms.hhs.gov/MedicaidGenInfo, you can find an excellent introduction to the plan as well as a link to "Medicaid Eligibility." Click that link, and then scroll down the page to find "Contact Information to State Medicaid Offices." The downloadable plan introduction, "Medicaid At-A-Glance 2005" (www.cms.hhs.gov/MedicaidGenInfo/Downloads/MedicaidAtAGlance2005.pdf), is the basic resource for understanding the plan.

Drug company resources

Every drug company that provides a drug for diabetes has a plan for people who can't afford their drug. Here's a rundown of the programs (including Web sites to visit for full details) of some major providers of insulin:

- ✔ Eli Lilly and Company has a program called Lilly Cares that offers free medication through physicians if the patient meets the eligibility criteria. You can find out more by visiting `www.lilly.com/products/access`.

- ✔ Novo-Nordisk has a Patient Assistance Program that gives you a 90-day supply of medication free if you meet eligibility criteria. You can download the guidelines and application for this program at `www.novonordisk-us.com/documents/pdf/2007NovoNordiskPAPGuidelines.pdf`.

- ✔ Sanofi-Aventis operates a Patient Assistance Program that distributes free medications, including insulins, to patients who meet eligibility criteria. You can find out more about this program at `www.rxassist.org/pap-info/company_detail.cfm?CmpId=49`.

- ✔ Pfizer's program, Connection to Care, offers 75 of the company's medications, including their insulin, free through your doctor. You have to fill out a form, and Pfizer provides the medication to your doctor for you. For information and an application, visit `www.pfizerhelpfulanswers.com/pages/Programs/programdetails.aspx?p=2`.

Part V
The Part of Tens

The 5ᵗʰ Wave   By Rich Tennant

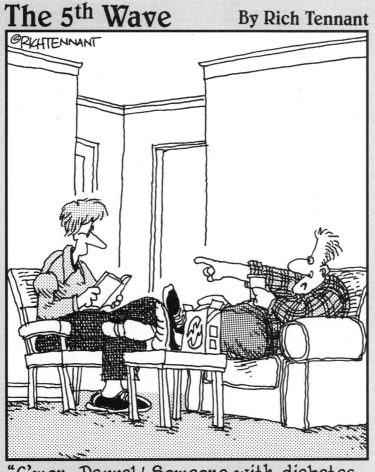

"C'mon, Darrel! Someone with diabetes shouldn't be lying around all day. Whereas someone with no life, like myself, has a very good reason."

In this part . . .

Children develop type 1 diabetes more often than adults, and it sometimes comes at a very young age. Parents can take care of their children in the early stages of the disease, but kids eventually must learn to manage their disease on their own. The first chapter in this Part of Tens provides ten ways to involve kids in their own treatment, the sooner the better. In the second chapter, I present ten key tools of management of type 1 diabetes as commandments, which isn't far from the truth. The third chapter dispels some common myths about type 1 diabetes, and the final chapter gives you some insight into the amazing strides being made toward finding a cure for type 1 diabetes. Hang in there; hope is on the way!

Chapter 18

Ten Ways to Involve Kids in Their Own Diabetes Care

*I*nvolving children in their own diabetes care is critical. Sooner or later, as a parent or caretaker, you have to give up your control of food, injection amount and timing, blood glucose testing, and all the other tasks that are required for good diabetes care. When you do so, you want to know that you're turning over the care to a highly qualified individual, your child with T1DM.

Before you turn over the care, you can do a lot to prepare your child by letting him participate in what you do for him. Start by asking for his ideas and views about how you take care of his diabetes. Be sure to listen to what he says and show that you take him seriously by turning his reasonable suggestions into reality. This collaboration will have many benefits for your child, including the following:

✔ It will increase his self-confidence.

✔ It will improve his communication skills.

✔ It will expand his knowledge as you discuss his ideas and why they're appropriate or not.

✔ It will make him ready to take over his diabetes care when you think the time is right.

This chapter covers ten ways that you can progressively involve your child with T1DM so that he's ready, willing, and able to care for himself.

Set Some Goals for Care with Your Child

Your child probably doesn't know if he wants to be a doctor or lawyer at the age of 8, but by this time, he may have an idea of how to handle his diabetes. If not, this is a good opportunity to discuss the subject with him and to really listen and learn. You'll quickly find out how he feels about having diabetes — whether it's a major burden on him and if he's coming to terms with it. You also may find out what he's willing to do for himself and whether you need to keep charge of his diabetes until he's more reconciled to it.

If your child doesn't have goals for his diabetes care, this is a time to set some with him. You can start by asking the following questions:

✔ When does he feel he can start doing his own blood glucose testing and administering his own insulin? (I discuss these tasks later in this chapter.)

✔ Does he understand the consequences of not taking good care of himself, for example, eating right and exercising? (I talk about the importance of good food and regular exercise later in this chapter.)

✔ Is he willing to share his diagnosis with other family and friends so that they can help when necessary? This should be done when the diagnosis is first made because their help may be needed even more at the beginning than later on, after you and your child have a better understanding of diabetes care.

These are all important issues. The way he manages them will determine if he'll earn a Joslin medal for diabetic longevity in 50 years (see Chapter 17 for more about this award).

Show Your Child How to Test His Blood Glucose

Unfortunately, at least at present, testing blood glucose means sticking your finger. And that can hurt, although modern testing devices (see Chapter 7) keep the pain to a minimum. As soon as your child has good hand-eye coordination (around age 7 to 10), start letting him stick his own finger for blood glucose testing. Remember, he may have to do this for the next 50 or 60 years. He needs to find out how to produce a drop of blood with little effort, to get the test strip ready for testing, and to get the blood on the strip with minimal effort.

Doing his own testing will give him a lot of confidence about his diabetes. You want to emphasize the key role that testing plays in the management of his diabetes and the significance of the numbers that appear on the monitor. The more willing he is to test, the better his diabetes control. And the better his control, the fewer complications (if any) he'll experience later in life.

The short-term benefits of letting your child do his own glucose testing also are clear. He'll always be on top of his blood glucose, and ketoacidosis (high blood glucose) should be unusual. Hypoglycemia (low blood glucose) should be rare as well because he'll know in advance when his glucose is dropping. (Flip to Chapter 4 for more about hypoglycemia and ketoacidosis.)

Shop for Food Together

Although your child may initially think that all food originates in the supermarket, having him join you there can be a very valuable lesson in choosing good foods and avoiding bad foods. Start this practice at age 4 or 5 because he'll soon have to make his own food choices at school.

It's best to eat before you and your child hit the store. A full stomach will lessen but not entirely eliminate his requests for all the goodies that are available at the supermarket.

Show your child the foods that are part of his healthy diet, going from the things he eats the most to the things he should avoid. Teach him what's what as follows:

- ✔ Begin with carbohydrates and emphasize low glycemic choices and whole grains. Show him how the label tells him about the amounts of calories, salt, fiber, and so forth.

- ✔ Go to the vegetable area and tell him to eat plenty of dark green vegetables, orange vegetables, dry beans, and peas. Teach him to keep the amount of starchy vegetables he eats reduced compared to the others.

- ✔ Head to the fruit bins and tell him to eat a variety of them as they become available through the seasons. Tell him to drink less fruit juices and eat more whole fruit.

- ✔ Point out the fats and tell him to get his fats from fish, nuts, and vegetable oil rather than solid fats like butter and margarine.

- ✔ In the milk area, show him the low-fat or fat-free choices as well as other sources of calcium like yogurt. Point out that hard cheese has lots of fat, so lower-fat versions are better for him.

- ✔ In the meats section, point out the lean choices, like chicken and turkey. Tell him that he should eat less meat and more fish, beans, peas, nuts, and seeds, which contain healthier oils.

Make food shopping a great adventure. And make it more fun by taking your child along with you the next time and letting him guide you through the store and point out the best choices that you've taught him. Check out Chapter 8 for the full scoop on eating a healthy diet.

Plant a Garden Together

If you have a little space in your backyard, plant a garden with your child. He'll be amazed to find out that he can start with one small plant and end up with boxes of tomatoes! If you don't have the space, go cherry picking or apple picking or some other fruit or vegetable picking so that your child realizes that food comes from the soil.

If there's no nearby farm and you don't have property for planting, take your child to a farmers' market. (They're popping up in almost every community, so it shouldn't be difficult to find one near you.) He'll understand that the real source of food is the farm rather than the supermarket.

Gardening is another opportunity to find out what your child wants and likes as well as to show that you aren't just asking but intend to act on his request. Get the seeds and plants he wants and let him plant them, be responsible for them, and be the first to taste the result.

Explain how the seed of good diabetes control, when carefully planted, watered, and tended, can lead to a healthy and fruitful life, just as a garden plant produces its fruit. Furthermore, he's responsible for the outcome; whether he has a plant full of delicious fruit or a few scrawny results is entirely in his hands.

Have Your Child Help with the Cooking

Food is such a major part of diabetes care that it's essential that your child be able to cook for himself and prepare healthy food. Letting your child help you cook has many benefits, including the following:

- ✔ It represents quality time between you and your child.
- ✔ It's a chance for your child to learn to cook and pick up new skills.
- ✔ It's an opportunity for you to introduce new healthy foods that he's more willing to try because he had a hand in the preparation.

Even at a very young age, your child can do something to participate.

✔ At age 2, he can scrub fruit and vegetables, tear lettuce, and break bread.

✔ At age 3, he can pour liquids, mix batter, spread butter, and knead bread.

✔ At age 4 to 5, he can juice different fruits, mash soft fruits, measure dry and liquid ingredients, and beat eggs.

As your child grows older, give him more complex cooking tasks.

Although you encourage cleanliness, you have to be willing to accept some mess when you first start cooking with your child. But definitely give him a share of the cleanup jobs. Also, it's critical that you supervise and instruct. And don't forget to praise him as you eat the food you cooked together so that he associates good food with positive feelings.

Exercise as a Family

Exercise, as you know, plays a key role in your and your child's health. You can't expect your child to want to exercise if he sees his parent sitting in front of the computer (as I'm doing right now — fortunately my kids are grown).

Regardless of their diagnosis, I encourage my patients to exercise daily — kids with parents and vice versa. I could tell you many happy stories of the closeness that has developed between parents and children who jog together, not to mention the stories of chubby, shy children who grew up into lean, assertive adolescents because they exercised with their parents.

Chapter 9 tells you what you need to do to get started exercising with your child. Let him decide where you'll go sometimes. You may discover that he wants to show you off to his friends (or hide you).

Show Your Child How to Administer Insulin

You may want to delay the time when your child calculates his own insulin dosage until you're certain he can do it properly, but teaching him to administer the insulin is also something that should be done early (around age 10). Fortunately, this is even less painful than finger sticking for the blood glucose (which I discuss earlier in this chapter).

When he has sufficient hand-eye coordination, he must learn to take the correct dose of insulin into the syringe and inject it under his skin properly. (Of course, if your child uses a different method of insulin delivery, be sure to fully explain the process.) You want to explain how you established his dose every time so that dosage also becomes second nature. (Turn to Chapters 10 and 11 for full details on using insulin.)

Keep up the positive reinforcement with praise, and minimize your response to mistakes if they aren't serious. For example, a tiny bubble in the syringe isn't a serious mistake; taking double the dose of insulin is. Your child will be eager to take over the task of calculating his insulin as well, but don't be in a hurry to let him until you're totally confident that he can do it properly.

Plan a Trip Together

Planning a trip is another chance to get good feedback from your child while you teach him what to be aware of when traveling with T1DM (which I discuss in Chapter 15). He can start participating in the planning when he's old enough to go to school. Here are a few guidelines:

- Find out where he wants to go and what he wants to do there. Let him make the preparations that are required to ensure that he has enough insulin and testing materials.
- He should know how to maintain the potency of his insulin regardless of the climate at your destination.
- He should begin to understand what to do as he travels through time zones.
- He should already know about eating wisely for his diabetes. The principles of eating are the same whether at home or on a trip.
- He should know about security at airports and how to take diabetes supplies through. He must be aware not to make any remarks about explosives, even in a joking manner.

Have Your Child Do Household Chores

Studies by Marty Rossen at the University of Minnesota have shown that one of the best predictors of general success at age 20 and up was whether a child performed household tasks at age 3 to 4. Involving your child in such tasks teaches him

- A sense of responsibility
- A sense of competence
- A sense of self-reliance
- A sense of self-worth

These positive traits stay with the child throughout life, and they transfer over to his care of his diabetes. The messages that you want to give your child are that work is important and that he's capable of doing it competently. It's amazing what helping out around the house can do for your child, not to mention the benefits for you.

There are tasks that a child can do at every age. For example:

- The 2- to 3-year-old can pick up his toys, help sweep the floor, help set the table, undress himself, and dress himself with help.

- The 4-year-old can set the table, put away groceries, help with yard and garden work, help make the beds, and spread butter on bread.

- The 5-year-old can help with meal planning and grocery shopping (as I explain earlier in this chapter), pour his own drink, set the table, pick up his clothes, fold clean clothes, and do yard work like collecting leaves or clippings.

- The 6-year-old can choose his own clothing, water flowers and vegetables, cook simple foods like hot dogs, walk a pet, and tie his shoes.

- The 7-year-old can take phone messages, wash the dog, carry groceries in from the car and put them away, get up and go to bed on his own, and run simple errands for his parents.

- The 8- to 9-year-old can fold napkins and set the table, mop the floor, run his bathwater, fold blankets, cut flowers, paint a fence, and write a simple thank-you note.

- The 10- to 11-year-old can earn his own money for doing yard work, be home alone, stay overnight with a friend, and be responsible for his own hobby.

- The 12-year-old and up can join clubs and organizations, help with errands, mow the lawn, clean the oven and stove, help his parents with household repairs, and be responsible for part-time jobs like a paper route.

Encourage Your Child to Play Video Games (Really!)

Video games are a favorite pursuit of today's kids, and they have so many different games to choose from. Now there are video games that teach about T1DM! Two of the top games are *Starbright Life Adventure Series: Diabetes* and *Packy and Marlon*.

- *Starbright Life Adventure Series: Diabetes* comes from the Starbright Foundation, a nonprofit organization that develops programs to help seriously ill children cope with the challenges of their illnesses. This particular program uses interactive adventures to teach children to manage their diabetes properly. There are exercises, quizzes, and arcade games, and the program is available in Spanish. It's available on CD-ROM free of charge for a family that has a child with T1DM between the ages of 5 and 13. Call 800-760-3818 for more information.

- *Packy and Marlon* is a role-playing game used with Super-Nintendo. Children learn to plan meals, calculate and administer insulin, and test the blood glucose of two elephants with T1DM. Players get points for properly accomplishing these tasks. The game is available for around $60 from the Boehringer Mannheim Corp.; call 800-428-5076 for more information.

  Children who played *Packy and Marlon* were found to have more self-confidence about managing their diabetes and better communication with friends and care providers. During the six-month trial period, there was a 77 percent reduction in acute care visits because of diabetes.

If it can be said that T1DM may be fun, these games are the basis for that statement.

Chapter 19

Ten Commandments for Good Diabetes Management

*T*ype 1 diabetes (T1DM) isn't a religion, despite the title of this chapter. In fact, it can be a real pain at times. However, there's a lot that you can do to minimize that pain. Everything you need to get your child started properly with the things he must do to keep his disease under control and minimize its impact is available.

The ten commandments discussed in this chapter are a major part of what excellent care for T1DM is all about. Other things need to be done as well, but if you follow through on these ten, whether you're the parent or the patient, the others will fall into place.

Everything discussed here is described much more extensively in previous chapters. I bring it all together here to give you the total picture of essential diabetes care. Keep in mind that nothing in this chapter is more or less important than anything else. Each action is like a piece of a puzzle; individually, the pieces don't provide much clarity, but together, they tell you how to get your child to the point that he's able to put the puzzle together on his own.

An Affirmative Attitude

If I were to tell you that all patients with T1DM are destined to be blind or have their kidneys fail (for the record, I'd never tell you that), you'd have little incentive to do much of anything to help your child. Fortunately, it's not true. Everything you do for your child (or yourself, if you're the patient) makes a difference.

To manage T1DM, you and your child have to do so much on a daily basis, and so little of it seems to have an immediate effect. The positive belief that what you're doing is helpful to your child in the long-run is what keeps you doing it. The power of positive thinking is an important tool that helps you do everything you must do for your child, knowing that your efforts will bear fruit in the form of a long and healthy life. I discuss the details of coping with T1DM positively in Chapter 6.

Total Testing

With modern methods available for management of the long-term complications of diabetes (see Chapter 5), it's sad, unfortunate, and unnecessary for a patient with T1DM to lose his sight or his kidney function because he wasn't tested early. For every potential long-term complication due to T1DM, there's an excellent test or study that can discover it when it's still at a reversible stage. In Chapter 7, I go over the routine tests that must be done to prevent irreversible damage to your child's eyes, kidneys, or nervous system. More and more, these tests are available as home kits that you can complete at home, like the hemoglobin A1c, or send to a lab that returns the result, like the urine microalbumin test.

Make a copy of the test table on the Cheat Sheet and make sure to keep it up-to-date with your child's test results. Don't depend on your child's pediatrician to get these tests when they're due; he has numerous other patients to think about, but your child is your one and only, so be an advocate for your child.

The importance of continued testing is also something that you must teach your child when he takes over management of his T1DM. By then he'll probably have had diabetes for ten years or more, and regular tests are even more important for adults than they are for younger folks because the long-term complications of diabetes begin to appear after ten years.

Extraordinary Eye Care

The eye is the one organ that allows doctors to see directly into the brain what they see happening in the tissues of the eye is probably happening in the brain as well. Doctors have wonderful tools for viewing and photographing the eyes and for treating any damage that occurs to them. What can you do to reduce the risk of eye damage (see Chapter 5) in your child?

✔ **Make sure that your child has yearly eye examinations from an eye doctor or optometrist beginning a few years after he develops his diabetes.** Abnormalities can be spotted early, and treatment preserves vision. (See Chapter 7 for more about eye exams.)

✔ **Make sure that your child understands the connection between his blood glucose and his eyes.** (In a nutshell, the higher the level of blood glucose, the greater likelihood of eye damage.) The Joslin Medalist Study of T1DM of extreme duration (see Chapter 17) shows that eye disease doesn't have to happen — even after 50 years of living with diabetes.

The picture used to be a lot bleaker because almost every patient with T1DM developed serious eye disease, and many went blind. Now, with careful monitoring of the blood glucose and the eyes, blindness need never occur. At worst, the patient may need treatment with laser therapy to the eyes, a very effective form of treatment that prevents blindness.

✔ **Make sure that your child takes care of his eyes and gets annual eye examinations as an adult.** I want him to be able to continue to read my books far into the future!

Foolproof Foot Care

One of the sad consequences of T1DM that should never occur is an amputation of the foot. Amputations are preventable, but they occur when relatively minor foot problems, especially ulcers of the foot, aren't caught and managed early. Ultimately, foot ulcers should never develop in the first place.

Your child's doctor should inspect his feet at every examination (see Chapter 7 for more information). Although it's very unlikely that there will be anything wrong with your child's feet in the early years of T1DM, it's good to get the child thinking about his feet and examining them himself from an early age. Here are a few guidelines for home foot care:

✔ **Keep the skin lubricated if it tends to be dry.**

✔ **Trim toenails carefully.**

> ✔ **Visually inspect the feet every day, looking for any small cut or other abrasion.**
>
> ✔ **Choose footwear carefully, both to prevent blisters and sores and to decrease pressure on any existing foot problems or deformities.**

It's essential that the foot doctor is consulted immediately when there's any sign of a new abnormality of the feet. Waiting a few days can make an enormous difference in the outcome.

Mega-Monitoring

Home testing of the blood glucose (see Chapter 7) is a truly valuable tool that has made an enormous difference in the successful management of T1DM. It's truly amazing that you can know your child's blood glucose in 5 seconds with less than a drop of blood. At first, your child won't like it, but with repetition, blood glucose testing hurts less and less and becomes more and more routine.

Monitoring the blood glucose provides a snapshot of your child's metabolism at a given instant in time. It provides the critical information that allows you to choose the proper dose of insulin to keep the blood glucose in a range of 80 to 140 mg/dl. A patient with an average blood glucose in that range will never suffer from diabetic complications.

How much testing should you do? The more, the merrier, as they say. There's no doubt that a major difference between my patients with T1DM who successfully manage their diabetes and those who have difficulty doing so is that the former test their blood sugar far more than the latter. I recommend testing at the following times:

> ✔ **Before meals** to figure out the bolus of insulin to give for the meal, depending upon the current blood glucose and the amount of carbohydrates about to be eaten (see Chapter 10 for more about insulin dosages)
>
> ✔ **An hour after eating** to gauge the rise in blood glucose with food and to respond with extra insulin before that meal next time
>
> ✔ **At bedtime** to see if your child is going to sleep with a low blood glucose, in which case a bedtime snack is in order to prevent hypoglycemia
>
> ✔ **Frequently when your child's sick** because illness causes major changes in blood glucose (see Chapter 15 for more about handling sick days)
>
> ✔ **Occasionally at other times** just to see how a given food or a certain amount of exercise affects your child's blood glucose

The other kind of monitoring that you can do is monitoring of the ketones in the blood. It requires a specific monitor but can give you a very early clue that your child is headed for diabetic ketoacidosis. I describe this test more extensively in Chapter 15. Testing the blood for ketones has resulted in earlier admissions to hospitals when necessary and shorter hospital stays.

Dedicated Dieting

Careful management of the diet in T1DM has been shown repeatedly to lower the hemoglobin A1c (see Chapter 7) by 1 percent or more. And every 1 percent drop in hemoglobin A1c causes a large decrease in the risk of microvascular complications that I describe in Chapter 5: retinopathy, nephropathy, and neuropathy.

Here are a few diet guidelines for a person with T1DM (see Chapter 8 for full details on eating sensibly):

✔ Because carbohydrates are the only macronutrients that directly and immediately raise blood glucose (unlike protein and fat), it makes sense either to limit the amount of carbohydrate in your child's meals or to choose carbohydrates that are absorbed more slowly (meaning those that aren't highly processed).

✔ Don't limit the amount of food your child eats, but make the good food choices that will control his blood glucose. He'll stop eating when he's full, and his growing body needs the extra calories.

✔ Definitely get your child involved in choosing good food and food preparation as described in Chapter 18. At some point, he'll go off to college or move out on his own, and then he must have these skills. A dependence on restaurant food or food ordered in like pizza is likely to result in fairly poor control of the blood glucose.

✔ Don't abandon a careful nutritional program when you eat outside your home. You can find out what's available at most restaurants by finding them on the Internet and glancing at their menus. Fast-food places serve the same food everywhere, and the nutritional content of their food is available on the Internet as well.

✔ If you're really stuck and have no idea of the nutritional value of what your child is eating, use blood glucose monitoring to measure his blood glucose (see the previous section), and treat the result as necessary.

Emphatic Exercising

As evidenced in a survey article, the fortunate folks who have received medals from the Joslin Diabetes Center for having lived with diabetes on insulin for 50 years or more have several things in common (see Chapter 17 for the full story). One is that they exercise more than most other people at their age. The authors conclude that "exercise may be an important protective factor." You can say that again!

The T1DM patients in my practice with the lowest hemoglobin A1c, the least need for insulin, and the fewest complications are the ones who do the most exercise. Exercise has so many positive aspects to it and such a minimal downside that it should be as routine for your child as brushing his teeth. I discuss exercise in detail in Chapter 9.

Don't expect your child to become physically active on his own. Unfortunately, schools are reducing physical education programs in favor of varsity football and basketball. Your child needs your example to start an exercise program. Get out and walk with him at first, then jog, swim, bike, or ski (or do a combination of these). There will come a day when your child will beat you to the end of the pool or down the ski slope and that should be a day of celebration because you know you've done your job right.

Mindful Medicating

Every time I see a high blood glucose result and my patient tells me it happened because he forgot to take his insulin shot, I feel like screaming (but I never do). The stakes are too high to allow that to occur. Most of the time poor diabetic control has little to do with problems that are outside the control of the person with diabetes and has everything to do with not taking medications, not testing the blood glucose, not following a nutritional plan, and not exercising (all of which I discuss earlier in this chapter). There are all kinds of alarms and monitors you can set up to prompt your child to take his insulin (or to prompt you to give it to him) if he has trouble remembering, but the bottom line is that the best treatments in the world are of little value if your child doesn't use them.

Not only do some people forget to take their insulin entirely, but insulin also is consistently in the list of the top ten medications associated with administration errors. At the present time, all people with T1DM take two kinds of insulin, long-acting and rapid-acting. Almost once a week I get a call from a patient who has taken the rapid-acting when he should have taken the long-acting, and vice versa. What can you do to make sure that you and your child avoid this mistake?

✔ One of the great benefits of inhaled insulin is that adult patients who take it never mistake it for something else. Insulin from an inhaler is always rapid-acting insulin and therefore is unlikely to be confused with long-acting insulin from a shot. At the present time, inhaled insulin isn't recommended for children. But if you're an adult patient, you may want to talk to your doctor about this option; see Chapter 10 for more information.

✔ Before insulin glargine became the long-acting insulin of choice, patients used intermediate (NPH) insulin. It was cloudy compared to clear rapid-acting insulin, so the two were rarely confused. Glargine, by contrast, is clear, so you can see where there may be confusion. One possible solution is to administer the rapid-acting insulin with an insulin pen and the glargine from a bottle with a syringe.

I explain the particulars of insulin in Chapters 10 and 11, including the kinds of insulin available, calculating insulin doses correctly, and various methods for delivering insulin.

Planning for Potential Problems

Planning is key if you're going to keep your child's diabetes under excellent control. Think about what your child will be exposed to in advance, and smooth the way. Consider doing dry runs to prepare for potentially difficult situations. Practicing how you'll handle situations before they arise makes it a lot easier to function when you're faced with the real thing. For example:

✔ When it comes to food, you can eat at places you know, inform your hostess that your child has diabetes and help her to prepare something he can eat (if possible), bring the food for your child with diabetes, and/or check the fast-food recipes on the Internet. If you've been invited to a new restaurant, visit it in advance and simply read the menu. Carefully select the foods that will help your child to stay in control of his T1DM.

✔ Plan for the times when your child's blood glucose is low. Have glucose tablets or any of the other treatments recommended in Chapter 4 available to bring the blood glucose up but not too high. An emergency glucagon kit is another valuable item to have on hand.

You may want to create checklists because remembering everything you have to do can be difficult. Have an eating-out checklist, a visiting-others checklist, a travel checklist, and so forth. You'll be so glad you did when you discover that you have the thing you need at that moment you need it.

Lifelong Learning

Diabetes is a "hot" disease right now, mostly because of the surge in cases of type 2 diabetes. As a result, a huge amount of money is directed at the disease, and T1DM is getting its share. Diabetes journals that used to be thin are now thick with new information. For example, the number of publications that I get in my office with "diabetes" somewhere in the title has become so great that I can't keep up with them and have to pick and choose what to read.

Use the following tips to ensure a lifetime of learning about your child's condition:

✔ As soon as you can after you've gotten over the initial shock of having a child with T1DM, sign up for a course on diabetes with a Certified Diabetes Educator. Make sure it's focused on T1DM because a lot of the information about T2DM has little relevance to your child's disease. (I explain how to find a diabetes educator in Chapter 2.)

✔ The fact that you're reading this book indicates how much you want to learn about T1DM. But don't stop with this book. There are other excellent publications available, many offered by the American Diabetes Association. Appendix B is chock-full of resources to help you find the latest information.

✔ When your child is old enough (around age 10), take him with you to a refresher course on T1DM. You'll be amazed at how much new material is offered. Encourage him to continue learning. As you see in Chapter 21, there are some incredible new approaches to the treatment of T1DM; one of them may turn out to be the "cure" you're looking for.

Chapter 20

Ten Myths about Type 1 Diabetes

*A*s you would expect for a disease that has been around for several thousand years, there are plenty of myths about diabetes. Some of them have a tiny bit of truth to them, so they keep being passed around. Unfortunately, thanks to the Internet, a myth can pop up on 10 million computer screens in two hours. But just because so many diabetes myths have been heard and read about doesn't make them true.

In this book, you find everything of importance that you need to know to help your child (or yourself, if you're an adult patient) live a long and healthy life with type 1 diabetes (or T1DM for short). If you don't read about something in one of the chapters on diagnosis and treatment, it's unlikely that it plays an important role in diabetes care. So if you hear about some great breakthrough in T1DM and it isn't in this book, consider it a myth until proven otherwise. You can even drop me an e-mail and tell me about it at diabetes@drrubin.com. I'm happy to either confirm or deny it.

Because insulin and food are key components of diabetes care, it's no surprise that a lot of myths in T1DM revolve around these two topics. There's also a lot of confusion about the difference between T1DM and T2DM. You may even encounter myths about the direction of science in curing T1DM. I break down all these myths in this chapter.

No Symptoms of Type 1 Diabetes Appear before Damage Has Occurred

Diabetes is sometimes called "the Silent Disease," but that nickname just isn't true. T1DM actually has plenty of symptoms — if you know where to look. Some of the symptoms that children complain of early in the disease include:

- ✔ Increased urination
- ✔ Increased thirst
- ✔ Dry skin
- ✔ Fatigue
- ✔ Blurry vision
- ✔ Irritability
- ✔ Extreme hunger
- ✔ Eating without weight gain
- ✔ Unexpected and unusual weight loss

These symptoms aren't severe, so they often go unnoticed by parents and caretakers. Put simply, it's hard to accept the fact that there's something seriously wrong with your 10-year-old. However, with so much emphasis on diabetes in general because of the huge increase in cases of T2DM, people are more aware of a diabetes diagnosis and are having their children checked earlier, long before they reach the stage of complete lack of insulin and ketoacidosis (see Chapter 4).

Flip to Chapter 2 for the basics of T1DM, its symptoms, and its diagnosis.

Type 1 Diabetes and Type 2 Diabetes Are the Same

Parents of children with T1DM would love for their children's disease to be called by another name so it isn't confused with type 2 diabetes (or T2DM). Although T1DM and T2DM share some of the same characteristics, they are hardly the same disease. They differ in the following ways:

- ✔ The cause of T1DM is a genetic tendency plus a virus. The cause of T2DM is heredity plus obesity plus a sedentary lifestyle.

- ✔ Patients with T1DM have an absolute lack of insulin when the disease strikes. Patients with T2DM may actually have too much measurable insulin when the disease strikes; they have insulin resistance.

- ✔ Most cases of T1DM occur in childhood. Most cases of T2DM occur after age 35.

- ✔ T2DM can be controlled with diet and exercise alone. T1DM can't be controlled in that way.

- ✔ Diabetic ketoacidosis (see Chapter 4) is often the first complaint in T1DM. It doesn't occur in patients with T2DM.

- ✔ Most patients with T1DM are thin. Patients with T2DM are generally (but not always) fat.

T1DM and T2DM are similar in the following ways:

- ✔ The clinical problem in both begins when the blood glucose rises too high.

- ✔ High blood glucose acts as a toxin in both forms.

- ✔ Complications of eye disease, kidney disease, nerve disease, and cardio-vascular disease (see Chapter 5) are similar for both kinds.

See Chapter 3 for more about the differences between T1DM and T2DM.

You Can't Eat Sugar with Type 1 Diabetes

This myth goes back to the time before insulin became available in 1921. At that time, there was nothing that could force glucose into the cells of the body where insulin was required, so the treatment was the elimination of all carbohydrates. The reasoning was that, if a patient didn't consume carbohydrates, then the blood glucose couldn't rise to the high levels that resulted in excessive urination, thirst, confusion, coma, and death. That approach worked for a time, but the liver is fully capable of making glucose from protein despite the fact that the glucose can't get into liver cells to be stored as glycogen once it's made.

Today, there are probably more types of insulin available than are needed. A little injected insulin can take care of lots of sugar or other carbohydrates.

A corollary to this myth is that T1DM is caused by consuming too many sweets. Doctors have a pretty good idea of the cause of T1DM, and sweets have nothing to do with it. As I explain in Chapter 2, the cause of T1DM is believed to be a combination of a hereditary tendency and infection with a virus that has characteristics similar to insulin-producing beta cells. As the body destroys the virus, it mistakenly destroys the beta cells as well.

All in all, some glucose as part of a good overall diet is definitely acceptable. Let your child enjoy a little sugar. Just don't let him overdo it. Eating anything in excess is discouraged, whether it's carbohydrate, protein, or fat. See Chapter 8 for the full details on eating a healthy, sensible diet.

You Have to Eat Special Foods When You Have Type 1 Diabetes

With T1DM, there's no advantage to eating special diabetic foods. It's difficult enough to deal with all the requirements for good diabetes care to have to eat boring tasteless foods! Food is one of life's great pleasures, and your child can have excellent glucose control with regular food so long as you account for the carbohydrate in it. Need some help?

- ✔ I provide resources for great recipes in Appendix B.
- ✔ In my book *Diabetes Cookbook For Dummies,* 2nd Edition (Wiley), I offer page after page of recipes for delicious meals that fit into a nutritional plan for patients with T1DM. These recipes come from some of the best restaurants in America.
- ✔ Books that feature good, nutritious food for children with T1DM fill the shelves of many bookstores.

Show your child that he can eat delicious meals and still follow his nutritional plan. Prepare meals that the whole family can eat. With food this good, there's no reason that everyone in the family shouldn't eat the same meals as your child with T1DM.

If You Take Insulin, You Must Have Type 1 Diabetes

In T1DM, insulin is an essential part of diabetes care because the disease is characterized by a total lack of insulin in the body. On the other hand, in T2DM, insulin is a tool to get the blood glucose to a level at which diet and exercise can work. T2DM is a lifestyle disease, not a disease of lack of insulin. When someone with T2DM improves his diet, exercise regimen, and weight, he can manage T2DM without insulin.

So how do patients with T2DM wind up on insulin? They initially have resistance to their own insulin. As time passes, many of them also seem to lose the ability to make enough insulin to control their blood glucose at their current weight. Then they must be put on insulin.

Many of those patients with T2DM could come off the insulin with proper diet and exercise. The diagnosis remains T2DM whether they are on insulin or not.

In my practice, I've seen many patients with T2DM who have been put on insulin by other doctors and still have poor control of their diabetes. When I successfully get them to lose 5 to 10 percent of their body weight, their need for insulin diminishes and sometimes even goes away. My patients can hardly believe that they can get off the insulin and have even better control of their blood glucose than they did when they were on it. These aren't true T1DM patients — they actually have T2DM. Their own bodies' insulin does a much better job of regulating their metabolism than any insulin shot I could give them.

I go over the basics of insulin for folks with T1DM in Chapters 10 and 11. To find out much more about the basics and treatment of T2DM, check out my book *Diabetes For Dummies,* 2nd Edition (Wiley).

Insulin Causes Atherosclerosis

This myth probably arose because insulin is often given in situations where atherosclerosis (narrowing of the arteries) is already present but not clinically evident. Atherosclerosis takes years to develop, so a medication like insulin that has been started in the last few months is hardly to blame. Want an example? When young men killed in combat during the Korean War were carefully examined, they already had evidence of early atherosclerosis that probably wouldn't have been clinically evident for decades.

The fact is that insulin actually causes a decline in atherosclerosis by reversing the processes that lead to elevated blood glucose levels and elevated fatty acids in the blood.

Insulin Cures Type 1 Diabetes

Doctors and researches are coming close to developing a cure for T1DM (see Chapter 21), but it won't involve patients using insulin. Insulin helps to control the blood glucose, but so far it's impossible to deliver insulin in the body in the same way that it comes from the pancreas. It also isn't possible to fine-tune the insulin dose like the body can, releasing and destroying insulin to maintain a blood glucose no lower than 80 mg/dl and no higher than 120 mg/dl.

Insulin tried on kids with a high risk of T1DM in the Diabetes Prevention Trials (ongoing trials of various drugs that may prevent T1DM) wasn't successful in preventing the disease. Insulin is a powerful drug that has saved the lives of hundreds of thousands of people with diabetes, but none of them has been cured. The most to hope for is that insulin keeps the blood glucose sufficiently low so complications of diabetes don't develop.

Many myths concern great new cures for T1DM with this medication or that medication. Ignore them. At the present time, no single medication can cure T1DM.

You're More Prone to Illness When You Have Type 1 Diabetes

If you compare frequency of illness in the population with T1DM with that of people who don't have diabetes, there's no difference between them. This myth about being prone to illness is a popular one that originated when T1DM was so hard to treat before 1921. Back then, kids with T1DM were a very sick bunch.

People with T1DM get viral illnesses no more often than those without T1DM. They need to take a flu shot every year to prevent the severe illness that may be associated with that disease. Elderly people with T1DM especially should get shots for pneumonia and shingles. But if someone with T1DM comes down with a bug, he has to adjust his insulin intake, modify his diet, and take medications carefully. See Chapter 15 for details.

Women with Type 1 Diabetes Shouldn't Get Pregnant

A woman with T1DM must take a number of precautions when dealing with pregnancy, like checking for any diabetic complications before she conceives and throughout the pregnancy, but besides that, she can have a textbook pregnancy and baby. Healthy, happy babies are born to women with T1DM every day. Much of Chapter 16 is devoted to how they do it.

The woman with T1DM who's even thinking about a pregnancy must improve her glucose control so that she has a hemoglobin A1c below 7 percent before she conceives. (See Chapter 7 for more about hemoglobin A1c.) She also must keep her blood glucose below 90 mg/dl before a meal and below 120 mg/dl an hour after the meal throughout the pregnancy.

Doctors Are Hiding the Cure for Type 1 Diabetes So They Can Make More Money

This myth sounds so silly, but I've heard it from people I respect. They think there's a hidden agreement that the cure for T1DM, which has already been found, won't be made available so that doctors and drug and device companies can continue to profit from caring for patients with T1DM.

There's nothing further from the truth than this myth. Scientists are a highly competitive bunch. None of them is holding back a T1DM cure because they can feel the others breathing down their necks! Thousands of hard-working doctors and other scientists have dedicated their lives to finding a cure for T1DM. (Chapter 21 features just a few of them.) I attend conferences on diabetes regularly, and at each one, I see numerous presentations showing just how close researchers are to a cure for T1DM.

Chapter 21

Ten of the Latest Discoveries in Type 1 Diabetes

. . . .

In This Chapter

▶ Possibly preventing type 1 diabetes with vaccines and insulin

▶ Monitoring blood glucose in new ways

▶ Fighting the complications of type 1 diabetes

▶ Reversing the loss of beta cells

. . . .

So much is being discovered every day in T1DM that I could write this whole book on that aspect rather than limiting it to a chapter of ten items. It's a very exciting time! I'll even go so far as to predict that you'll see your child cured of T1DM in your lifetime.

The work is occurring in every phase of T1DM.

✔ **In the area of prevention and diagnosis,** T1DM is being broken down into subgroups based on new findings in genetics. New substances are being found in patients' blood that suggest the diagnosis much earlier.

✔ **In the area of monitoring,** new tests are being developed to show much earlier responses to treatment. New devices are coming on the market for testing the blood glucose continuously and painlessly.

✔ **In the area of complications,** doctors' understanding of the mechanism of complications is expanding. They're getting down to the details of the transition from normal tissue to damaged tissue, and new substances are being found in the blood that point to the earliest development of complications.

Perhaps the most work is focused on finding a way to reverse the loss of beta cells that make insulin in T1DM. Doctors and researchers are taking all kinds of approaches, from restoring the beta cells with injections of fresh beta cells from an outside source to trying to get various cells to transform themselves into beta cells. The trouble is that these new cells are still subject to the destructive effects of the same substances in the body that destroyed the beta cells in the first place, so new drugs are being offered to overcome that difficulty. Another approach is to eliminate all the immunologic cells in the child's body by irradiation and then to restore them with new cells that may not kill the beta cells that produce insulin.

In this chapter, I provide you with ten of the latest discoveries in T1DM. Knowing that you're most interested in a cure, I discuss the most likely directions from which that cure will come. Not every approach will bear fruit, but you only need one to work in order for your child to be free of his least desired role: a person with T1DM. (See Appendix B for a list of resources that can help you keep up with the latest discoveries.)

Doctors are well on the way to major advances in type 1 diabetes prevention and treatment. It's definitely a good move for you to keep your child as well controlled as possible (or to do the same for yourself if you're the patient). After all, you want your child's body to be in perfect condition when the cure becomes available.

The Development of the GAD Vaccine

In 1988, two scientists at UCLA were studying genes involved in brain development and function, and they discovered the genes that caused the production of glutamic acid decarboxylase (GAD). GAD is an enzyme that leads to the production of an important *neurotransmitter,* a chemical that transmits information from one nerve to another. At the time, it wasn't known that GAD is also made in the beta cells of the pancreas — the same cells that produce and store insulin.

One of the original investigators then read a report about a connection between autoimmunity to an unknown protein in insulin-producing cells and diabetes. Somehow he realized that the protein was probably GAD, so he went to work to prove his hypothesis.

First he found that patients with T1DM had high levels of GAD autoantibody. Then he discovered that mice prone to develop T1DM could be protected from the disease by receiving small amounts of GAD. He and his colleagues then created a vaccine using GAD that could slow the development of T1DM even after the immune response had begun.

The next step was trying the GAD vaccine on humans, which happened in a study in which neither patient nor doctor knew whether the patient was getting GAD vaccine or a placebo. The result was that the GAD vaccine preserved insulin production without any adverse effects. The vaccine is called Diamyd and may prove to be very valuable in protecting high-risk children from developing T1DM. See Chapter 2 for more about GAD.

The Possible Prevention of Type 1 Diabetes with Oral Insulin

The Diabetes Prevention Trials in 2002 showed that oral insulin could delay or prevent the onset of T1DM. Now a much larger study is underway (it began in February 2007 and will end in seven or eight years) based on the theory that oral insulin quiets the immune system. It's set up as follows:

- Half the patients get oral insulin in a capsule.
- The other half get a placebo.
- Neither the patient nor the doctor knows what's in the capsule.

The patients in this study are relatives of patients with known T1DM. Those who may develop diabetes are found to have positive tests for autoantibodies against insulin and another substance called glutamate decarboxylate. If autoantibodies are found, they're asked to enroll in the study.

The study will follow the patients to see if and when they develop T1DM. If nothing else, the participants will know that they may develop T1DM much earlier than they normally would know.

If oral insulin works as the researchers hope, those who get it in their capsules will get T1DM later or not at all compared to those who get the placebo capsules.

The Possible Prevention of Type 1 Diabetes with Intranasal Insulin

The basis of this treatment is the theory that exposing the mucous membranes of the nose to insulin will act like a virus to stimulate protective immune cells. These protective cells will counteract the damaging cells that destroy the beta cells that produce and store insulin (or so researchers hope).

The patients in the study will be relatives of people with T1DM who are found to have positive autoantibodies against insulin or GAD and therefore have a greater chance of developing T1DM than those who don't have the antibodies. Some patients will get insulin, and some will get a placebo, but neither the patients nor the doctors will know who got what until the study ends.

In this study, 264 people are scheduled to be enrolled by 2007, and it isn't due for completion until 2012. The patients will be studied for the development of

T1DM as well as evaluated for the development of more evidence of immunity. (This study is taking place in Australia, so it's a long way to go if you're interested.)

Another study of intranasal insulin called Pre-POINT will involve giving the insulin to children at high risk of T1DM (because they have relatives with T1DM) even before they've developed antibodies.

The Study of Continuous Glucose Monitoring

The Diabetes Control and Complications Trial (DCCT) published in 1993 revealed that tight control of the blood glucose could prevent complications of T1DM. Here it is about 15 years later, and most patients with T1DM still don't meet the targets of glucose control shown to be necessary by the DCCT.

The Juvenile Diabetes Research Foundation (JDRF) is funding a study of continuous glucose monitoring (CGM) to see if the technique leads to better control. The authors believe that CGM decreases anxiety about hypoglycemic attacks but may increase stress when the CGM doesn't agree with a finger stick. (The discrepancy in results occurs when there's a rapid fall or rise in the blood glucose.) The authors also are concerned that the amount of blood glucose data from CGM will overwhelm the patient and family.

CGM is also being used in a JDRF-funded study with an insulin pump wherein the pump responds to the CGM reading by supplying insulin to the patient. This is the *closed-loop system* that's the ultimate goal of treatment, a working "pancreas." So far the system has worked very well. It may be the temporary solution for T1DM until there's a way to replace and restore the beta cells destroyed in T1DM.

See Chapter 7 for details on home systems for continuous glucose monitoring and Chapter 11 for more about insulin pumps.

Contact Lenses That Indicate Your Glucose Level

If this device pans out, you'll be looking in the mirror every time you want to know your blood glucose. Researchers at the University of Pittsburgh have developed plastic contact lenses that change color depending upon the amount of glucose in body fluids.

The glucose sensor could be embedded in regular contact lenses or worn as separate contact lenses for people without vision problems. It would change from red, indicating dangerously low blood glucose, to violet, indicating dangerously high blood glucose. A normal blood glucose level produces a green lens.

The device works by combining moisture from the tear ducts with molecules of boronic acid in the sensor to create fluorescence. A potential problem is the delay between the level of glucose in the blood and its reflection in tear ducts. This work is ongoing and may reach the market in the next few years.

A Drug to Fight Diabetic Neuropathy

Diabetic neuropathy causes pain and discomfort in the feet. Numerous drugs have been used in an attempt to reverse the neuropathy, but nothing has worked consistently until the introduction of SB-509. The drug currently called SB-509 has been found to cause the production of a protein called vascular endothelial growth factor, which helps to improve the structure and function of nerves.

In a study conducted by JDRF, SB-509 is being injected into both legs of patients who have T1DM and neuropathy three times over four months. Some people will receive the actual drug, and some will receive a placebo. The authors plan to look at pain intensity and nerve conduction velocity to look for recovery from neuropathy. They'll also look at the nerves under a microscope to see if repair of nerves damaged by T1DM is possible. The study began in 2006 and is scheduled to end in 2008.

Flip to Chapter 5 for details on diabetic neuropathy and other long-term complications that your child can avoid with tight control of T1DM.

Drugs to Block the Immunity That Kills Beta Cells

T1DM results when the process of autoimmunity (immune damage directed back at the person rather than at an outside invader) destroys the beta cells that produce insulin. Two types of cells in the body are responsible for the immune destruction: T cells and B cells. T cells are the ones that actually attack and destroy the beta cells. B cells somehow promote the attack by the T cells.

When symptoms develop in T1DM, within three months of the diagnosis, up to 80 to 90 percent of beta cells are destroyed but 10 to 20 percent remain. The purpose of a study conducted by diabetes clinics throughout the country is to see whether it's possible to stop further loss of beta cells by giving a drug called rituximab to patients. Rituximab is to lower B cells.

The authors plan to measure whether the beta cells that are left when the drug is given at or before three months of T1DM continue to exist and produce insulin. They'll check hemoglobin A1c measurements and insulin doses. As of this writing, the results of this study are expected to be published very soon.

Another drug that's undergoing the same study is TRX4; the study is also being conducted by diabetes clinics throughout the country. The intention is to see if TRX4 can preserve or even improve beta cell function and reduce the amount of insulin that the patient has to take. Results should be available soon for this study as well.

The Regeneration of Beta Cells with a Protein

One of the most exciting approaches that I've come across regarding T1DM is the work of Dr. Lijun Yang, an associate professor at the University of Florida College of Medicine. She's found that she can infuse a protein called recombinant Pdx1 into mice with T1DM and no beta cell function, and it both regenerates beta cells in their pancreas and turns liver cells into insulin-producing beta cells. The mice no longer have diabetes after this treatment, and the Pdx1 protein isn't toxic to the mice in substantial doses.

As of this writing, Dr. Yang is working on a study of humans with T1DM to see if she can accomplish the same thing in human volunteers. The patients will be given human Pdx1 protein. As of this writing, this study hasn't begun.

It remains to be seen whether the beta cells, however they're regenerated, will be subject to the immune rejection of the original beta cells that turned the patients into people with T1DM in the first place.

The Infusion of Stem Cells

One approach to preventing further loss of insulin production in newly diagnosed patients with T1DM is suppression of the immune response that's destroying the beta cells. A group in Brazil took this treatment a little further, and their work was published in *The Journal of the American Medical Association* in April 2007.

The scientists began by obtaining *stem cells,* which are cells that haven't become any particular kind of cell like white blood cells or red blood cells, from each newly diagnosed patient with T1DM. (The stem cells were taken within six weeks of the patients' diagnoses.) The patients received a high dose of an immunosuppressive drug to prevent the immune response that's believed to cause the destruction of beta cells. Then the scientists gave the stem cells back to the respective patients.

Of the 15 patients who received this treatment, 14 became able to control their blood glucose without insulin for different lengths of time: one patient for 35 months, four patients for at least 21 months, seven patients for at least 6 months, and two patients who were late responders and were insulin-free for one and five months, respectively. Levels of hemoglobin A1c were maintained at less than 7 percent in 13 of 14 patients, and only one patient needed to resume insulin after a year.

The Use of Cord Blood to Regenerate Beta Cells

As of this writing, a study going on at the University of Florida is using the stem cells found in umbilical cord blood to attempt to regenerate beta cells. Cord blood has the advantage of containing a large number of cells that decrease immunity.

The plan is to enlist 23 children with T1DM over the age of 1 whose parents had the foresight to store their cord blood at birth. The cord blood is infused back into the child from whom it was taken.

The study, which is to be completed by 2009, will determine if the cells in the cord blood can change into insulin-producing cells and/or provide immune tolerance that will permit regeneration of beta cells.

Part VI
Appendixes

The 5th Wave — By Rich Tennant

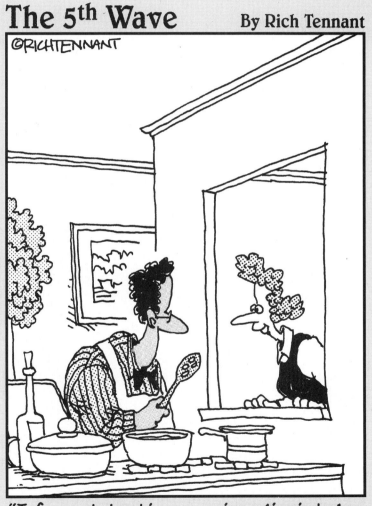

"I forgot to time my insulin intake correctly, so if you don't mind, I'll just nibble on the centerpiece until dinner's served."

In this part . . .

In this part, I leave you with a bit more information to help you deal with type 1 diabetes. First, I don't want you to go away not understanding any term in the book; therefore I provide a glossary in Appendix A where you can look up every perplexing term. I also don't believe that this book is the last word on the subject of type 1 diabetes. Fortunately, doctors and other scientists are working day and night to make it easier for you to care for your child (or yourself) and to find a cure. Appendix B directs you to what I consider the best sources of the latest information on every aspect of type 1 diabetes.

Appendix A

Glossary

ACE (angiotensin converting enzyme) inhibitor: A drug that lowers blood pressure but is especially useful when diabetes affects the kidneys.

Acetone: A breakdown product of fat formed when fat rather than glucose is being used for energy.

Adrenal glands: Organs sitting on top of each kidney, producing cortisol and adrenaline, which oppose insulin.

Adrenaline: Hormone from the adrenal gland that increases blood glucose.

Advanced glycated end products (AGEs): Combinations of glucose and other substances in the body; too much may damage various organs.

Alpha cells: Cells in the islets of Langerhans within the pancreas that make glucagon, which raises blood glucose.

Amyotrophy: A form of diabetic neuropathy causing muscle wasting and weakness.

Anorexia: Lack of appetite; also used in anorexia nervosa, an eating disorder in which the patient eats little or nothing.

Antibodies: Substances formed when the body detects something foreign, such as bacteria.

Antigens: Substances against which an antibody forms.

Artificial pancreas: A machine that measures blood glucose and releases appropriate insulin.

Aspart insulin: a rapid-acting insulin; also known by its brand name, NovoLog.

Atherosclerosis: Narrowing of arteries due to deposits of cholesterol and other factors; also called coronary artery disease or arteriosclerosis.

Autoimmune disorder: Disease in which the body mistakenly attacks its own tissues.

Autonomic neuropathy: Diseases of nerves that affect organs not under conscious control, such as the heart, lungs, and intestines.

Background retinopathy: An early stage of diabetic eye involvement that doesn't reduce vision; signs include retinal aneurysms, retinal hemorrhages, hard exudates, and soft exudates.

Basal insulin: The small amount of insulin always present in the bloodstream; also the continuous insulin provided by an insulin pump.

Beta cells: Cells in the islets of Langerhans in the pancreas that make the key hormone insulin.

Blood urea nitrogen (BUN): A substance in blood that reflects kidney function.

Body mass index (BMI): An indicator of appropriate weight for a person's height; derived by dividing your weight (in kilograms) by your height (in meters), and dividing that number by your height (in meters) again; alternately, you can multiply your weight in pounds by 703, divide that by your height in inches, and divide that result by your height in inches again.

Bolus insulin: The amount of insulin taken before meals.

Carbohydrate: One of the three major energy sources; the one most responsible for raising the blood glucose; usually found in grain, fruits, and vegetables.

Carbohydrate counting: Estimating the amount of carbohydrate in food to determine insulin needs.

Cataract: A clouding of the lens of the eye often found earlier and more commonly in people with diabetes.

Celiac disease: Intolerance of gluten found in barley, oats, rye, and wheat.

Charcot's foot: Destruction of joints and soft tissue in the foot leading to an unusable foot as a result of diabetic neuropathy.

Cholesterol: A form of fat that's needed in the body for production of certain hormones; it can lead to atherosclerosis if present in excessive levels.

Coronary artery disease: Narrowing of arteries due to deposits of cholesterol and other factors; also called atherosclerosis or arteriosclerosis.

Cortisol: An adrenal hormone released during times of stress.

Creatinine: A substance in blood that's measured to reflect the level of kidney function.

Dawn phenomenon: The tendency of blood glucose to rise early in the morning due to secretion of hormones that counteract insulin.

Diabetes Control and Complications Trial (DCCT): The decisive study of type 1 diabetes that showed that intensive control of blood glucose prevents or delays complications of diabetes.

Diabetic ketoacidosis: An acute loss of control of diabetes with high blood glucose levels and breakdown of fat leading to acidification of the blood; symptoms are nausea, vomiting, and dehydration; this condition can lead to coma and death.

Diabetologist: A physician who specializes in diabetes treatment.

Dialysis: Artificial cleaning of the blood when the kidneys aren't working.

Distal polyneuropathy: A disease of many nerves noticed in the hands and feet; associated with loss of sensation.

Endocrinologist: A physician who specializes in diseases of the glands, including the adrenals, thyroid, pituitary, parathyroids, ovaries, testicles, and pancreas.

Fasting blood glucose: The blood glucose measured after fasting overnight.

Fiber: A substance in plants that can't be digested; it provides no energy but can lower fat and blood glucose if it dissolves in water and is absorbed; it can help prevent constipation if it doesn't dissolve in water and remains in the intestine.

Fructose: The sugar found in fruits, vegetables, and honey; it has calories but is absorbed more slowly than glucose.

Gastroparesis: A form of autonomic neuropathy involving nerves to the stomach; results in food being held in the stomach.

Gestational diabetes mellitus: Diabetes that occurs during a pregnancy, usually ending at delivery.

Glucagon: A hormone made in the alpha cells of the pancreas that raises glucose and can be injected to treat severe hypoglycemia.

Glucophage: An oral agent for diabetes that lowers glucose by blocking glucose release from the liver.

Glucose: A sugar that's the body's main source of energy in the blood and cells.

Glulisine insulin: A rapid-acting insulin; also known by its brand name, Apidra.

Glycemic index: The extent to which a given food raises blood glucose usually compared to table sugar; low glycemic index foods are preferred in diabetes management.

Glycogen: The storage form of glucose in the liver and muscles.

Hemoglobin A1c: A measurement of blood glucose control reflecting the average blood glucose for the last 60 to 90 days.

High density lipoprotein (HDL): A particle in blood that carries cholesterol and helps reduce atherosclerosis.

Honeymoon phase: A period of variable duration (usually less than a year) after a diagnosis of type 1 diabetes when the need for insulin injections is reduced or eliminated.

Hyperglycemia: Levels of blood glucose greater than 100 mg/dl fasting or 140 mg/dl in the fed state.

Hyperthyroidism: An overactive thyroid; sometimes found in people with type 1 diabetes.

Hypoglycemia: Levels of blood glucose lower than normal, usually less than 60 mg/dl.

Hypothyroidism: An underactive thyroid; sometimes found in people with type 1 diabetes.

Insulin: The key hormone that permits glucose to enter cells.

Insulin detemir: A long-acting insulin; also known by its brand name, Levemir.

Insulin glargine: An insulin that provides a constant basal level 24 hours a day; also known by its brand name, Lantus.

Insulin pump: Device that slowly pushes insulin through a catheter under the skin but also can be used to give a large dose before meals.

Insulin resistance: Decreased response to insulin; found early in people with type 2 diabetes.

Insulin-dependent diabetes: Former name for type 1 diabetes.

Islet cells: The cells in the pancreas that make insulin, glucagon, and other hormones.

Juvenile diabetes mellitus: Former name for type 1 diabetes.

Ketones or ketone bodies: The breakdown products of fat metabolism.

Lancet: A sharp needle that pricks the skin for a blood glucose test.

Lipoatrophy: Indented areas where insulin is constantly injected into the body.

Lipohypertrophy: Nodular swelling of the skin where insulin is constantly injected.

Lispro insulin: A very rapid-acting form of insulin that's active within 15 minutes of injection; also known by its brand name, Humalog.

Long-acting insulin: Insulin that has glucose-lowering activity for 24 hours or more.

Low density lipoprotein (LDL): A particle in the blood containing cholesterol and thought to be responsible for atherosclerosis.

Macrosomia: The condition of a large baby born when the mother's diabetes isn't controlled.

Macrovascular complications: Heart attack, stroke, or diminished blood flow to the legs in people with diabetes.

Microalbuminuria: A finding of small but abnormal amounts of protein in the urine.

Microvascular complications: Eye disease, nerve disease, or kidney disease in people with diabetes.

Mononeuropathy: A sudden inability to move or use a muscle controlled by a single nerve.

Monounsaturated fat: One form of fat from vegetable sources like olives and nuts that doesn't raise cholesterol.

Nephropathy: Damage to the kidneys.

Neuropathic ulcer: An infected area, usually on the leg or foot, resulting from damage that wasn't felt.

Neuropathy: Damage to parts of the nervous system.

NPH insulin: An intermediate-acting insulin that starts to work in 4 to 6 hours and ends within 12 hours; also known by its brand names, Humulin N and Novolin N.

Pancreas: The organ behind the stomach that contains the islets of Langerhans, where insulin is produced.

Periodontal disease: Gum damage; common in patients with uncontrolled diabetes.

Peripheral neuropathy: Pain, numbness, and tingling, usually in the legs and feet.

Polyunsaturated fat: A form of fat from vegetables that may not raise cholesterol but lowers HDL.

Pramlintide: A drug that blocks the secretion of glucagon, a major hormone that tends to raise blood glucose; it slows the emptying of the stomach so that glucose is absorbed more slowly; also known by its brand name, Symlin.

Proliferative retinopathy: Undesirable production of blood vessels in front of the retina; left untreated, this conditions results in partial or complete loss of vision.

Protein: A source of energy for the body made up of amino acids and found in meat, fish, poultry, and beans.

Radiculopathy-nerve root involvement: A form of neuropathy in which the root of a nerve is damaged as it leaves the spinal column.

Rapid-acting insulin: Insulin given just before a meal in order to manage the carbohydrate in that meal.

Rebound phenomenon: The significant increase in blood glucose that results from the body's response after low blood glucose.

Regular insulin: A fast-acting form of insulin that's active in 1 to 2 hours and gone within 4 to 6 hours; also known by its brand names, Humulin R and Novlin R.

Retina: The part of the eye that senses light.

Retinopathy: Disease of the retina.

Saturated fat: A form of fat from animals that raises cholesterol.

Somogyi effect: A morning increase in blood glucose in response to overtreatment with insulin resulting in hypoglycemia during the night.

Trans fatty acid: A form of fat that not only raises LDL (bad) cholesterol but also lowers HDL (good) cholesterol at the same time.

Triglycerides: The main form of fat in animals.

Very low density lipoprotein (VLDL): The main particle in the blood that carries triglyceride.

Visceral fat: The fat accumulation that results in increased waist measurement.

Vitrectomy: Removal of the gel in the center of the eyeball because of leakage of blood and formation of scar tissue.

Resources for the Latest Information

• •

*T*here's so much information available on the Internet about T1DM that it's almost overwhelming. In fact, it is overwhelming! That's why I've checked out all the resources for you and collected the best ones in this appendix. You can count on every Web site on this list to be authoritative, accurate, and free of bias (mostly). (Some aren't worth your time, and I've left them off this list.)

The Web sites in this list are divided into general sites, government sites, company sites (here's where you find a bit of bias but also some good information), sites offering great recipes for people with diabetes, and sites for the visually impaired.

If you don't have Internet access, I have to say that you're missing out on the greatest collection of information ever assembled in one place — your home. Visit your local library and get on the Internet there to check out all the fabulous resources in this appendix. (All I can say is that without the Internet, this book could never have been written. And if this book hadn't been written, what would I have done with all my free time for the past six months?)

My Web Site

My Web site, `www.drrubin.com`, is a good place to start because it has links to all the sites listed here. You don't have to copy Web addresses; just click on the link and go.

You may want to stop at my Web site look around for a bit because it contains a lot of content in addition to links. For example, I've posted many articles about diabetes as well as podcasts, recorded discussions of many issues in diabetes and other medical problems that you can download to your computer or MP3 player to listen to later.

General Web Sites

You can find out about everything from antibodies to zinc preparations at the sites listed in this section. They offer in-depth discussions of all aspects of diabetes as well as assistance in finding specialists.

- ✔ **American Association of Diabetes Educators (AADE):** This organization for all diabetes educators in the United States maintains a Web site with information about diabetes education plus a way to find a diabetes educator for yourself or your child. Just click "Find an Educator" on the home page. www.diabeteseducator.org

- ✔ **American Diabetes Association:** The American Diabetes Association is, for better or for worse, the major player in diabetes in the United States. It conducts numerous programs for professionals and the public, and they're generally very good. The information about diabetes that this site provides is all-encompassing. In addition, the association publishes numerous books and pamphlets covering everything you want or need to know. You can order all publications off the site. www.diabetes.org

- ✔ **Canadian Diabetes Association:** This association's Web site has a lot of information that (obviously) pertains to the special needs of Canadians with diabetes. However, much of the information is general and of use to everyone. A major bonus on this site is that the information is in French as well as English; also, several of its valuable publications are available in other languages. www.diabetes.ca

- ✔ **Children with Diabetes:** This site is the creation of a father of a diabetic child and is an enormous database of information for the parents of children with diabetes. www.childrenwithdiabetes.com

- ✔ **The Diabetes Exercise and Sports Association:** The association's Web site is a place where you can find out about many different kinds of exercise, how much you (or your child) can and should do, and whether there are any limitations because of diabetes. You can also find others who share your interests. www.diabetes-exercise.org/about.asp

- ✔ **The Diabetes Monitor:** The Diabetes Monitor is the creation of diabetes specialist Dr. William Quick. On this Web site, he discusses every aspect of diabetes, including the latest discoveries. www.diabetes monitor.com

- ✔ **The International Diabetes Federation:** This organization, representing more than 100 countries, meets every three years and supports many studies aimed at diabetes prevention. At this site, you can locate knowledgeable diabetes experts around the world and discover information about diabetes prevention. The federation recently launched a $10 million program to improve diabetes care. www.idf.org

✔ **Joslin Diabetes Center:** The Joslin Diabetes Center is one of the world's leading pioneers in diabetes care, and the information on this site reflects that fact. The site also tells you how you can join Joslin, do research, or go to diabetes camp. www.joslin.org

✔ **Juvenile Diabetes Research Foundation:** The foundation prides itself on its contribution to research in diabetes, and this site reflects that. You can find what you want to know about the latest government programs that emphasize finding a cure for diabetes. The site also tells you how to get into an ongoing or beginning study (or get your child into one). www.jdf.org

✔ **New York Online Access to Health:** New York Online Access to Health, or NOAH, is a partnership of New York institutions. The organization's Web site provides extensive diabetes information in both English and Spanish. On the home page, search the term "type 1 diabetes." http://www.noah-health.org

✔ **Online Diabetes Resources by Rick Mendosa:** Rick Mendosa, a medical writer who has type 2 diabetes, has cataloged just about everything there is on the Web concerning diabetes. This is a huge undertaking, and he's managed to pull it off beautifully. He's also written some excellent articles on various topics related to diabetes. The site is well organized and constantly updated. You won't miss much in diabetes if you visit this Web site on a regular basis. www.mendosa.com/diabetes.htm

Government Web Sites

The Web sites listed in this section provide lots of authoritative information in their many online publications about diabetes. They also tell you about the latest government programs working to eradicate the disease.

✔ **Centers for Disease Control:** If you want to know all the latest statistics about every aspect of diabetes, go to this site. www.cdc.gov/doc.do/id/0900f3ec802723eb

✔ **Healthfinder:** A service of the U.S. Department of Health and Human Services, Healthfinder has information about many important diseases and has a large section about diabetes. Simply enter "type 1 diabetes" into the search box on the home page. www.healthfinder.gov

✔ **MedFetch:** MedFetch is a nongovernment Web site that allows you to search the national library. It's an excellent site for creating repeated searches over time on a topic like diabetes. The information arrives by e-mail, and the results are delivered in one of six languages: English, Spanish, French, Italian, German, or Portuguese. www.medfetch.com

✔ **National Diabetes Education Initiative:** With the National Diabetes Education Initiative, the federal government is determined to teach physicians about the importance of meeting the standards of diabetes care and how to go about doing this. The site for the initiative contains case studies, a slide library, and podcasts that you can listen to. As someone with T1DM or the parent of a child with T1DM, you can learn a lot by looking at its programs; they aren't too difficult for the educated non-physician to understand. www.ndei.org/website

✔ **National Diabetes Education Program:** The federal government sponsors the National Diabetes Education Program to improve treatments and outcomes for people with diabetes, to promote early diagnosis, and to prevent the onset of diabetes. It's a vast undertaking. The Web site for the program contains access to all kinds of free publications. (The site is also available in Spanish.) ndep.nih.gov

✔ **National Diabetes Information Clearinghouse:** The Internet clearing-house for information from the Institute of Diabetes and Digestive and Kidney Disease is loaded with great publications about diabetes. diabetes.niddk.nih.gov

✔ **PubMed Search Service of the National Library of Medicine:** This is where you go to use the National Library of Medicine. The site is easy to use and gives you free access to a large number of the latest scientific papers on any medical topic of interest. Simply search PubMed for "type 1 diabetes" on the home page. www.ncbi.nlm.nih.gov/PubMed

The U.S. Government also provides numerous links to diabetes information in other languages at www.cdc.gov/diabetes/ndep/lang.htm.

Companies That Make Diabetes Products

The following sections help you find companies that make the products needed to control your child's diabetes (or your own). If you have questions about the proper use of a drug or a device, you can usually find answers at these Web sites.

Companies are very limited (by the FDA) with respect to the uses of their products, and often doctors use drugs in ways that have proven successful but haven't yet received FDA approval. So you may not find the answers you need online, in which case you should talk to your child's doctor.

Glucose meters

The following companies make the meters used by the majority of people with diabetes. You can expect that these companies will still be around when your child starts having problems with his meter after a year or two of use.

- ✔ **Abbott Laboratories:** www.abbott.com
- ✔ **Bayer:** bayercarediabetes.com
- ✔ **LifeScan:** www.lifescan.com
- ✔ **Medtronic:** www.medtronic.com
- ✔ **Roche:** www.roche.com

Lancing devices

A company with a very large share of the market for lancing devices is **Owen Mumford,** which you can find at www.owenmumford.com. You can get the SoftClix lancet at the Roche site (www.roche.com) or at pharmacies and online diabetes suppliers. The BD lancet is also generally available.

Insulin

These four companies dominate the insulin market in the United States:

- ✔ **Eli Lilly and Company:** www.lilly.com
- ✔ **Novo Nordisk:** www.novo-nordisk.com
- ✔ **Pfizer:** www.pfizer.com
- ✔ **Sanofi-Aventis:** www.sanofi-aventis.us/live/us/en

Insulin syringes

The major manufacturer of insulin syringes is **Becton, Dickinson and Company** (also known as BD), www.bddiabetes.com.

Insulin jet injection devices

Jet injection devices provide relatively painless insulin injection because they don't use needles. A number of companies are leading in this market, including the following:

- ✔ **AdvantaJet:** www.advantajet.com/mainsite.htm
- ✔ **Antares Pharma (formerly Medi-Ject Corp.):** www.mediject.com
- ✔ **Bioject Medical Technologies, Inc.:** www.bioject.com

Insulin pumps

Six companies dominate the market for insulin pump devices. The pumps they make are found at the following sites:

- **AccuChek Spirit Insulin Pump System:** www.disetronic-usa.com/dstrnc_us
- **Animas:** www.animascorp.com
- **CozMore Insulin Technology System:** www.cozmore.com
- **DANA Diabecare II Pump:** www.sooil.com/NEW/eng/main.htm
- **MiniMed Paradigm REAL-time Insulin Pump:** www.minimed.com
- **OmniPod Insulin Management System:** www.myomnipod.com

Recipes for People with Diabetes

You can find a number of excellent recipes on the Web, but approach them with caution. Whereas you can generally count on getting accurate nutritional content information for recipes in cookbooks, when you find a recipe on the Web, you need to evaluate its source to be sure that the listed nutritional content is accurate.

You can trust the sites that I list here. These are the best of the currently available Web sites that provide recipes appropriate for a person with diabetes. Things change so frequently on the Web that it's difficult to keep up-to-date, so check the sites often.

- **American Diabetes Association:** The nutrition section of the American Diabetes Association Web site begins at www.diabetes.org/nutrition-and-recipes/nutrition/overview.jsp. Here you find discussions of nutrition as well as lots of diabetes-friendly recipes.
- **Ask NOAH About Diabetes:** NOAH supplies links to many important articles about diabetic nutrition as well as diabetes-friendly recipes at www.noah-health.org/en/endocrine/diabetes/nutrion/index.html.
- **Children with Diabetes:** The Children with Diabetes site includes a large amount of information on meal planning, sugar substitutes, and the food guide pyramid as well as many recipes (click "Readers' Favorite Recipes"). Find it all at www.childrenwithdiabetes.com/d_08_000.htm.

- **Diabetic Gourmet Magazine:** The magazine maintains an archive of its recipes in all categories, from side dishes to regional and ethnic cuisine to sauces and condiments; visit diabeticgourmet.com/recipes.

- **Diabetic-Recipes.com:** This site has more than 800 recipes for people with diabetes at www.diabetic-recipes.com.

- **Joslin Diabetes Center:** The Joslin Diabetes Center points out that "there is no such thing as a diabetic diet." That's one of many statements about nutrition you can find, along with recipes, at www.joslin.org/managing_your_diabetes_709.asp.

- **The Vegetarian Resource Group:** This organization maintains a site filled with information for vegetarians who have developed diabetes; along with suggested menus, you can find recipes at www.vrg.org/journal/vj2003issue2/vj2003issue2diabetes.htm.

- **3 Fat Chicks on a Diet:** This site has complete calorie counts for most fast-food restaurants at www.3fatchicks.com. The site doesn't contain recipes, but the popularity of fast food makes this site a must-have resource.

Web Sites for Diabetes Complications

Diabetes has a major impact on vision, the kidneys, and the nervous system, not to mention the heart, when the disease isn't controlled (see Chapter 5). Here are the best sites on the Web to explore those problems further.

Vision

You can find information on every issue relating to visual impairment at the following sites:

- **American Foundation for the Blind:** The foundation has resources, information, reports, recorded books, and limitless other facts and wisdom about dealing with visual impairment. www.afb.org

- **Blindness Resource Center:** This site points you in the right direction for information on every aspect of blindness. It's a fantastic guide to other sites about visual impairment. www.nyise.org/text/blindness.htm

- **National Federation of the Blind:** This national organization is another major source of information about every aspect of blindness. www.nfb.org/nfb/Default.asp

Kidneys

The best site for everything you want or need to know about kidney failure — whether it's associated with T1DM or not — is the **National Kidney Foundation's** site at www.kidney.org. Head to the "A to Z Health Guide" under "Kidney Disease" to get started.

Diabetic neuropathy

The government offers two extensive sites for information on diabetic neuropathy:

- ✔ **National Diabetes Information Clearinghouse:** diabetes.niddk. nih.gov/dm/pubs/neuropathies
- ✔ **National Institute of Neurological Disorders and Stroke:** www.ninds. nih.gov/disorders/diabetic/diabetic.htm

Heart disease

The **American Heart Association's** Web site is loaded with information on all aspects of heart disease, including diabetic heart disease, at www.american heart.org. On the home page, select "Diseases & Conditions," and then click "Diabetes" from the drop-down menu.

Index

• E •

morning basal insulin, 178
morning highs of blood glucose levels, 48
myths about T1DM
  atherosclerosis is caused by insulin, 313
  cure for T1DM is hidden by doctors so
    they can make money, 315
  illness is more frequent with T1DM, 314
  insulin cures T1DM, 313–314
  insulin is only for T1DM, 312–313
  pregnancy should be avoided with T1DM,
    314–315
  special foods must be eaten, 312
  sugar can't be eaten, 311–312
  symptoms of T1DM do not appear before
    damage occurs, 310
  T2DM is the same disease as T1DM,
    310–311

• N •

National Association for Sport and
  Physical Education, 157
National Association of Anorexia Nervosa
  and Associated Disorders, 149
National Diabetes Education Initiative
  (Web site), 338
National Diabetes Education Program, 101,
  338
National Diabetes Information
  Clearinghouse, 338, 342
National Eating Disorders Association, 149
National Federation of the Blind, 341
National Institute of Neurological Disorders
  and Stroke, 342
National Kidney Foundation, 342
nausea
  as symptom of DKA, 57
  as symptom of T1DM, 28
necrobiosis lipoidica, 80
needles
  blocked needles, avoiding, 187
  changing, 198–199
  disposal of syringes and needles, 184
  insulin injections, 180–181
neotame, 143
nephropathy, 13, 162, 332

Neporent, Liz *(Weight Training For
  Dummies),* 165
nerve conduction velocity (NCV), 71
nerve disease
  disorders of automatic (autonomic)
    nerves, 75–76
  disorders of movement
    (mononeuropathy), 74
  disorders of sensation, 72–74
  factors contributing to, 71
  light touch testing for, 72
  overview, 71–72
  temperature testing for, 72
  testing for, 72
  vibration testing for, 72
  Web sites for, 342
neuroarthropathy, 73
neuroglycopenic symptoms of
  hypoglycemia, 48–49
neuropathic ulcer, 332
neuropathy
  acupuncture for, 209
  defined, 332
  described, 13
  drug for, 321
The New England Journal of Medicine, 51, 62
New York Online Access to Health (Web
  site), 337
newborns
  diet, 140
  exercise, 157
The New Glucose Revolution, 130
*The New Glucose Revolution, Shopper's
  Guide to GI Values,* 130
niacin, 138
nicotine gum, 217
nicotine inhaler, 217
nicotine nasal spray, 217
nicotine patches, 217
nicotine replacement therapy, 217
nicotinic acid, 42
non-insulin dependent diabetes. *See* type 2
  diabetes
non-nutritive sweeteners, 143
Novo Nordisk (Web site), 339
NPH insulin, 332
nutrition. *See* diet

• *Q* •

• *R* •

• *S* •

Notes

Notes

BUSINESS, CAREERS & PERSONAL FINANCE

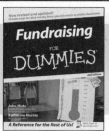

0-7645-9847-3

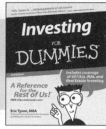

0-7645-2431-3

Also available:
- Business Plans Kit For Dummies
  0-7645-9794-9
- Economics For Dummies
  0-7645-5726-2
- Grant Writing For Dummies
  0-7645-8416-2
- Home Buying For Dummies
  0-7645-5331-3
- Managing For Dummies
  0-7645-1771-6
- Marketing For Dummies
  0-7645-5600-2

- Personal Finance For Dummies
  0-7645-2590-5*
- Resumes For Dummies
  0-7645-5471-9
- Selling For Dummies
  0-7645-5363-1
- Six Sigma For Dummies
  0-7645-6798-5
- Small Business Kit For Dummies
  0-7645-5984-2
- Starting an eBay Business For Dummies
  0-7645-6924-4
- Your Dream Career For Dummies
  0-7645-9795-7

HOME & BUSINESS COMPUTER BASICS

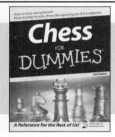

0-470-05432-8

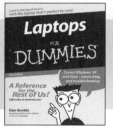

0-471-75421-8

Also available:
- Cleaning Windows Vista For Dummies
  0-471-78293-9
- Excel 2007 For Dummies
  0-470-03737-7
- Mac OS X Tiger For Dummies
  0-7645-7675-5
- MacBook For Dummies
  0-470-04859-X
- Macs For Dummies
  0-470-04849-2
- Office 2007 For Dummies
  0-470-00923-3

- Outlook 2007 For Dummies
  0-470-03830-6
- PCs For Dummies
  0-7645-8958-X
- Salesforce.com For Dummies
  0-470-04893-X
- Upgrading & Fixing Laptops For Dummies
  0-7645-8959-8
- Word 2007 For Dummies
  0-470-03658-3
- Quicken 2007 For Dummies
  0-470-04600-7

FOOD, HOME, GARDEN, HOBBIES, MUSIC & PETS

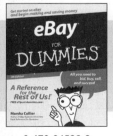

0-7645-8404-9

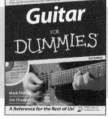

0-7645-9904-6

Also available:
- Candy Making For Dummies
  0-7645-9734-5
- Card Games For Dummies
  0-7645-9910-0
- Crocheting For Dummies
  0-7645-4151-X
- Dog Training For Dummies
  0-7645-8418-9
- Healthy Carb Cookbook For Dummies
  0-7645-8476-6
- Home Maintenance For Dummies
  0-7645-5215-5

- Horses For Dummies
  0-7645-9797-3
- Jewelry Making & Beading For Dummies
  0-7645-2571-9
- Orchids For Dummies
  0-7645-6759-4
- Puppies For Dummies
  0-7645-5255-4
- Rock Guitar For Dummies
  0-7645-5356-9
- Sewing For Dummies
  0-7645-6847-7
- Singing For Dummies
  0-7645-2475-5

INTERNET & DIGITAL MEDIA

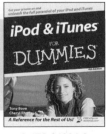

0-470-04529-9

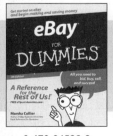

0-470-04894-8

Also available:
- Blogging For Dummies
  0-471-77084-1
- Digital Photography For Dummies
  0-7645-9802-3
- Digital Photography All-in-One Desk Reference For Dummies
  0-470-03743-1
- Digital SLR Cameras and Photography For Dummies
  0-7645-9803-1
- eBay Business All-in-One Desk Reference For Dummies
  0-7645-8438-3
- HDTV For Dummies
  0-470-09673-X

- Home Entertainment PCs For Dummies
  0-470-05523-5
- MySpace For Dummies
  0-470-09529-6
- Search Engine Optimization For Dummies
  0-471-97998-8
- Skype For Dummies
  0-470-04891-3
- The Internet For Dummies
  0-7645-8996-2
- Wiring Your Digital Home For Dummies
  0-471-91830-X

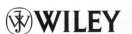

SPORTS, FITNESS, PARENTING, RELIGION & SPIRITUALITY

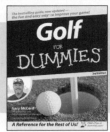

0-471-76871-5

0-7645-7841-3

Also available:

- Catholicism For Dummies
  0-7645-5391-7
- Exercise Balls For Dummies
  0-7645-5623-1
- Fitness For Dummies
  0-7645-7851-0
- Football For Dummies
  0-7645-3936-1
- Judaism For Dummies
  0-7645-5299-6
- Potty Training For Dummies
  0-7645-5417-4
- Buddhism For Dummies
  0-7645-5359-3

- Pregnancy For Dummies
  0-7645-4483-7 †
- Ten Minute Tone-Ups For Dummies
  0-7645-7207-5
- NASCAR For Dummies
  0-7645-7681-X
- Religion For Dummies
  0-7645-5264-3
- Soccer For Dummies
  0-7645-5229-5
- Women in the Bible For Dummies
  0-7645-8475-8

TRAVEL

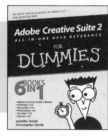

0-7645-7749-2

0-7645-6945-7

Also available:

- Alaska For Dummies
  0-7645-7746-8
- Cruise Vacations For Dummies
  0-7645-6941-4
- England For Dummies
  0-7645-4276-1
- Europe For Dummies
  0-7645-7529-5
- Germany For Dummies
  0-7645-7823-5
- Hawaii For Dummies
  0-7645-7402-7

- Italy For Dummies
  0-7645-7386-1
- Las Vegas For Dummies
  0-7645-7382-9
- London For Dummies
  0-7645-4277-X
- Paris For Dummies
  0-7645-7630-5
- RV Vacations For Dummies
  0-7645-4442-X
- Walt Disney World & Orlando
  For Dummies
  0-7645-9660-8

GRAPHICS, DESIGN & WEB DEVELOPMENT

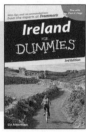

0-7645-8815-X

0-7645-9571-7

Also available:

- 3D Game Animation For Dummies
  0-7645-8789-7
- AutoCAD 2006 For Dummies
  0-7645-8925-3
- Building a Web Site For Dummies
  0-7645-7144-3
- Creating Web Pages For Dummies
  0-470-08030-2
- Creating Web Pages All-in-One Desk
  Reference For Dummies
  0-7645-4345-8
- Dreamweaver 8 For Dummies
  0-7645-9649-7

- InDesign CS2 For Dummies
  0-7645-9572-5
- Macromedia Flash 8 For Dummies
  0-7645-9691-8
- Photoshop CS2 and Digital
  Photography For Dummies
  0-7645-9580-6
- Photoshop Elements 4 For Dummies
  0-471-77483-9
- Syndicating Web Sites with RSS Feeds
  For Dummies
  0-7645-8848-6
- Yahoo! SiteBuilder For Dummies
  0-7645-9800-7

NETWORKING, SECURITY, PROGRAMMING & DATABASES

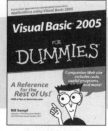

0-7645-7728-X

0-471-74940-0

Also available:

- Access 2007 For Dummies
  0-470-04612-0
- ASP.NET 2 For Dummies
  0-7645-7907-X
- C# 2005 For Dummies
  0-7645-9704-3
- Hacking For Dummies
  0-470-05235-X
- Hacking Wireless Networks
  For Dummies
  0-7645-9730-2
- Java For Dummies
  0-470-08716-1

- Microsoft SQL Server 2005 For Dummies
  0-7645-7755-7
- Networking All-in-One Desk Reference
  For Dummies
  0-7645-9939-9
- Preventing Identity Theft For Dummies
  0-7645-7336-5
- Telecom For Dummies
  0-471-77085-X
- Visual Studio 2005 All-in-One Desk
  Reference For Dummies
  0-7645-9775-2
- XML For Dummies
  0-7645-8845-1

HEALTH & SELF-HELP

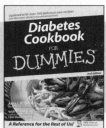

0-7645-8450-2

0-7645-4149-8

Also available:
- Bipolar Disorder For Dummies
  0-7645-8451-0
- Chemotherapy and Radiation
  For Dummies
  0-7645-7832-4
- Controlling Cholesterol For Dummies
  0-7645-5440-9
- Diabetes For Dummies
  0-7645-6820-5* †
- Divorce For Dummies
  0-7645-8417-0 †

- Fibromyalgia For Dummies
  0-7645-5441-7
- Low-Calorie Dieting For Dummies
  0-7645-9905-4
- Meditation For Dummies
  0-471-77774-9
- Osteoporosis For Dummies
  0-7645-7621-6
- Overcoming Anxiety For Dummies
  0-7645-5447-6
- Reiki For Dummies
  0-7645-9907-0
- Stress Management For Dummies
  0-7645-5144-2

EDUCATION, HISTORY, REFERENCE & TEST PREPARATION

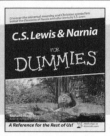

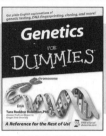

0-7645-8381-6

0-7645-9554-7

Also available:
- The ACT For Dummies
  0-7645-9652-7
- Algebra For Dummies
  0-7645-5325-9
- Algebra Workbook For Dummies
  0-7645-8467-7
- Astronomy For Dummies
  0-7645-8465-0
- Calculus For Dummies
  0-7645-2498-4
- Chemistry For Dummies
  0-7645-5430-1
- Forensics For Dummies
  0-7645-5580-4

- Freemasons For Dummies
  0-7645-9796-5
- French For Dummies
  0-7645-5193-0
- Geometry For Dummies
  0-7645-5324-0
- Organic Chemistry I For Dummies
  0-7645-6902-3
- The SAT I For Dummies
  0-7645-7193-1
- Spanish For Dummies
  0-7645-5194-9
- Statistics For Dummies
  0-7645-5423-9

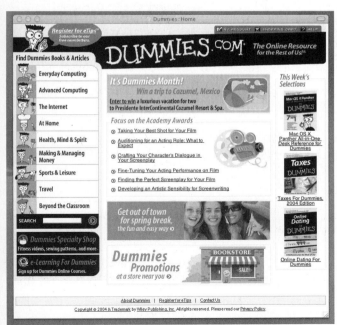

Get smart @ dummies.com®

- **Find a full list of Dummies titles**
- **Look into loads of FREE on-site articles**
- **Sign up for FREE eTips e-mailed to you weekly**
- **See what other products carry the Dummies name**
- **Shop directly from the Dummies bookstore**
- **Enter to win new prizes every month!**

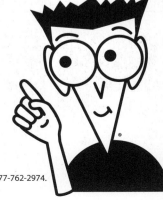

* Separate Canadian edition also available
† Separate U.K. edition also available

Available wherever books are sold. For more information or to order direct: U.S. customers visit www.dummies.com or call 1-877-762-2974.
U.K. customers visit www.wileyeurope.com or call 0800 243407. Canadian customers visit www.wiley.ca or call 1-800-567-4797.

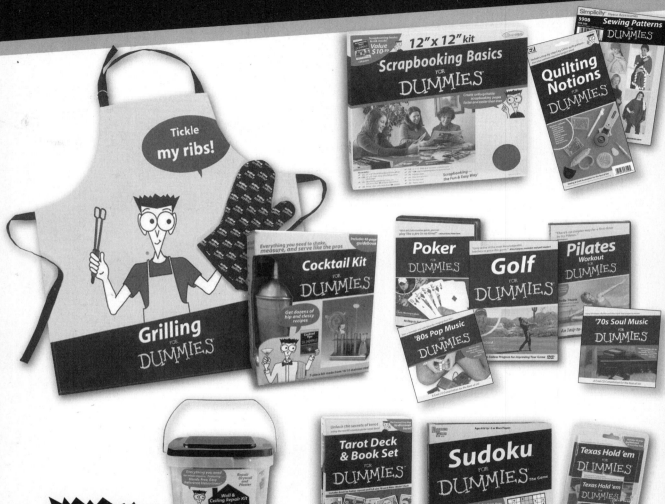
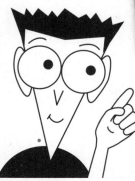
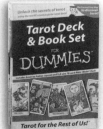
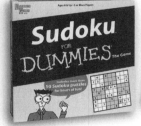
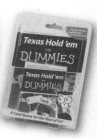
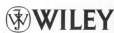